Treatment of metastasis:
Problems and prospects
PROCEEDINGS

Treatment of metastasis:
Problems and prospects
PROCEEDINGS

Strand Palace Hotel, London
15-17 October 1984

Edited by
K. Hellmann
Imperial Cancer Research Fund, London
and
S.A. Eccles
Institute of Cancer Research, Sutton, UK

Taylor & Francis
London and Philadelphia
1985

UK   Taylor & Francis Ltd, 4 John St, London WC1N 2ET

USA   Taylor & Francis Inc., 242 Cherry St,
              Philadelphia, PA 19106-1906

British Library Cataloguing in Publication Data
Treatment of metastasis: problems and prospects.
    proceedings
    Metastasis
    I. Hellmann, K. II. Eccles, S.
    616.99'4   RC269

    ISBN 0-85066-294-X

Library of Congress Cataloging in Publication Data
Main entry under title:

Treatment of metastasis: problems and prospects:
    proceedings: Strand Palace Hotel, London, 15-17
    October 1984.

    Includes bibliographies and index.
    1. Metastasis—Treatment—Congresses. I. Hellmann,
    K. (Kurt). II. Eccles, S. [DNLM: 1. Neoplasm Metastasis
    —congresses. 2. Neoplasms—therapy—congresses.
    QZ 202 T7841 1984]
    RC270.8.T74 1985   616.99'4   84-24066
    ISBN 0-85066-294-X

Abstracts of the papers and posters presented at the
conference are also available, published as *Treatment of
Metastasis: Problems and prospects. Abstracts* (edited by
K. Hellmann and S.A. Eccles) by Taylor & Francis
ISBN 0-85066-293-1.

**Printed in Great Britain by Taylor & Francis (Printers) Ltd,
Basingstoke, Hants.**

CONTENTS

Contents ix

PREFACE

The papers in this volume represent the proceedings of a meeting on
TREATMENT OF METASTASIS: PROBLEMS AND PROSPECTS held at the Strand Palace
Hotel, London 15-17 October, 1984. The meeting was in essence a follow-
up of a conference on Clinical and Experimental Aspects of Metastasis held
under the auspices of the EORTC Metastasis Group in London in 1980, since
at that time many had expressed a desire for further similar international
conferences. It was also intended to have a meeting that would firstly
provide an open forum for all those working in the metastasis research
field; allow presentation of recent results, and furnish opportunities for
the exchange of ideas, and secondly to found a METASTASIS RESEARCH SOCIETY.

The organisation of the meeting differed from the previous EORTC
meeting and that of many other conferences, in that there were no invited
speakers, and papers were selected for presentation on the basis of the
quality of abstracts submitted. The papers represent a fair cross-
section of the current interests in experimental and clinical metastasis
research. Recently, a number of new metastasis research laboratories
have been established, and we can therefore predict with some confidence
an acceleration in our understanding of the complex process of metastasis.
The advances which have already taken place, some of which are described
in this volume, have not yet been reflected in improved diagnosis or
treatment of cancer patients, but it is to be hoped that by the time the
proceedings of the next metastasis meeting appear there will be more
clinically valuable progress to report.

ACKNOWLEDGEMENTS

The Organizing Committee wishes to express its appreciation of the support which made this Conference possible. It is particularly grateful to:

      Taylor & Francis Limited
        (publishers of Clinical & Experimental Metastasis)
      Imperial Cancer Research Fund
      Boehringer Ingelheim Limited (Hospital Division)
      Lederle Laboratories Limited
      Janssen Pharmaceutical Limited
      Sera-Lab Limited

The Organizing Committee would also like to place on record the invaluable administration and co-ordinating efforts made by the conference manager and editorial secretary of CEM, Mrs. Jean Hartley, and her assistants, Mrs. M. Evans and Mrs. G. Hutchinson. They also wish to thank Mr. Roger Butler for his help with the meeting.

PULMONARY METASTASECTOMY - REAPPRAISAL OF SELECTION CRITERIA

J.A. VAN DONGEN

Netherlands Cancer Institute, Plesmanlaan 121, 1066 CX Amsterdam,

The Netherlands

Keywords : Pulmonary metastasectomy; selection criteria

Most malignant tumours follow the vena cava type of metastatic pathway and, postulating the cascade sequence, the lung may be an efficient filter organ. Incidentally, depending on the time of suppression of the primary, the type of the primary and certain soil properties, pulmonary metastases may present themselves as solitary lesions or may be very few in number. Resection, aiming at cure is then to be considered.

Close observation of patients, logical thinking and experimental data guide the policy in selecting patients for such operations.

Slow tumour growth, disease-free interval between treatment of the primary and appearance of the metastases, the number and size of the metastases and certain primary tumour types have been thought to be main prognostic factors and are therefore used as selection criteria (Van Dongen & Van Slooten 1978; Van Zandwijk 1983).

Cell kinetic studies and clinical observations linked slow growth with better prognosis (Gentili et al. 1981; Tubiana et al. 1984). It seems reasonable to postulate in slow growing tumours the shedding of tumour emboli to be scanty and late in the course of the disease. Tumour doubling time (TDT) measurements can be used to express tumour growth and when measured in pulmonary metastases it can give important information of the gain in survival time which can be expected and it may be an important predictor of the chance of being cured after matastasectomy.

Easier and more widely used for patient selection is the interval between tumour treatment and presentation of the metastases. A long interval is a major indicator of slow growth; moreover in such cases there is a chance that the metastasis is really a solitary lesion, originating only shortly before the removal of the primary. In contrast in synchronous cases there is a fair chance that other metastases are already present.

1

Data from the first published series of metastasectomies showed relatively favourable results so the selection criteria were extended to include cases with short disease-free intervals or with other unfavourable prognostic factors.

We studied the metastasectomy cases treated in the Netherlands Cancer Institute with special references to the classic prognostic criteria. In the period 1964 to 1984 107 cases were operated; the largest subgroups were bone tumours (24), soft tissue sarcoma cases (16) and patients treated for renal carcinoma (12).

A very unexpected finding was that the cases with short interval, including many synchronous cases, followed the same survival curve as patients presenting after longer intervals (see Figure 1). This phenomenon is now also being found in liver metastasectomy studies in gastrointestinal tumours.

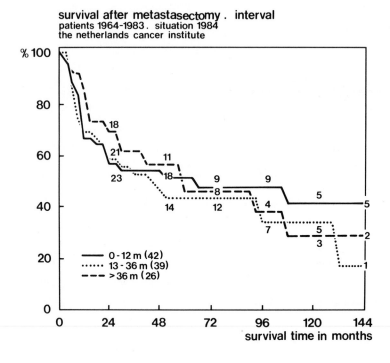

Figure 1. Survival curves of patients with short, with moderate and with long intervals between treatment of primary tumour and detection of metastasis; better survival in the long interval group is not seen.

We may explain these findings by realizing that in patients with slow

tumour growth the time factor may be rather important. The slower the
tumour growth the longer the time available to disseminate. In an experimental setting, using tail implants and having the possibility to accelerate
tumour growth by subcutaneous fixation of the tail, we could also demonstrate for many mouse tumours that the duration of growth dominated the
factors which influence bad prognosis (Van Dongen 1961).

    More recently supposedly worse prognostic factors were accepted when
considering patients for pulmonary metastasectomy. Previous adjuvant
therapy, earlier described as a bad prognostic factor when considering the
results after metastasectomy (Van Dongen 1980), was now rather frequently
given and also, comparing two 10 year periods in our Institute, more
patients with multiple metastases are being operated in the more recent
years. Now more that half of the patients have multiple metastases from
the beginning. However, the survival curves given in Figure 2 indicate
that the prognosis in recent years is equal to that in the earlier period.
So the validity of the classic prognostic factors is challenged.

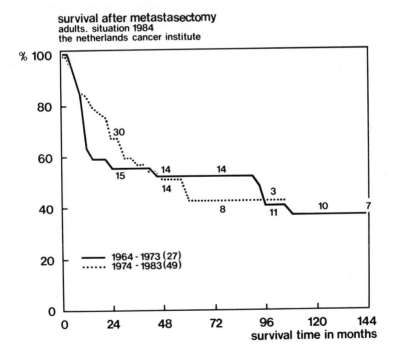

Figure 2. Survival curves of adult patients treated in 1963-1974 and in
1974-1983. The prognosis seems equally good in both periods, despite that
in the more recent period more patients with supposed bad prognostic
characteristics were operated.

To understand better the mechanisms involved in prognosis in these
patients large patient groups are needed. Only then is multivariate
analysis possible. Pooling of data of different centres should be organized.

REFERENCES

Dongen, J.A. van, 1980, Changing aspects in the surgical approach to
    metastatic disease; influence of chemotherapy on indications for and
    results of metastasectomies. In Metastasis, Clinical and Experimental
    Aspects. Edited by K. Hellmann, P. Hilgard & S Eccles, M. Nijhoff,
    The Hague, Boston, London. p. 381.
Dongen, J.A. van, 1961, Haematogenous metastases. Thesis, Scheltema &
    Holkema, Amsterdam.
Dongen, J.A. van & Slooten, E.A. van, 1978, The surgical treatment of
    pulmonary metastasis. Cancer Treatment Reviews, 5, 29.
Gentili C et al., 1981 Cell proliferation and its relationship to clinical
    features and relapse in breast cancers. Cancer, 48, 974.
Tubiana, M. et al., 1984, The long-term prognostic significance of the
    thymidine labelling index in breast cancer. International Journal of
    Cancer, 33, 441.
Zandwijk, N. van, et al., 1983, Pulmonary metastasectomy. Indication and
    policy adapted to different primary tumors. Workshop Report. In
    Proceedings ESSO Workshops, Amsterdam.

SURGICAL TREATMENT OF PULMONARY METASTASES CONCERNING 68 PATIENTS OPERATED ON BETWEEN 1962 AND 1982

G. DEPADT, R. DELACROIX, J. MEURETTE, L. ADENIS

Centre Oscar Lambret (Directeur : Pr. A. DEMAILLE) Rue F. Combemale, BP 307, 59020 LILLE Cédex (France)

KEY WORDS : Lung - pulmonary metastases - surgical treatment

INTRODUCTION

Currently, we no longer have the right to prescribe systematic chemotherapy without histological proof when faced with isolated pulmonary opacity in a patient treated for cancer. Indeed this opacity may be a metastasis but also a primary cancer, a benign tumor or an inflammatory lesion. And if it is a metastasis, a resection may be carried out in certain cases. Thus, it is indispensable to perform a thoracotomy for every pulmonary opacity without histological proof.

MATERIALS AND METHODS

Sex and age

This study concerned 30 males and 38 females. Patients ranged between the second and the eighth decade of life with a peak between 41 and 60 years.

Characteristics of the primary tumor (Table 1)

Table 1. Primary tumor sites

Breast	14	20.6 %	Lung	2	2.9 %
Colo-rectum	9	13. %	Skin	2	2.9 %
Kidney	8	11.8 %	Soft tissue	2	2.9 %
Bones	6	8.8 %	Placenta	1	1.4 %
Head and neck	5	7.3 %	Uterine cervix	1	1.4 %
Endometrium	3	4.4 %	Ovarian cancer	1	1.4 %
Parotid gland	3	4.4 %	Thyroid	1	1.4 %
Testicular cancer	2	2.9 %	Unknown	8	11.8 %

52 cases were carcinomas (76,5 %) and 8 cases were sarcomas (11,7 %). In 8 cases, metastases revealed an unknown primary tumor. Among the carcinomas could be found in order of frequency : breast, colo-rectal, kidney cancer.

Among the sarcomas, 6 developed in bones and 2 in soft-tissue.

Circumstances of discovery

75 % of the metastases were discovered by routine chest X-ray. In 25 % of the cases, metastasis was symptomatic (cough, dyspnea, hemoptysis).

Disease free interval between diagnosis of primary tumor and of the metastasis

In 33 cases, this was less than 2 years : 8 revealing metastases, 11 synchronous metastases, 14 metastases discovered within 2 years after treatment of the primary tumor. In 35 cases, the disease free interval was over 2 years.

Paraclinical investigations

Radiological features : in 52 cases the metastases were single (76,5 %), in 16 cases they were multiple (23,5 %). In 28 cases the right side was affected, in 36 cases the left side. Metastases were bilateral in 4 cases. 8 patients presented ventilation problems.

Tumor doubling time could seldom be observed. It was short for one patient, long for 12 patients but unknown in 55 cases.

22 bronchoscopies were performed (7 were positive), 17 cytologies (5 positive), 12 biopsies (5 positive). We can notice the relative lack of histological proof obtained by paraclinical investigations. This is normal since pulmonary metastases rarely give bronchus symptoms.

Necessary conditions for resection

They were : successful treatment of the primary tumor or likely success of the treatment, no other metastatic locations, good operative risk. The multiplicity of metastatic lesions as well as their uni- or bilateral nature were not automatically contra-indications.

Operations performed (Table 2)

Table 2. Operations

Exploratory thoracotomies	10	14.7 %
Wedge resections	10	14.7 %
Segmental resections	8	
Lobectomies	31	
Bilobectomies	5	70.6 %
Pneumonectomies	4	

Ten thoracotomies were merely exploratory. Resections concerned 58 patients. In 48 cases, they were "regular" but in ten cases a Wedge resection was performed. We observed one post-operative death due to cardiac insufficiency after exploratory thoracotomy in a 20 year old patient who had received doxorubicin.

Post-operative treatment

3 patients received additional radiotherapy, 41 chemotherapy and 2 received radiotherapy plus chemotherapy.

RESULTS

Survival

This was calculated according to the Kaplan-Meier method. The future is known for 64 patients. Survival rates at 1, 3 and 5 years were respectively 80, 45 and 25 % (Figure 1). 49 survived over 1 year, 32 over 2, 26 over 3, 13 over 4, 9 over 5 years.

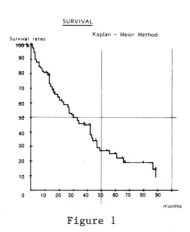

Figure 1

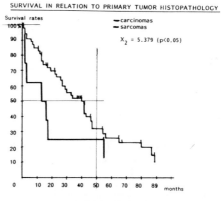

Figure 2

Second operations for pulmonary recurrence

We reoperated on 2 men (70 and 22 years old). One had been operated on for a rectum cancer, the other for an osteosarcoma of the femur. A first pulmonary resection had been performed for metastases. A further resection was performed due to the appearance of a second metastasis, in one case 3 years after, in the other 2 years after the first resection. It is interesting to note the survival since the treatment of the first metastasis: for one 5 years (but now presents a recurrence) for the other 6 years (NED).

DISCUSSION

Factors influencing survival

- Survival in relation to primary tumor histopathology (fig 2). In our study carcinomas had a better prognosis than sarcomas, the difference was significant (p<0.05).
- Survival in relation to disease free interval (fig 3). The difference is significant for a disease free interval of over 2 years compared with one of under 2 years (p<0.01). It must noted that survival rate of patients with revealing metastases was not lower than that of all the patients with a disease free interval of less than 2 years.

- Survival in relation to operation (fig 4). The difference was significant
(p<0.05) for resections compared with exploratory thoracotomies. Median
survival was 38 months in the case of resections and only 14 months in the
case of exploratory thoracotomies. On the other hand, there was no significant difference between lobectomies or pneumonectomies and wedge resections.

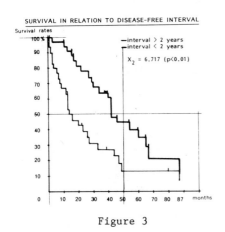

Figure 3   Figure 4

- Survival in relation to number of metastases. We did not observe any
significant difference for survival in relation to the number of metastases
although we are approaching this if we compare single and multiple metastases. The X_2 is 3.242 while significance is reached at 3.841.
- Survival in relation to post-operative chemotherapy. In our study, we
found no significant difference whether patients received surgical chemotherapy or not.

CONCLUSION

   Surgery is an efficient weapon against pulmonary metastases. Most often
it is performed after the treatment of the primary tumor. It may be performed at the same time, when the metastasis is synchronous, and even before
when the metastasis is revealing. Multiple metastases are not an absolute
contra-indication but it is always necessary to spare the pulmonary parenchyma. Firstly because there is no survival difference between Wedge resection and segmental resection or lobectomy and secondly because reoperations
are feasible in certain cases.

SURGICAL TREATMENT OF HEPATIC METASTASES

R. DOCI, P. BIGNAMI, F. BOZZETTI and L. GENNARI

Istituto Nazionale per lo Studio e la Cura dei Tumori, Milan, Italy

Keywords: Hepatic metastases; Hepatic surgery

INTRODUCTION

During the last two decades the surgical approach to hepatic metastases from solid tumours has become a reasonable option for treating selected patients. Operative mortality is reported to range from 1.7 (Wilson & Adson 1976) to 10% (Cady et al. 1979), with a 5-year survival of more than 20% (Foster 1970, Wanebo et al. 1978, Wilson & Adson 1976, Fortner et al. 1984) in patients with solitary metastasis from colorectal cancer. However, the indications to hepatic surgery are controversial regarding metastases from primary sites other than the large bowel, the extent of liver involvement, and the multiplicity of metastases. Here we report our surgical experience with hepatic metastases from different primaries.

CASE MATERIAL

From January 1980 to April 1984, 53 patients have undergone hepatic resection for metastases; the site and the histologic type of the primary are reported in Table 1. The extent of resection is reported in Table 2. In most of the patients a typical resection (lobectomy or segmentectomy) was the procedure of choice. Wedge resections were preferred when the metastatic lesion was marginal or situated in the residual lobe (bilateral metastases).

RESULTS

Two patients died postoperatively; one because of ischemic colitis and the other, whose primary was testicular embryonal carcinoma, because of neoplastic embolism into the pulmonary artery; thus the mortality rate was 3.8%. Major complications were observed in 3 patients: two of them

Table 1. Site and histologic type of the primary tumour.

Site and histology	No. of patients
Colorectal adenocarcinoma	37
Gastrointestinal carcinoid	3
Bronchial carcinoid	2
Gastric carcinoma	2
Gastric leiomyosarcoma	2
Testicular embryonal carcinoma	2
Melanoma of the eye	1
Cutaneous melanoma	1
Breast carcinoma	1
Ovarian adenocarcinoma	1
Cervical carcinoma	1
Total	52

Table 2. Extent of liver resection.

Procedure	No. of patients
Right extended lobectomy	5
Right lobectomy	20
Left lobectomy	1
Left lateral lobectomy	8
Segmentectomy	13
Wedge resection	6

developed a subphrenic abscess that required surgical drainage; the third had a biliary fistula. Twenty patients had mild complications (pleural effusion or pneumonia).

The overall actuarial survival of patients with colorectal adenocarcinoma and that of patients with different primaries is reported in Fig. 1. All but one of the second group of metastatic patients died within 2 years of the operation, whereas 40% of colorectal cancer patients are still alive.

Among these patients it is interesting to distinguish survival according to the extent of liver involvement and the number of metastases. Patients with a single metastasis involving less than 25% of the liver (H_{1s} patients according to our clinical classification; Gennari et al. 1982) had a prognosis consistently better than that of other patients with more extensive involvement (> 25%) or multiple metastases (Fig. 2).

As regards disease-free survival, all patients with multiple metastases developed distant or liver recurrence within 2 years of the hepatic resection; 40% of patients with a single metastasis are still disease free at 30 months after surgery. In total, 18 patients developed a recurrence, which was at distant organs in half of them.

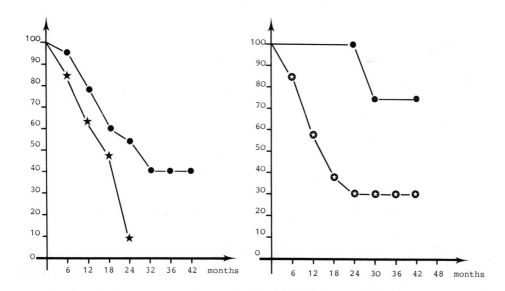

Figure 1.   Actuarial survival of 36 patients resected for hepatic
metastases from colorectal cancer (●) in comparison with the survival of
15 patients (o) with hepatic metastases from a different primary.

Figure 2.   Actuarial survival of 16 patients (●) with single metastases
involving less than 25% of liver parenchyma (H_{1s}) vs. actuarial survival of
all others (o , 20 patients). Results after liver resection.

Survival of patients with liver metastases from different primaries was
consistently different according to the site and histologic type of tumour
(Table 3).

The prognosis of carcinoid tumour is by far the best: all patients
actually living are disease free in spite of the fact that none of them had
a single metastasis. Among the others, the sole long-surviving patient had
a single metastasis from adenocarcinoma.

DISCUSSION

The results observed in our consecutive series of hepatic resections for
liver metastases from colorectal cancer are not dissimilar from those
reported in the literature. At present, actuarial analysis estimates the
overall 3-year survival rate of our resected patients to be 40%; nevertheless, the figure rises to 75% when a single metastasis involving less than
25% of liver parenchyma was detected and resected.   However, it is

Table 3.   Survival after liver resection of patients with metastases from
different primaries.

Primary	Alive (mos)	Died (mos)
Carcinoid	4, 14, 15, 26	22
Melanoma		2, 7
Gynecologic tumour	4	6
Testis	3	
Gastric carcinoma	3	23
Gastric sarcoma	6	14

difficult to compare this group of patients with those reported by other
authors who did not consider the extent of liver involvement.

However, the excellent results observed in these cases are undoubted, and
if the low operative mortality and morbidity is also considered, the indication to hepatic resection for solitary metastasis is categoric. It may
seem questionable whether multiple metastases should be treated by surgery:
in agreement with Wilson and Adson (1976), our data suggest a substantial
improvement in survival also in these patients. Therefore we believe that,
when feasible, a surgical procedure affected by 4% mortality and 6% morbidity may be considered a useful "palliative" treatment that, in selected
cases, might result in a real chance of cure. The indication to resect
liver metastases from different primaries is difficult to assess, and the
overall experience is too limited for drawing conclusions. Postoperative
survival observed for carcinoid liver metastases could induce one to
consider this tumour candidate to surgical treatment; however, it is well
known that carcinoid is often a slow-growing tumour, and untreated long
survivors have been reported. The poor results observed do not support the
indication to resect hepatic metastases from other primaries, in spite of
the fact that occasional patients have survived longer than expected.

REFERENCES
Cady, B., Bonneval, M. & Fender, H., 1979, Am. J. Surg. 137, 514.
Fortner, J. G., Silva, J. S. et al., 1984, Ann. Surg. 199, 306.
Foster, J. A., 1970, Cancer 26, 493.
Gennari, L., Doci, R., Bozzetti, F. & Veronesi, U., 1982, Tumori 68, 443.
Wanebo, H. J. et al., 1978, Am. J. Surg. 135, 81.
Wilson, S. M. & Adson, M. A., 1976, Arch. Surg. 111, 330.

HEPATIC ARTERIAL INFUSION FOR METASTATIC COLORECTAL CARCINOMA IN THE LIVER

Paola BIGNAMI, Roberto DOCI and Federico BOZZETTI

Istituto Nazionale per lo Studio e la Cura dei Tumori, Milan, Italy

Keywords: Intrahepatic   infusion;   Colorectal   hepatic   metastases

INTRODUCTION

The purpose of this paper is to report the experience of the Istituto Nazionale Tumori of Milan, with hepatic intraarterial infusion of cytotoxic drugs for metastases from a colorectal cancer.

PATIENTS AND METHODS

From 1970 to 1980 61 patients with metastases confined to the liver from a previously operated colorectal cancer were treated with intrahepatic arterial infusion of 5-fluorouracil (5-FU) (53 patients) or adriamycin (8 patients). The main characteristics of the series are reported in Table 1. The stage of metastases, according to the clinical classification proposed by Gennari et al. (1982) is reported in Table 2. Catheterization of the hepatic artery was performed by surgical approach and placement of a poly- ethylene or polyvinylchloride catheter in the hepatic artery through the gastroepiploic artery (17 patients) or by a transfemoral approach, accord- ing to the Seldinger technique (44 patients).   Therapy consisted of the continuous administration of 5-FU or adriamycin, according to a schedule reported in Table 3.

RESULTS

Complications due to drug toxicity or to the arterial access are reported in Table 4. Drug side effects were observed in 22/61 (36%) of cases and consisted mainly of upper gastrointestinal distress after 5-FU infusion and bone marrow toxicity after adriamycin administration.

Table 1.   Characteristics of 61 patients with metastatic liver from colorectal cancer.

Males (no.)	29
Females (no.)	32
Mean age (years)	57
Interval between primary and secondary (months)	15

Table 2.   Stage of liver metastases in 61 patients.

H_1 (< 25% liver involvement),	16 patients;	s (single),	7 patients
H_2 ($\overline{25}$–50% liver involvement),	13 patients;	m (multiple),	10 patients
H_3 (> 50% liver involvement),	32 patients;	b (bilateral),	44 patients

Table 3.   Hepatic arterial infusion: treatment schedule.*

Drug	No. of patients	Treatment
5-FU	33	20 mg/kg^{-1} day^{-1} x 8 days
5-FU	20	12 mg/kg^{-1} day^{-1} x 21 days
Adriamycin	8	0.3 mg/kg^{-1} day^{-1} x 8 days

* Thirty-three patients received more than 1 cycle (range 2–7).   Median interval between cycles, 12 weeks; overall number of cycles, 154.

Table 4.   Hepatic arterial infusion: toxicity.

Toxicity	5-FU (53 pts)	Adriamycin (8 pts)
Bone marrow (grade 1)	–	8
Severe stomatitis	–	1
Upper abdominal pain	10	–
Duodenal ulcer	2	–
Mental confusion	1	–
Thrombosis of hepatic artery	20	–
Sepsis of catheter	2	–
Aneurysm of femoral artery	1	–
Total	35	9

Catheter complications accounted for a further 23 complications (37%) and necessitated cessation of the therapy in a high number of cases. However, no mortality related to the treatment was observed, and drug toxicity was always transient and reversed by withdrawal from the therapy.

     Partial regression (i.e., a reduction ranging from 25 to 50% of hepato-megaly measured on two vertical lines starting from the xyphoid apophysis or the middle clavicle) was observed in 12 of 27 patients with hepatomegaly (median duration 2 months). However, only two responding patients showed a decrease in tumour size and vascularity at the angiographic examination.

Survival is reported in Figs. 1-3, where the survival of untreated patients of the same H category is shown for comparison. The median survival of H_1, H_2 and H_3 infused patients was respectively 22, 14 and 10 months, compared to 4, 6 and 5 months survival in untreated patients. It appears that the higher the extent of metastatic involvement the lesser the efficacy of the arterial infusion.

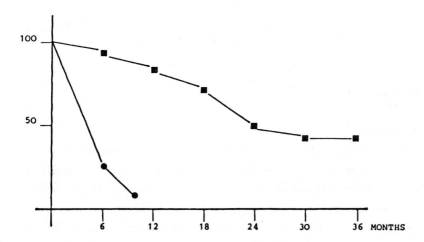

Figure 1. (r)H_1 Hepatic metastases from colorectal cancer. Survival of patients untreated (●, 8 patients) or treated by locoregional chemotherapy (■, 16 patients).

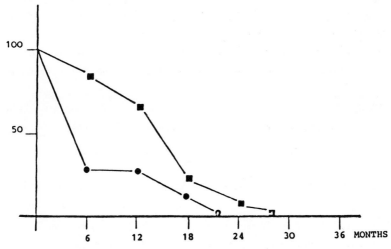

Figure 2. (r)H_2 Hepatic metastases from colorectal cancer. Survival of patients untreated (●, 7 patients) or treated by locoregional chemotherapy (■, 13 patients).

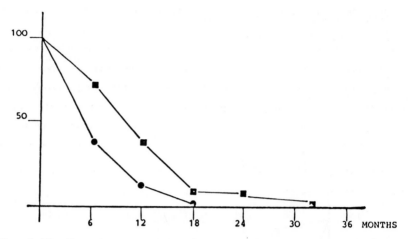

Figure 3. (r)H$_3$ Hepatic metastases from colorectal cancer. Survival of patients untreated (● , 8 patients) or treated by locoregional chemotherapy (■ , 32 patients).

CONCLUSIONS

Chemotherapy delivered through the arterial route by continuous infusion appears to be an effective palliative treatment. It probably slows tumour growth without producing an evident clinical regression in most cases. The advantage of a local infusion over no treatment is apparent when liver involvement is limited. However, complications related to the vascular access are unacceptable and suggest that amelioration of the technique is necessary.

In prospective, we can recommend intraarterial infusion in patients with unresectable liver metastases involving no more than 50% of the parenchyma. The use of implantable pumps and silicone catheters can improve the local tolerance of the treatment. Also, a more adequate dosage and use of new drugs or combination chemotherapy could improve the final results.

REFERENCES

Gennari, L., Doci, R., Bozzetti, F. & Veronesi, U., 1982, Tumori, 68, 443.

PROSPECTIVE SERIAL LIVER ULTRASOUND SCANNING IN RESECTABLE COLORECTAL
CANCER TREATED WITH ADJUVANT RAZOXANE

R.H. TAYLOR[1], J.M. GILBERT[2], M.G.C. EVANS[3], H.G. LANE[1],
P.G. CASSELL[4], and K. HELLMANN[3]

[1]Central Middlesex Hospital, Acton Lane, London, NW10
[2]University College Hospital, Gower Street, London, WCl
[3]Imperial Cancer Research Fund, Lincoln's Inn Fields, London, WC2
[4]Wexham Park Hospital, Slough, Berks.

Keyword: Liver metastases, razoxane, ultrasound

INTRODUCTION

　　Razoxane (Rz) has a number of characteristics which make it of interest
as an adjuvant drug for resectable colorectal cancer (CRC).　　It is:

　　　　1.　active in advanced CRC (Marciniak et al., 1975)

　　　　2.　taken orally

　　　　3.　well tolerated

　　　　4.　antimetastatic in 6/8 experimental tumours

　　A prospective randomized controlled clinical trial of adjuvant Rz for
resectable CRC was therefore started at the end of 1976.　Two years later
this trial indicated that a statistically significant benefit in terms of
recurrence free interval and survival had been obtained by the Rz treated
group (Gilbert et al., 1982).　Since some 50% of CRC patients who die of
the disease die of liver metastases and perhaps a further 20-25% die with
metastases it seemed of interest to see whether the clinical advantage
seen with Rz treatment could have been due to a lower incidence rate of
liver metastases.　We therefore decided to follow all further entrants to
the trial by serial liver ultrasound scans.

PATIENTS AND METHODS

　　The scans were done at 3 monthly intervals and were carried out by one
person (RHT) using a Nuclear Enterprises Diasonograph for the first half of
the study (until June 1981) and a Philips Sono Diagnost for the second half.
A total of more than 1,000 ultrasound scans were done on these patients.
Patients in whom the ultrasound was doubtful were investigated by other
means.　Patients were well matched for age, sex, Dukes' staging and site
of tumour.　The study which is now closed was in progress for 6 years and

17

followed the clinical course of 126 patients of which 65 were controls and 61 treated with 125 mgs Rz b.d. for 5 consecutive days per week.

RESULTS

Only one patient had liver metastases on the first scan and two had probable metastases which became definite later on.   All other patients had clear ultrasounds and the development of liver metastases could therefore be followed in all except one patient.   In total, 12/61 patients in the Rz treated Dukes' A, B, and C groups developed liver metastases compared with 16/65 who received no Rz (Table 1).

Ultrasound failed to pick up liver metastases in 8 of the 28 patients who developed them, giving a 71% detection rate.

Although there were no significant differences in the incidence rate of liver metastases between controls and Rz treated patients the median time from operation to first detection of liver metastases was 60 weeks for those who had no Rz and 87 weeks for those who received it (p=0.055).   In the total series of patients from first entry in 1976, the difference in time to development of metastases was even greater.   Here too the incidence rate of the combined B & C groups is not very different.   However, when Dukes' groups were analysed separately it transpired that there were twice as many patients with liver metastases in Dukes' C patients amongst controls as amongst those who took Rz.

Details on the number, size, distribution, character or change of these parameters with time are not available.   It is possible however that these parameters could give considerable information and ought to be examined in any further investigation.

Table 1.   Liver metastases detected by serial ultrasound.

Dukes'	Control	Treated
A	2/9 (22%)	1/10 (10%)
B	4/33 (12%)	4/29 (14%)
C	10/23 (43%)	7/22 (32%)
Total	16/65 (25%)	12/61 (20%)

Toxicity due to Rz was confined to leukopenia which occurred in more than half of the patients and always required dose modification either on a transient or permanent basis.   The drug was otherwise extremely well tolerated and nausea and vomiting were conspicuous by their virtual complete absence.   Thinning of the hair was apparent in a few patients, though none had alopecia requiring wigs.   During the course of this trial our attention was drawn to 2 psoriasis patients treated with Rz for varying periods of time and in whom acute myeloblastic leukaemia developed. Up to that time only one of our patients had developed acute leukaemia, but subsequently 2 more patients who had taken Rz developed AML giving an incidence of 3 in 122 (2.5%).

DISCUSSION

Although there is no difference between controls and Rz treated patients in the ultrasound detected incidence of liver metastases there has been a significant delay in their appearance and this delay may well account for the increase in recurrence free interval as well as the increase in survival of the CRC patients treated with Rz. Neither an increase in survival nor delay in metastases appearance in a critical organ has previously been observed after adjuvant treatment.

When the whole trial (from its start in 1976) is considered and this trial has accrued 272 patients, it is worth noting that in the Dukes' C group, 7/38 (18%) of the Rz treated patients developed liver metastases compared with 17/50 (34%) who had no Rz. Moreover the median time to development of these metastases was also twice as long (20 months) in the Rz treated group compared with 10 months for those who had no Rz.

For the Dukes' B patients differences were not as marked in the incidence, but numbers are small 7% against 12% and 12.5 months compared with 17 months.

The occurrence of 3 AMLs in the Rz treated group makes it seem likely, though not completely certain, that these leukaemias are drug related. The Committee on Safety of Medicines of the UK has therefore requested that no further clinical trials with Rz be done. It may be worth comparing the present results with those recently reported by the G.I. Tumor Study Group (1984), which showed that 5-Fu + semustine ± immunotherapy not only did not produce any statistically significant benefit in terms of survival or recurrence free interval, but was associated with the appearance of 7 AMLs amongst 288 patients who had the chemotherapy, giving an incidence that is identical to that observed here.

Long term treatment by compounds having an influence on bone marrow (as judged by the production of leukopenia) may well be responsible for the development of AML no matter what the chemical may be or whether or not it has any mutagenic or carcinogenic activity. Rz has no mutagenic action and is only weakly, if at all carcinogenic. If it were given at a dose causing no leukopenia and over a limited period of time it might well be that the activity and the bone marrow remained unaffected. This might well be put to the test in poor risk, i.e. Dukes' C colorectal cancer patients.

REFERENCES

Gilbert, J.M., Hellmann, K., Evans, M. et al., 1982, Cancer Chemotherapy & Pharmacology, 10, 228-229.

G.I. Tumor Study Group, 1984, The New England Journal of Medicine, 310, 737-743.

Marciniak, T.A., Moertel, C.G., Schutt, A.J., et al., 1975, Cancer Chemotherapy Reports, 59, 761.

FUNCTIONAL AND MORPHOLOGICAL CHARACTERISATION OF COLORECTAL CARCINOMA AND ITS LIVER METASTASES

P. HOHENBERGER[1], F. LIEWALD[2], D. LORKE[2], P. SCHLAG[1], P. MÖLLER[2]
[1]Department of Surgery and [2]Department of Pathology,
University of Heidelberg, Im Neuenheimer Feld 110, West Germany

Keywords: morphological characterisation; colorectal carcinoma; liver
    metastases

INTRODUCTION

Variation in behaviour of experimental metastases derived from the same primary led Fidler to suppose that clonal selection in the primary tumour was a prerequisite for differences in the clinical course of disseminating cancers.

On the other hand differences in the response to cytostatic agents shows that treatment of colorectal cancer or its metastases is tantamount to treating a group of heterogenous tumours. Taken together with the results of tumour cell growth in vitro it is evident that the tumour itself has a heterogenous pattern.

We were therefore interested to know whether metastases from the same primary tumour have a more homogenous functional and morphological pattern compared to their primaries as would be expected if clonal selection had really taken place.

PATIENTS AND METHODS

We examined 16 colorectal primaries and their corresponding liver metastases. To characterize the tumours both morphologically and functionally we used 6 lectins and 3 tissue antigens (Table 1) by means of immunoperoxidase technique in normal, orthotopic colonic mucosa, primary tumour and metastases.

The patients' characteristics are shown in Table 2. There was one case of loss of differentiation from the primary to the metastasis.

Table 1. Lectins and Antigens used to characterize colorectal carcinoma.

Lectin/Antigen Abbr.	Lectins derived from	Specificity
PNL	Arachis hypogaea	D-Gal-β-(1-3)-GalNAc
UEA	Ulex europaeus I	α-L-Fuc
HPA	Helix pomatia	α-D-GalNAc
SBA	Glycine max	α-D-GalNAc/D-Gal
WGA	Triticum vulgaris	β (1-4)-D-GlcNAc
RCA	Ricinus communis	β-D-Gal
	Antigen	
CEA	Carcinoembryonic Antigen	
SP	Secretory piece of IgA	
ACT	α-1-anti-Chymotrypsin	

Table 2. Patient Characteristics.

Total No.:   16

Sex   :   M - 11; F - 5

Age   :   40 - 76 years

Primary

  Site   :   rectum - 13; descending col. - 2; caecum - 1

  Type   :   adeno Ca.- 12; mucinous adeno Ca.- 4

  Grade   :   well/moderately well diff. - 12; poorly diff.- 4

Metastases

  Chronologic : synchronous - 6; metachronous - 10

  Time to   : 3 - 48 mths, mean - 16 mths

  Grade   : well/moderately well diff. - 11; poorly diff.-5

The presence and distribution of lectins and antigens was analysed and the morphology of the binding sites classified with respect to the cellular structure of mucosal and tumour glands.

The classification recognized several groups viz; luminal staining (L), diffuse staining (D), a combination of both (LD) and secretory staining (S) if there was supranuclear vesiculous staining at the region of Golgi particles. If less than 10% of the cells were stained, the specimen was classified as negative (N).

RESULTS

The overall picture is difficult to analyse statistically. A number of problems were encountered.

The normal orthotopic mucosa was stained in almost every case by all lectins and antigens except α-1-ACT in a constant, homogenous way.

In the primary tumours, different lectins bind to different parts of the cells. Some markers such as PNL and SP are not detectable in all cases and a different morphology of binding pattern therefore results.

An individual marker map is therefore obtained for each tumour and there is no conformity between individual cases. One of the most impressive findings was the occurrence of mosaic structures; areas with and without expression of the same antigen in one and the same tumour, sometimes even within one tumour gland.

Neither grading of the primary nor localisation within the large bowel, nor mucus production had any influence on the presence and distribution of lectins and antigens.

Moreover there was no preferred morphological staining in any of the liver metastases. All kinds of staining patterns occurred, for example positive staining at the border of the metastasis where it invaded normal liver tissue corresponded with negative staining in the more central, but non-necrotic parts.

Neither the synchronous nor metachronous character of the metastases had any influence on binding sites.

Comparing primary tumours and their corresponding liver metastases, there was no consistant relationship in antigen- and lectin distribution. New expression, loss and stability of markers were all observed. Four different basic relationships were found:

- identical expression of markers
- loss of markers in the metastases compared to the primary
- expression of markers by metastases in negative primaries
- change in marker morphology between primary and secondary,
  e.g. change from extensive diffuse to slight luminal pattern

With regard to Fidler's hypothesis of clonal selection; one would expect that in cases of mosaic structure in the primary if one of the pre-existing clones was selected, either expression or loss of this marker will occur in the metastases. But we found all possible relationships in our material:

- mosaic structure in primary and stable negative staining in
  the metastases, i.e. marker lost
- mosaic structure in primary and stable positive staining in
  the metastases, i.e. marker was selected. But
- stable mosaic in primary and metastases and
- stable negative primary and mosaic structure in the metastases
  seem not to support the hypothesis of clonal selection, because
  the secondary seems to have more clones compared to the primary.

CONCLUSIONS

Differentiation of the tumours does not correspond with expression
or loss of lectins and antigens. The 4 poorly differentiated primaries
showed less positive marker staining than the metastases. Nor was there
any loss in marker-expression in the one case where a change occurred from
a well to a poorly differentiated tumour from primary to metastases.

The heterogeneity of primary tumours and metastases can account for
a different clinical course, response to therapy and in vitro growth rates.

Our method of characterising tumour cells, lends no support to the
hypothesis of clonal selection as a presupposition of the metastatic
process, but neither does it refute it.

PREVENTION OF METASTASIS : A NEW TARGET

G. STORME[1], D. SCHALLIER[1], W. DE NEVE[1], J. DE GREVE[1], S. VAN BELLE[1],
G. DEWASCH [1] and S. DOTREMONT[2]

[1]Oncology Centre A.Z.-V.U.B., Laarbeeklaan 101, 1090 Brussels, Belgium
[2]Department of Internal Medicine and Pneumology, A.Z.-Sint Lucas Hospital
Sint Lucaslaan 29, 8320 Assebroeck-Brugge 4, Belgium

Keyword: anti-invasive, anti-metastatic, lung cancer

INTRODUCTION

Data obtained from in vitro experiments have shown that microtubule
inhibitors (MTI) such as the vinca alkaloids possess, not only anti-
proliferative and anti-migratory, but also anti-invasive properties
(Mareel & De Brabander 1978, Storme & Mareel 1980, Schallier et al. 1981,
Mareel et al. 1982). In animal experiments, MTI have an antimetastatic
activity suggesting therefore an indirect proof of the anti-invasive
activity (Hart et al. 1980, Atassi et al. 1982). However until now, no
clinical trial studied this action in humans. We therefore initiated a
randomised trial to evaluate the possibility of an increase in the metastatic free survival (MFS) of lung cancer patients with limited operable
disease by adding a vinca alkaloid, vinblastine (VLB) to standard
radiotherapy.

PATIENTS AND METHODS

Forty-eight patients with limited inoperable squamous cell lung
cancer, staged clinically and/or surgically with or without involvement
of the mediastinal nodes were randomised for local RT to tumor and
mediastinum (55 Gy in 6 weeks) with VLB (6 mg/m^2 in weekly IV bolus injection) (group A) or without VLB (group B). Patients with a performance
status (PS) less than 60 on the Karnofsky scale, age over 70, second
neoplasia, other debilitating disease, pleural effusion and/or chest wall
invasion, abnormal hematological and/or neurological signs were excluded.
Follow-up was performed monthly in both groups by clinical examination
with routine blood chemistry and chest X-ray. Every 6 months a complete
initial work up including brain-, bone scintigraphy and liver echography
was performed. Complementary investigations to rule out metastatic disease
were allowed. Patients who developed metastases could be treated with

combination chemotherapy or other palliative measures. VLB was reduced following myelosuppression and/or neurotoxicity according to standard criteria. Neurotoxicity was evaluated according to the WHO criteria. To score esophagitis a scale from 0 to 5 was taken (0 : no complaints; 1 : slight dysphagia for less than 1 month after RT; 2 : dysphagia for more than one month after RT and requiring semiliquid food; 3 : severe dysphagia for less than one month after RT capable only of liquid food; 4 : severe dysphagia requiring hospitalisation and parenteral nutrition; 5 : lethal complication). The local response was evaluated three months after randomisation by means of chest X-ray and was defined as follows : complete remission (CR) meant disappearance of all tumor; partial remission (PR) required decrease of tumor; stable disease (SD) was essentially status quo and evolving disease (ED) was local evolution and/or appearance of metastasis. All patients were evaluated for the MFS and survival (S). MFS and S were computed by the life table method. Logrank test was used for statistics. Twenty-five patients were randomised to group A and 23 to group B. Both groups were homogenous with respect to P.S./tumor stage (TNM) and age (Table 1). Patients were evaluable for MFS and S. In group A there were : 25, 25 and in group B : 23, 23 respectively; for local response there were 16 in group A and 16 in group B.

Table 1. Patient characteristics.

	RT + VLB	RT
Randomised	25	25
P.S.	range : 70 - 100	range : 70 - 100
	median : 90	median : 90
Age (y)	range : 37 - 69	range : 52 - 70
	median : 60	median : 62
TNM*		
Tis	1	–
1	5	2
2	7	11
3	12	10
N		
0	5	4
1	1	3
2	16	13
x	3	3

*Includes in RT + VLB : 2 thoracotomies with heavy debulking and 2 exploratory thoracotomies; in RT : 3 thoracotomies with heavy debulking and 2 exploratory thoracotomies. The post surgical stages are reported for these patients.

RESULTS

<u>Response</u>

The response rate is presented in Table II.

Table II. Response.

	RT + VLB	RT	
Responders	11 (5CR + 6PR)	6 (1CR + 5P5)	p = .08
Non responders	5 (5SD)	10 (9SD + 1ED)	(Chi square)

<u>Metastatic free survival and survival</u>

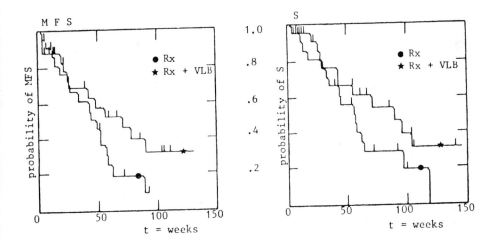

To the small group of patients we find only a trend to a better MFS
(p 0.14) and S (p 0.2).

<u>Toxicity</u>

Myelosuppression was rather moderate since approximately 70 % and
± 50 % of the expected VLB dosage could be administered respectively
during RT and long term treatment. Dysphagia was higher in group A, with
a median value between grade 2 and 3, versus 0 to 1 in group B.

Neurotoxicity was acceptable in all evaluable patients (median value 1)
except for one who developed a severe paralytic ileus at 25 weeks.

DISCUSSION

The hypothesis that MTI such as the vinca alkaloids are able to prevent metastasis in man has never been investigated. To evaluate the antimetastatic potential of VLB, we have chosen squamous cell lung cancer because this tumor ends frequently by metastatic spread (Kjaer 1982). Two investigators (Crosbie et al. 1966, Coy 1970) added VLB to surgery and RT, but were not able to demonstrate any effect on long term survival. The antimetastatic action could however not be evaluated adequately since VLB was only administered for 3 months and 4 weeks. Only in the EORTC Hodgkin trial (Tubiana et al. 1979) was VLB administered for a period of 2 years. The overall disease free survival was significantly higher in patients treated with VLB. Relapses mainly in the adjacent irradiated area were significantly decreased. However it was concluded that this favorable result was due to the cytostatic action of VLB on small tumor deposits not detectable by clinical evaluation. It seems to us worthwhile to go on with this trial considering the promising preliminary results with acceptable toxicity.

REFERENCES

Atassi, G., Dumont, P. & Vandendris, M./ 1982, Invasion and Metastasis 2, 217.
Coy, P., 1970, Cancer 26, 803.
Crosbie, W.A., Belcher, J.R. & Kamdar, H.H., 1966, British Journal Disease Chest 60, 28.
Hart, I.R., Raz, A. & Fidler, I.J., 1980, Journal National Cancer Institute 64, 891.
Kjaer, M., 1982, Cancer Treatment Reviews 9, 1.
Mareel, M. & De Brabander, M., 1978, Journal National Cancer Institute 61, 787.
Mareel, M., Storme, G., De Bruyne, G. & Van Cauwenberghe, R., 1982, European Journal of Cancer and Clinical Oncology 18 (2), 199.
Schallier, D., Storme, G., De Bruyne, G. & Mareel, M., 1981, Tumour Progression and Markers, 33, Ed. Kugler.
Storme, G. & Mareel, M., 1980, Cancer Research 40, 943.
Tubiana, M., Henry-Amae, M., Hayat, M., Breur, K., Vander Werf-Messing, B. & Burgers, M., 1979, European Journal of Cancer and Clinical Oncology 15, 645.

This work was supported by a grant of : Belgische Sportvereniging tegen Kanker.

BREAST CANCER RELAPSES AND GROWTH RATE

E. GALANTE, A. BONO, S. CATANIA, I. BETTONI, L. De FLAVIIS, S. Di PIETRO

Istituto Nazionale per lo Studio e la Cura dei Tumori, Via Venezian 1,
20133 Milan, Italy

Keywords: breast cancer, growth rate, relapse risk, prognosis

INTRODUCTION

This study concerns a population of 180 breast cancers for which the growth rate of the primary tumour, expressed as doubling time (DT), was evaluated by means of a double mammographic examination performed before the surgical treatment (Galante et al. 1981). The DT value was calculated by applying the formula of exponential growth (Spratt et al. 1977):

$$DT = \frac{0.6931}{b} \qquad \text{where} \quad b = \frac{\ln V_1 - \ln V_0}{T_1 - T_0}$$

V_0 is the mammographic volume of the tumour at the time, T_0, of the first examination; V_1 is the mammographic volume at the time, T_1, of the second examination; and T_1-T_0 is the interval between the two radiological examinations. On the basis of the DT values, three subsets of growth were defined: fast (DT up to 30 days), intermediate (DT from 31 to 90 days) and slow (DT more than 90 days). There were 31 (15.8%) fast-growing tumors, 84 (42.9%) intermediate, and 81 (41.3%) slow-growing tumors.

The distribution of the three subsets of growth according to lymph node involvement (N-, N+ (1-3), N+ (> 3)) showed that slow-growing tumours represented half of the N- cases, intermediate represented half of the N+ cases, and fast-growing tumours were equally distributed between N- and N+ cases. These differences in distribution were statistically significant (Table 1).

Table 1. Doubling time versus lymph node involvement.

Doubling time	N−		N+ (1–3)		N+ (> 3)		Total
Fast	16	(19)*	7	(11)	7	(19)	30
Intermediate	25	(30)	35	(56.5)	18	(48.6)	78
Slow	43	(51)	20	(32.3)	12	(32.4)	75
Total	84		62		37		183

*Number of cases; in parenthesis, percentage values. $p < 0.02$.

In contrast, the distribution of the three subsets of growth according to mammographic size (T_1 and T_2) did not show any statistically significant difference, although slow-growing cases prevailed in the T_1 group and intermediate cases in the T_2 group (Table 2).

Table 2. Doubling time versus mammographic T.

Doubling time	T1	T2	T3	T4	Total
Fast	8 (14.5)	22 (16.4)	1	0	31
Intermediate	20 (36.5)	61 (45.0)	0	3	84
Slow	27 (49.0)	51 (38.6)	0	3	81
Total	55	134	1	6	196

*Number of cases; in parenthesis, percentage values.

The follow-up from 3 to 7 years of 180 evaluable cases showed that there was no statistically significant difference among the free-disease probabilities of the three subsets of growth in N− and N+ (1–3) groups of lymph node involvement. In contrast, the differences among the free-disease probabilities of three subsets of growth N+ (> 3) were statistically significant (Table 3). Moreover, there was a highly significant difference among the free-disease probabilities of the three N groups of fast- and intermediate-growing tumours, but there was no statistically significant difference among the free-disease probabilities of the slow-growing subset.

The Cox model (1972) applied to two parameters, lymph node involvement and growth rate, showed a statistically significant relationship between them. On the basis of this test, relapse risk (RR) of a cancer population distributed according to lymph node involvement and growth rate was calculated. Starting with the RR of fast-growing N− tumours = 1 (the course of this tumour was the most favourable), fast-growing N+ (> 3) tumours showed

Table 3. Free disease probabilities of 180 cancers after 36–85 months of follow-up (growth rate vs lymph node involvement).

Doubling time	N–		N+ (1–3)		N+ (> 3)		P*
	Rel	FD(%)	Rel	FD(%)	Rel	FD(%)	
Fast	3/16	80	2/6	66	6/6	0	0.0001
Intermediate	4/23	80	11/35	59	13/19	31	0.001
Slow	7/23	77	4/21	68	5/11	51	0.2
P**		0.9		0.7		0.01	

Rel, relapses; FD, free disease probability.
* P values refer to the comparison among values of the FD line.
** P values refer to the comparison among values of the FD column.

the highest RR, which was 15 times the RR of fast-growing N– tumours. It is noteworthy that the RR of fast-growing N+ (> 3) tumours was six times the RR of slow-growing tumours of the same N class, but the RR of the latter tumours was only twice that of slow-growing N– tumours (Fig. 1).

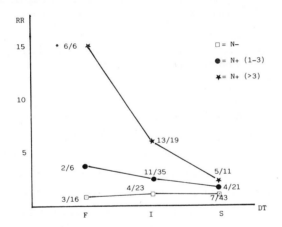

Figure 1. Relapse risk (RR) of 180 breast cancers distributed according to the doubling time (DT) and lymph node involvement (N). * Number of cases at risk. F, fast; I, intermediate; S, slow. □, N–; ●, N+ (1–3); ★, N+ (> 3).

Since there is a relationship between the growth characteristics of the primary tumour and relapse of the disease, the question is whether the behaviour of relapses is also influenced by the growth rate of the tumour. Our analysis concerned 52 evaluable first metastases of 56 relapses occurring in the 180 studied breast cancers. Bone metastases were the most frequent compared to the other sites. Table 4 shows the sites of the first metastases according to the growth rate of the primary tumour. Considering the limited case material, the relapses were consequently distributed into

Table 4.   Site of first metastases of 55 breast cancers distributed
according to the growth rate of the primary tumor.

Growth rate	Bone	Lung	Skin	Lymph nodes	Liver	Pleura	Multiple sites	Total
Fast	7	2	–	–	1	–	1	11
Intermediate	8	5	3	2	1	2	8	29
Slow	5	1	3	–	1	–	5	15
Total	20	8	6	2	3	2	14	55

osseous, non-osseous, and osseous + non-osseous (Table 5). This distribution showed that 60% of the first metastases of fast-growing tumours were
osseous; in contrast, 69% of first metastases of intermediate tumours were
non-osseous, whereas slow-growing tumours showed only a slight prevalence
of non-osseous metastases.

Table 5.   Characteristics of first metastases of 52 breast cancers
distributed according to the growth rate of the primary tumor.

Growth rate	Osseous		Non-osseous		Osseous + non-osseous	
	No.	%	No.	%	No.	%
Fast	7	(63.6)	3	(27.2)	1	(9.1)
Intermediate	8	(30.7)	18	(69.3)	–	
Slow	5	(33.3)	8	(53.3)	2	(13.3)
Total	20		29		3	

No statistical evaluation was made of these results, because the distribution of the case material was chosen for convenience, not according to a
biological criterion. Consequently two observations only will be made. In
our case material the osseous metastases of fast-growing tumours represented one-third of all the detected osseous metastases (Table 5), whereas the
fast-growing tumours represented less than one-sixth of the original series.

The high frequency of non-osseous metastases of intermediate-growing
tumours could be related to the high frequency of lymph node involvement of
these tumours (Table 1). The biological meaning of these behaviours and
their clinical implication could be better studied in the future on a more
substantial case material.

REFERENCES

Cox, D. R., 1972, Regression models and life tables (with discussion),
    J. R. Stat. Soc. B., 34, 187.
Galante, E., Guzzon, A., Gallus, G., Mauri, M., Bono, A., De Carli, A.,
    Merson, M. & Di Pietro, S., 1981, Prognostic significance of the growth
    rate of breast cancer: preliminary evaluation on the follow-up of 196
    breast cancers, Tumori, 67, 333.
Spratt, J. S. Jr., Kaltenbach, M. L. & Spratt, J. A., 1977, Cytokinetic
    definition of acute and chronic breast cancer, Cancer Research, 37, 226.

HUMAN MAMMARY CANCER INDUCED OSTEOLYSIS

C.S.B. GALASKO, STELLA RUSHTON, GAYE OLIVER, C. ELSWORTH and A.   HOWELL*

University of Manchester, Department of Orthopaedic Surgery, Clinical Sciences Building,

Hope Hospital, Eccles Old Road, Salford M6 8HD   * Christie Hospital, Manchester

Keywords: osteolysis, mammary carcinoma

Previous studies (Galasko, 1976) have shown that there are two phases to tumour-induced

osteolysis. The first and quantitatively more important is mediated via osteoclasts; in

the second phase malignant cells seem to be directly responsible for the bone destruction.

Our previous studies have also shown that PGE2 plays an important role in tumour-mediated

osteolysis (Galasko and Bennett, 1976; Galasko et al, 1979).

This study was carried out to determine whether PGE2 secretion by human mammary carcin-

oma was related to tumour-induced osteolysis, and to assess which agents may be useful in

the management of tumour-induced osteolysis.

The osteolytic activity of primary mammary carcinoma was measured in pieces of tumour

obtained at the time of mastectomy or excision biopsy in 161 patients using a mouse

calvarium/tumour co-culture system (Galasko et al, 1980). In 110 patients the prostaglandin

E2 activity of the tumour was also measured by radio immuno-assay. The effect of two

diphosphonates (EHDP and Cl_2MDP), three prostaglandin inhibitors (indomethacin, flurbi-

profen and ibuprofen) in three different doses, and the combination of indomethacin and

Cl_2MDP on tumour-induced osteolysis was measured in 30 tumours using the mouse calvarium/

tumour co-culture technique (Galasko et al, 1980). In a further 30 tumours the effect of

tamoxifen (in three different doses), flurbiprofen, Cl_2MDP and the combinations of

indomethacin + Cl_2MDP and flurbiprofen + Cl_2MDP was assessed.

The patients have been followed up and their survival rates measured.

RESULTS

The results showed that there were two types of primary mammary carcinoma. Approximately

55% of the tumours were osteolytically active in the mouse calvarium/tumour co-culture

system (Table 1), the remaining 45% of tumours being inactive. However, there was no

difference in PGE2 values between the two groups of tumours and both groups had

significantly higher PGE2 levels than normal breast tissue.

The results of the mouse calvarium/tumour co-culture experiments showed that when all

the tumours were included the effect of prostaglandin inhibitors, diphosphonates, their combination and tamoxifen were dampened by the inclusion of the osteolytically inactive tumours. The effect of these agents on reducing tumour-induced osteolysis could be more accurately assessed from the results obtained with osteolytically active tumours alone. The results of two protocols are shown in Tables 2 and 3. The combination of prostaglandin inhibitor and diphosphonate was more effective than either agent alone or tamoxifen.

The survival studies showed that the prognosis was better for those patients whose primary tumour contained larger amounts of PGE2 (Table 4) but there was no correlation between PGE2 and eostrogen receptor status. There was no difference in survival between patients with osteolytically active and those with osteolytically inactive tumours.

Table 1.   The Osteolytic activity and PGE2 levels in primary human mammary cancers.

	Osteolytic activity (mg/dl Ca)	PGE2 (ng/g)
Normal breast tissue	-0.091 ± 0.204	20.93 ± 2.04
All tumours	0.34 ± 0.08	88.17 ± 18.06
Osteolytically active	*0.62 ± 0.06	**85.48 ± 21.75
Osteolytically inactive	-0.08 ± 0.08	**93.54 ± 34.36
Compared with normal * p<0.0005	** p<0.005	

DISCUSSION

Our results show that tumour-induced osteolysis can be significantly inhibited by the combination of prostaglandin inhibitors and diphosphonates. Skeletal metastases can be associated with severe pain and these agents may have an important role to play in the treatment of early, but established skeletal metastases. However, our results also indicate that patients whose primary tumour contains large amounts of PGE2 have a better prognosis. This questions whether prostaglandin inhibitors should be used prophylactically, in an attempt to prevent the development of skeletal metastases, as it is theoretically possible that they may adversely affect the prognosis by reducing prostaglandin secretion in the primary tumour. Our results also show that there is no difference in survival between patients with osteolytically active and those with osteolytically inactive tumours. However, the follow-up is too short to determine whether there is a difference in the pattern of dissemination in these two groups of patients.

REFERENCES

Galasko, C.S.B., 1976, Nature, 263, 507.
Galasko, C.S.B., Bennett, A., 1976,Nature, 263, 508.
Galasko, C.S.B., Rawlins, R., Bennett, A., 1979, British Journal Cancer, 40, 360.
Galasko, C.S.B., Samuel, A.E., Rushton, S., Lacey, E., 1980, British Journal Surgery, 67, 493.

ACKNOWLEDGEMENTS

This work was supported by a grant from the Medical Research Council.

Table 2. Effect of prostaglandin inhibitors, diphosphonates and their combination on human mammary cancer induced osteolysis (protocol 1).

Agent*	Dose	Osteolytically Active Tumours	All Tumours	Osteolytically Inactive Tumours
Tumour only	–	0.62 ± 0.06	0.34 ± 0.08	-0.08 ± 0.08
EHDP	$2.4 \times 10^{-5}M$	0.35 ± 0.11	0.18 ± 0.09	-0.07 ± 0.11
Indomethacin	$2.4 \times 10^{-6}M$	0.32 ± 0.14	0.18 ± 0.11	-0.04 ± 0.14
Flurbiprofen	$2.4 \times 10^{-7}M$	0.32 ± 0.14	0.14 ± 0.11	-0.13 ± 0.17
Indomethacin	$2.4 \times 10^{-5}M$	0.31 ± 0.10	0.07 ± 0.10	-0.28 ± 0.16
Indomethacin	$2.4 \times 10^{-7}M$	0.30 ± 0.12	0.18 ± 0.09	0.01 ± 0.14
Flurbiprofen	$2.4 \times 10^{-5}M$	$0.22 \pm 0.15**$	0.10 ± 0.11	-0.09 ± 0.15
Cl_2MDP	$2.4 \times 10^{-5}M$	$0.18 \pm 0.08**$	0.06 ± 0.08	-0.13 ± 0.15
Ibuprofen	$2.4 \times 10^{-7}M$	$0.16 \pm 0.08**$	0.15 ± 0.08	0.15 ± 0.16
Indomethacin+ Cl_2MDP	$2.4 \times 10^{-7}M$) $2.4 \times 10^{-5}M$)	$0.13 \pm 0.10**$	0.05 ± 0.10	-0.07 ± 0.21
Ibuprofen	$2.4 \times 10^{-5}M$	$0.09 \pm 0.13**$	0.04 ± 0.11	-0.03 ± 0.20
Flurbiprofen	$2.4 \times 10^{-6}M$	$0.05 \pm 0.11**$	0.04 ± 0.10	0.03 ± 0.21
Ibuprofen	$2.4 \times 10^{-6}M$	$0.004 \pm 0.10**$	0.03 ± 0.10	0.06 ± 0.20
Indomethacin+ Cl_2MDP	$2.4 \times 10^{-5}M$) $2.4 \times 10^{-5}M$)	$-0.01 \pm 0.08**$	-0.02 ± 0.09	-0.04 ± 0.19
Indomethacin+ Cl_2MDP	$2.4 \times 10^{-6}M$) $2.4 \times 10^{-5}M$)	$-0.06 \pm 0.20**$	$-0.1 \pm 0.14**$	-0.15 ± 0.18
No. tumours		18	30	12

*The agents are listed in rank order; the results were analysed using analysis of variance followed by Duncan's multiple range test.

The osteolytic activity is in mgms Ca/dl. Figures are Mean $\pm$ SEM.** $p < 0.05$

Table 3. Effect of prostaglandin inhibitors, diphosphonates, their combination,
          and tamoxifen on human mammary cancer induced osteolysis (protocol 2).

Agent*	Dose	Osteolytically Active Tumours	All Tumours	Osteolytically Inactive Tumours
Tumour only	–	0.93 ± 0.11	0.19 ± 0.17	-0.54 ± 0.16
Cl_2MDP	$2.4 \times 10^{-5}M$	0.80 ± 0.11	0.42 ± 0.17	0.04 ± 0.34
Flurbiprofen	$2.4 \times 10^{-5}M$	0.64 ± 0.15	-0.02 ± 0.19	-0.68 ± 0.27
Flurbiprofen	$2.4 \times 10^{-6}M$	0.61 ± 0.16	-0.005 ± 0.16	-0.60 ± 0.18
Cl_2MDP	$2.4 \times 10^{-6}M$	$0.58 \pm 0.19**$	-0.09 ± 0.21	-0.75 ± 0.29
Tamoxifen	$2.4 \times 10^{-9}M$	$0.53 \pm 0.14**$	0.02 ± 0.18	-0.50 ± 0.28
Cl_2MDP	$2.4 \times 10^{-7}M$	$0.45 \pm 0.13**$	$-0.28 \pm 0.20**$	-0.98 ± 0.29
Flurbiprofen+ Cl_2MDP	$2.4 \times 10^{-6}M)$ $2.4 \times 10^{-7}M)$	$0.40 \pm 0.12**$	$-0.26 \pm 0.18**$	-0.93 ± 0.22
Indomethacin+ Cl_2MDP	$2.4 \times 10^{-6}M)$ $2.4 \times 10^{-6}M)$	$0.39 \pm 0.17**$	$-0.23 \pm 0.21**$	-0.86 ± 0.31
Tamoxifen	$2.4 \times 10^{-8}M$	$0.35 \pm 0.16**$	$-0.17 \pm 0.18**$	-0.68 ± 0.25
Flurbiprofen+ Cl_2MDP	$2.4 \times 10^{-7}M)$ $2.4 \times 10^{-7}M)$	$0.34 \pm 0.12**$	$-0.13 \pm 0.16**$	-0.71 ± 0.23
Flurbiprofen+ Cl_2MDP	$2.4 \times 10^{-7}M)$ $2.4 \times 10^{-6}M)$	$0.33 \pm 0.21**$	$-0.18 \pm 0.19**$	-0.68 ± 0.26
Tamoxifen	$2.4 \times 10^{-7}M$	$0.29 \pm 0.15**$	$-0.18 \pm 0.16**$	-0.64 ± 0.23
Indomethacin+ Cl_2MDP	$2.4 \times 10^{-7}M)$ $2.4 \times 10^{-7}M)$	$0.29 \pm 0.13**$	$-0.21 \pm 0.18**$	-0.72 ± 0.27
Flurbiprofen+ Cl_2MDP	$2.4 \times 10^{-6}M)$ $2.4 \times 10^{-5}M)$	$0.27 \pm 0.14**$	$-0.29 \pm 0.17**$	-0.85 ± 0.24
Flurbiprofen+ Cl_2MDP	$2.4 \times 10^{-7}M)$ $2.4 \times 10^{-5}M)$	$0.15 \pm 0.16**$	$-0.33 \pm 0.19**$	-0.08 ± 0.29
Flurbiprofen+ Cl_2MDP	$2.4 \times 10^{-6}M)$ $2.4 \times 10^{-6}M)$	$0.12 \pm 0.10**$	$-0.47 \pm 0.21**$	-1.05 ± 0.35
No tumours		15	30	30

*The agents are listed in rank order; the results were analysed using analysis of
variance followed by Duncan's multiple range test.

The osteolytic activity is in mgms Ca/dl. Figures are Mean $\pm$ SEM.** $p<0.05$.

Table 4. Effect of PGE2 level in primary human mammary cancer on prognosis.
          The difference is significant ($p<0.02$)

PGE2 level	No. patients	Observed deaths	Expected deaths	Observed/Expected
< 20 ng/g	37	15	8.70	1.72
> 20 ng/g	73	19	25.30	0.75

PROPOSAL FOR STAGING LIVER METASTASES

L. Gennari,   R. Doci, F. Bozzetti and P. Bignami
Istituto Nazionale per lo Studio e la Cura dei Tumori, Via Venezian 1,
20133 Milan, Italy

Keywords: Liver metastases; Classification

INTRODUCTION

In 1982 we reviewed the main prognostic factors in liver metastases and
the published main staging systems; we then proposed a new classification
(Gennari et al., 1982).   In spite of some criticism regarding the distribution by extent of liver involvement (< 25%; 25-50%; > 50%), the results
of our recent analysis of the prognosis of unresected liver metastases from
colorectal cancer confirm the significant trend among the 3 groups (Fig.
1). The time of diagnosis of liver metastases with respect to the primary
did not influence survival. Moreover, during the three-year experience we
have realized that cirrhosis was a rare finding in patients with liver
metastases; thus we suggest that both symbols (r = recurrences; c,
cirrhosis) be omitted.

The new simplified classification is presented in Table 1. For clinical
practice a further simplified system of classification seems necessary.
This system includes four stages, which are defined in Table 2.   The
rationale for such a distribution derived from the analysis of survival,
recurrence rate and distribution of recurrences.

Stage I.   When metastatic disease to the liver consists of a single
metastasis of limited size, the five-year survival after surgery ranges
from 20% (Foster and Berman 1977) to 42% (Wilson and Adson 1975).   In our
surgical series the actuarial survival at three years of H_{ls} patients
is 75% (Fig. 2). In unresected patients the three-year actuarial survival
was 20%.   It seems therefore justified to consider, irrespective of

37

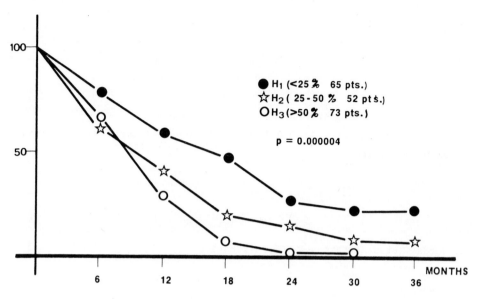

Figure 1. Actuarial survival of patients with unresected liver metastases from colorectal cancer, according to the extent of liver involvement.

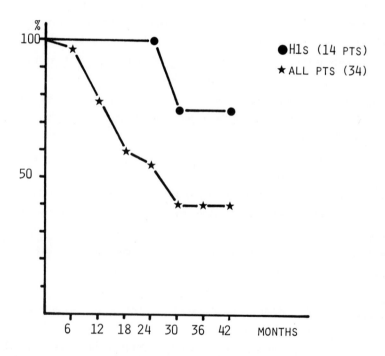

Fig. 2. Actuarial survival of patients with solitary metastasis involving <25% of liver (●, H_{1s}), and overall actuarial survival (*) after hepatic resection.

Table 1. Classification of hepatic metastases, 1984.

H_1	Liver involvement equal to or less than 25%
H_2	Liver involvement between 25-50%
H_3	Liver involvement more than 50%
s	Single metastasis
m	Multiple metastases to one surgical lobe
b	Bilateral metastases
i	Infiltration of adjacent organs or structures
F	Impairment of liver function

Table 2. Proposed staging.

Stage	
I	H_{1s}
II	$H_{1m,b}$ H_{2s}
III	$H_{2m,b}$ $H_{3s,m,b}$
IV	A) "Minimal" intraabdominal extrahepatic disease (detected only at laparotomy)
	B) Extrahepatic disease

treatment results, all patients with single metastasis of limited size in the best prognostic Stage I.

Stage II.   Patients included in this stage (i.e., $H_{1m,b}$, H_{2s}) had a median postoperative survival ranging from 10 to 14 months and a recurrence rate ranging from 50 to 75% (Table 3). The two-year actuarial survival of unresected H_{2s}, H_{1m} and H_{1b} patients was respectively 18%, 20% and 17%.

Stage III. Patients included in this stage have liver involvement of more than 25% (but with multiple metastases) or more than 50% (independently of the number of lesions). All these patients had a poor prognosis, with a recurrence rate approaching 100% and an almost constant hepatic relapse.

Stage IV.   The presence of extrahepatic metastases is generally considered a worsening prognostic factor. It seems reasonable to distinguish between "minimal" intraabdominal disease discovered only at laparotomy (lymph node metastases, peritoneal implants) and clinically evident growth (peritoneal diffuse carcinosis; lung, bone, soft-tissue metastases). A further analysis is required to confirm the prognostic value of both a and b subgroups.

Table 3.   Survival and recurrences in stage II patients.

	Median survival (mos)	% of recurrence		
		Local	Distant	Total
H_{1m}	13.5	75	25	75
H_{1b}	14	50	50	50
H_{2s}	10	–	50	50

In conclusion, we hope that the present staging system is favorably considered by oncologists and that constructive criticisms and suggestions might lead to a worldwide accepted common language.

REFERENCES

Foster, J.H. & Berman, M.M. (1977) Solid liver tumors. In Major problems in clinical surgery, edited by P.A. Ebert (WB Saunders, Philadelphia) p. 209.
Gennari, L., Doci, R., Bozzetti, F. & Veronesi, U. (1982) Tumori, 68, 443.
Pettavel, T., Leywraz, S. & Douglas, P. (1984) The necessity for staging liver metastases and standardizing treatment-response criteria. The case of secondaries of colo-rectal origin. In Liver metastasis, edited by C.J.H. Van De Valde & P.H. Sugarbaker (Martinus Nijhoff, Dordrecht), p. 154.
Wilson, S.M. & Adson, M.A. (1976) Archives of Surgery, 111, 330.

PATTERNS OF FAILURE AFTER HEPATIC RESECTION FOR METASTASES AND RATIONALE
FOR A MULTIMODAL APPROACH

Federico BOZZETTI, Roberto DOCI, Paola BIGNAMI and Leandro GENNARI

Istituto Nazionale per lo Studio e la Cura dei Tumori, Milan, Italy

Keywords: Failure: after hepatectomy; after metastasis resection

INTRODUCTION

Although surgical resection of hepatic metastases from a colorectal
cancer has gained worldwide acceptance as a therapeutic approach in
selected cases, there is considerable paucity of data concerning the
natural history of the resected patients and the areas of failure after
hepatic resection. We think that a deeper knowledge of the natural history
of these patients could help the oncologist to plan a multimodal approach
to patients with liver metastases from colorectal cancer.

PATIENTS AND METHODS

From October 1980 to May 1984, 35 patients radically operated on for a
colorectal cancer and with metastases confined to the liver were treated by
surgical liver resection.   The main characteristics of the series are
reported in Table 1.   Patients were staged according to the classification
proposed by Gennari et al. (1982) at the Istituto Nazionale Tumori of
Milan, which classifies the extent of liver resection as H_1 (liver involvement $\leq$ 25%), H_2 (liver involvement $>$ 25% $\leq$50%), and H_3 (liver involvement
$>$ 50%). There were 20 H_1, 8 H_2 and 6 H_3 patients. Metastases were also
classified as single (s), multiple (m) and bilateral (b), and included 18,
11, and 5 patients, respectively. The median postoperative follow-up was
16 months (range 5-36). The rate of total failure, local (hepatic)
failure, as the only failure or as a component of the total failure, and
distant failure (mainly lung), as the only failure or as a component of the
overall failure, is analyzed in Tables 2 and 3, and the differences were
tested according to the chi-square test.

Table 1.   Patients operated by hepatic resection of metastases from colorectal cancer.

No. of patients	35
Age (median)	51 (33-75)
Males	23
Females	12
Diagnosis of metastases	
Synchronous	9
Metachronous	26
Median interval (months)	21 (4-60)
Type of surgery	
Right lobectomy	14
Right extended lobectomy	3
Left lobectomy	1
Left lateral lobectomy	6
Segmentectomy (mono- or bilateral)	11
Total	35
Operative mortality (ischemic colitis)	1/35 = 2.8%

Table 2.   Areas of failure according to some characteristics of the primary tumor.

	Resect No	Fail No (%)	Liver Only No (%)	Liver Component No (%)	Distant Only No (%)	Distant Component No (%)	Both No (%)
Site of primary							
Rectum/sigmoid	24	15 (63)	6 (25)	10 (42)	5 (21)	9 (38)	4 (17)
Colon	10	4 (40)	2 (20)	3 (30)	1 (10)	2 (20)	1 (10)
Dukes primary							
Dukes B N-	8	5 (63)	2 (25)	4 (50)	1 (13)	3 (8)	2 (25)
Dukes C N+	14	7 (50)	4 (28)	6 (42)	1 (7)	3 (21)	2 (14)
Dukes D	12	7 (58)	2 (17)	3 (25)	4 (33)	5 (42)	1 (8)
Metastases onset							
Synchronous	9	7 (77)	4 (44)	6 (66)	1 (11)	3 (33)	2 (22)
Metachronous	25	12 (48)	4 (17)	7 (28)	5 (20)	8 (32)	3 (12)
Total	34	19 (55)	8 (24)	13 (39)	6 (17)	11 (32)	5 (15)

RESULTS

The median follow-up on the overall series was 16 months, and the recurrence rate was 55%. Approximately 1/4 and 1/5 of the patients had respectively only hepatic or lung involvement, and both these sites were involved as a component of metastatic spread in about 1/3 of the cases. Despite the limits due to the univariate analysis and to a relatively short follow-up, some categories of patients appear to have a different prognostic trend. A better prognosis seems to be related to the class H_1 vs H_2 and H_3 (p < 0.003) and s vs m + b (p < 0.003). An ominous prognosis is related to the class H_3 and class b. Patients classified as H_2 or m had

Table 3. Areas of failure according to some characteristics of the liver metastases.

	Resect No	Fail No (%)	Liver Only No (%)	Liver Component No (%)	Distant Only No (%)	Distant Component No (%)	Both No (%)
Stage							
H_1	20	8 (40)	3 (15)	6 (30)	2 (10)	5 (25)	3 (15)
H_2	8	5 (62)	1 (13)	2 (25)	3 (38)	4 (50)	1 (3)
H_3	6	6 (100)	4 (67)	5 (83)	1 (17)	2 (33)	1 (17)
Site & number metastases							
s	18	7 (38)	1 (6)	3 (17)	4 (22)	6 (33)	2 (11)
m	11	9 (82)	5 (45)	7 (63)	2 (18)	4 (36)	2 (18)
b	5	3 (60)	2 (40)	3 (60)	0	1 (20)	1 (20)
Preoperative CEA							
0-10	6	3 (50)	1 (17)	2 (33)	1 (16)	2 (33)	1 (17)
11-50	6	4 (66)	2 (33)	4 (67)	-	2 (33)	2 (3)
> 50	16	8 (50)	3 (19)	5 (31)	3 (19)	5 (31)	2 (13)
?	6	4 (66)	2 (33)	-	2 (33)	-	-
Surgery							
Lobectomy	23	15 (65)	6 (26)	10 (43)	5 (22)	9 (39)	4 (17)
Wedge resect.	11	4 (36)	2 (18)	3 (27)	1 (9)	2 (18)	1 (9)
Total	34	19 (55)	8 (24)	13 (38)	6 (18)	11 (32)	5 (14)

an intermediate prognosis. Other variables such as Dukes classification of the primary, site of origin of the primary, interval between primary and metastasis, preoperative CEA, and type of surgery failed to show any prognostic importance. A further evaluation of this series allowed us to identify three groups of patients with significantly different prognostic features (Table 4).

DISCUSSION

Since the final goal of this analysis was the identification of some prognostic variables and the recognition of the areas of failure, we can conclude with the following observations. 1) Relapses after hepatic resection for metastases mainly involve liver and lung. It is also possible that peritoneal spread is present but that it frequently goes undetected due to the lesser accuracy of routine sonography and CAT to identify it. 2) The presence of this "halfway" spread between the primary site of cancer and liver should favor an intraperitoneal infusion in patients candidate to adjuvant chemotherapy after hepatic resection. The median interval between liver resection and onset of metastases is 9.5 and 10 months for liver and lung relapses, respectively. This suggests that both a local

Table 4. Provisional staging of cancer with hepatic metastases.

	Re-sec-tion	Fail-ures	Mean follow-up (mos)	Liver Only No. %	Component No. %	Distant Only No %	Component No. %	Both No %
Group 1								
H_{1s}	14	4 (28%)	17.5	1 (7%)	2 (14%)	2 (14%)	3 (21%)	1 (7%)
Group 2								
H_{1m}	4							
H_{1s}	2	5 (62%)	14	2 (25%)	4 (50%)	1 (12%)	3 (37%)	2(25%)
H_{2b}	2							
Group 3								
H_{2m}	5							
H_{3s}	2							
H_{3m}	2	10 (83%)	12	5 (41%)	7 (58%)	3 (25%)	5 (41%)	2(16%)
H_{2b}	1							
H_{3b}	2							
Total	34	19 (56%)		8 (23%)	13 (38%)	6 (17%)	11 (32%)	5(14%)

(intraperitoneal or intrahepatic) or systemic treatment is necessary to attain control of the disease.

3) Since the reported doubling times of liver metastases range between 50 and 112 days, the onset of a detectable liver metastasis (≥ 1 cm^3 = 10^9 cells, after only 2 or 5 doublings) suggests a gross neoplastic residue within the liver (> 1 mm^3 = 10^6 cells) or an extremely accelerated post-operative growth rate, or both.

4) In group 1 patients the benefit/risk ratio of an adjuvant chemo-therapy should be carefully evaluated due to the limited risk of hepatic (14%) and distant (21%) recurrence.

5) In group 2 patients, due to the high recurrence rate, especially in the liver, a multimodal approach including surgery and a local infusional treatment is warranted.

6) In group 3 patients surgery alone is not a worthwhile approach and a local and systemic chemotherapy should be attempted after resection of monolateral lesions. In bilateral ones (H_{2-3b}), an intrahepatic adminis-tration of the drug is recommended.

REFERENCES

Gennari, L., Doci, R., Bozzetti, F. & Veronesi, U., 1982, <u>Tumori, 68, 443.</u>

OBSERVATIONS ON MALIGNANT MELANOMA METASTASES IN MAN

S. PLESNIČAR
The Institute of Oncology and Faculty of Medicine, Vrazov trg 2, 61000
Ljubljana, Yugoslavia

Keyword: malignant melanoma; metastases

INTRODUCTION

Malignant melanoma is a heterogenous tumor composed of cells with different metastatic potential. Clinical observations (Patel et al. 1978) and experimental data (Nicolson et al. 1976) suggest that the distribution of metastases is not random (de la Monte et al. 1983), and that metastases occur in a multistep sequence (Kržišnik-Logar & Plesničar 1980).

Therefore, the purpose of the present investigation was 1) to study the frequency distribution of metastatic involvement, which could indicate the existence of preferential organs and sites for metastases formation in malignant melanoma, and 2) to study the possible existence of the sequential spread of metastases in different sites.

MATERIAL

In the study 201 patients with cutaneous melanoma treated from 1965 to 1974 were included. Among them were 79 males and 122 females ranging in age from 29 to 79 years, the median being 48 years. The primary tumor was histologically verified in all instances, and the distribution of primary tumors was as follows: the skin of the lower extremities 37 % of cases, trunk 34 %, head 15 %, upper extremities 10 %, neck 4 %, and ano-genital region 1 % of cases. Patients were treated for their primary, and during the course of disease, predominately with surgery and radiotherapy. Chemotherapy was used only in six per cent of cases. Data concerning the metastatic dissemination of ocular melanoma were obtained from a series of 31 cases treated during the same period of time.

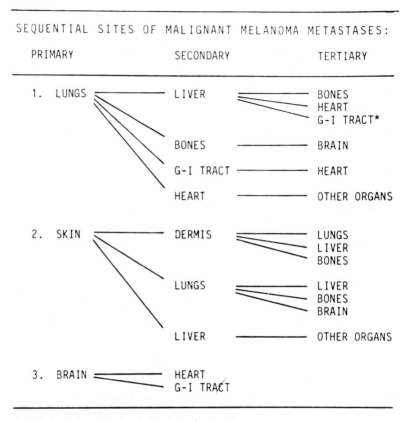

SEQUENTIAL SITES OF MALIGNANT MELANOMA METASTASES:

* G-I tract = Gastrointestinal tract

Figure 1. Possible model of a multistep cascade-like spread of hematogenous metastases originating from malignant melanoma.

RESULTS

The principal characteristics regarding 1) the incidence of metastases in different target organs, and 2) the sequential spread of metastases were reported:

1. Incidence of metastases from cutaneous malignant melanoma in target organs at autopsy:

70 - 90 % : Lung, liver, skin, lymph nodes.

50 - 69 % : Brain, heart muscle, kidney, adrenals, small intestine, pancreas.

20 - 49 % : Bones, thyroid, breast, spleen, stomach, colon.

10 - 19 % : Diaphragm, gall bladder, peritoneum with omentum and mesenterium, pericardium, bladder, ovaries.

under 10 %: Pituitary, parathyroid, esophagus, uterus, testis and prostate.

Less frequent sites were the major blood vessels, eye, bile ducts, larynx and pharynx. Occasionally metastases were found in placenta and fetus, and in bones without bone marrow, e.g. patella, scapula and others.

In ocular melanoma the observed distinct tendency to metastasize into the liver parenchyma (Davies 1849) was confirmed. Clinical incidence indicated that the liver is involved in 46 - 56 % of cases, lungs in 12 - 17 %, bones in 3 - 12 % and other sites (skin, lymph nodes, brain, gastrointestinal tract) were involved in 20 - 31 % of cases. As the sole initial site the liver was involved in 46 % of patients.

2. Time sequence in the appearance of metastases in malignant melanoma (Figure 1). In the present series it was found that the primary sites of metastatic involvement were the lungs (45 % of cases), epidermis of the skin (37 %) and brain (18 % of cases). The secondary and tertiary sites were numerous, however, it appears that the lungs, liver and bones are the three sites which are most commonly involved. Since the metastatic involvement of the brain could be considered as a terminal event, involvements of tertiary sites were not observed. Among other involved organs were the adrenals, pancreas, small intestine, thyroid, breast, spleen, stomach.

3. Unusual distribution of numerous metastases in one sole organ or area was observed, indicating the organotropic tendency of metastatic cells. Among the observed patterns were the metastatic involvement of the skin limited to one side of the body, roughly symetrical distribution of metastases over the skin of the trunk, and the involvement of the mucosa of the bile and pancreatic ducts, and the mucosa of the small intestine with numerous small metastatic lesions.

DISCUSSION

The organs and sites with the highest frequency of metastases are the lungs, liver and bones. However, in these organs extremely frequent are also metastases originating from tumors of epithelial and glandular origin. Therefore, in this respect, differences in the frequency and distribution were not found between the metastases from malignant melanoma and other tumors. When considering the metastatic spread in other organs and sites,it appears that the behaviour is different compared with metastatic dissemination from other tumors. In the first place, the high incidence in organs like the brain, the adrenals and the muscular substance of the heart should be noted. Further on, a tendency of metastasizing into a predetermined target organ is evident particularly in ocular melanoma with liver metastases, and cutaneous melanoma with skin metastases as the sole primary sites. It seems, therefore, that an organotropic distribution of metastases is apparent under given yet unknown conditions. Concluding, while the most frequently involved sites are similar for malignant melanoma and other tumor types, there are specific modes of spread indicating a patterned distribution of metastases.

Davies, H., 1849, Transactions of the Pathological Society of London, 2,128.

de la Monte, S.M., Moore, G.W., Hutchins, G.M., 1983, Cancer Research, 43, 3427.

Kržišnik-Logar, M., Plesničar, S., 1979, Zdravstveni Vestnik, 48, 701.

Nicolson, G.L., Brunson, K.W. & Fidler, I.J., 1976, Cancer Research, 38, 4111.

Patel, J.K., Didolkar, M.S., Pickren, J.W. & Moore, R.H., 1978, The American Journal of Surgery, 135, 807.

COMPARATIVE CONTROLLED STUDY OF ADJUVANT MELANOMA IMMUNOTHERAPY AND CHEMO-
IMMUNOTHERAPY.   EIGHT YEAR RESULTS

G. MATHÉ, J.L. MISSET   (Villejuif), B, SERROU (Montpellier), C. JEANNE (Rouen)
J. GUERRIN (Dijon), R. PLAGNE (Clermeont-Ferrand), M. SCHNEIDER (Nice),
B. LE MEVEL (Nantes), R. METZ (Nancy), Study analysis : M. DELGADO and
F. DE VASSAL (Villejuif), Statistical analysis : V. MORICE)Paris)

ONCOFRANCE COMPARATIVE TRIAL PROJECT, Institut de Cancerologie et d'Immuno-
genetique (INSERM, CNRS) et Service des Maladies Sanguines et Tumorales,
Groupe Hospitalier Paul-Brousse, 94804 Villejuif - France

Keywords : Melanoma; adjuvant immunotherapy; adjuvant chemo-immunotherapy

The Oncofrance Group initiated this trial on adjuvant treatment of melanoma
in 1975, when immunotherapy had recently been suggested as improving prognosis. (Eilber et al. 1976). Many studies of active immunotherapy were
conducted comparing chemo-immunotherapy to immunotherapy which we had
experimentally shown to be a non-valid method as chemotherapy can suppress
the possible benefit of immunotherapy (Mathé 1976). We set up the present
study to determine whether this effect, which had been observed in mice,
could be found in man.

PATIENTS AND METHODS

Eligibility

   The conditions for eligibility for the trial were : a) histologically
confirmed malignant melanoma, either of Clark Grade III, IV or V (MacGovern
 et al. 1973) or with any Clark grade and positive regional lymph nodes;
b) surgical removal of all detectable disease not more than 6 weeks before
randomization; lymph node dissection was mandatory only in cases of suspic-
ion of lymph node involvement; c) patients were less than 70 years old.

Stratification

   The patients were stratified according to lymph node status (stage I or
II), and to localisation of the primary tumour (head and neck, trunk, upper
limb, lower limb) (Table I).

Table I.

	IMMUNOTHERAPY 132	CHEMO-IMMUNOTHERAPY 146
SEX F	71	73
M	61	73
STAGE I	119	129
II	13	17
CLARK III	73	76
IV	43	56
V	11	12
UNKNOWN STAGE II	5	2
SITES head and neck	16	22
trunk	40	36
upper limb	15	22
lower limb	61	66

Treatment

The patients in each stratification category above mentioned were allo-
cated at random to be either in Group A (Immuno-BCG F Pasteur : 75 mg be
weekly scarification rotating on the four limbs for two years), or in Group
B (the same immunotherapy following six months of chemotherapy as follows :
Veham (VM26), 60 mg/m2 IV day 1 q 4 weeks, Deticene (DTIC), 150 mg/m2 days
2, 3, 4, 5 q 4 weeks, Belustine (CCNU), 60 mg/m2 days 2, 3 per os q 8 weeks.

Patients

278 patients (134 males and 144 females) were entered in the trial
between February 1975 and August 1980. 248 had stage I melanoma, 30 stage
II. 149 had a Clark III, 99 a Clark IV, 23 a Clark V and 7 a Clark level
unknown but stage II melanoma. Stage I primaries in 38 cases were located
in the head and neck, 76 in the trunk, 37 cases in the upper limb and 127
in the lower limb.

RESULTS

Tolerance of the regimen was good. No major toxicity occurred and the
chemotherapy as well as immunotherapy programs could be performed according
to the protocol schedule in most cases.

Overall survival and disease-free survival curves were drawn according
to the Kaplan Meier method and compared by the log-rank test. 48% of the
patients are in first complete remission and 63 alive at eight years. At
the median follow-up time, which is now in excess of 5 years, the probability of being free of disease is 52%, the probability of being alive is 63%.

Prognostic factors were studied : sex was significant in favour of females for disease-free survival (p=0.0001) and for survival (p=0.038). Clark level was significant in terms of survival with p=0.035. No prognostic value of the location of the primary tumour could be found (p=0.6). Node positive patients had a borderline worse disease-free survival (p=0.08) and a significantly poorer survival (0.3). According to the treatment arm, the analysis performed in March 1984 with an eight year follow-up, gave no difference between group A and group B for disease-free survival (fig. 1), and a significant difference (p=0.02) for survival after relapse (fig. 2).

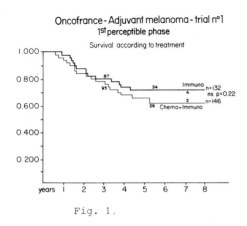

Fig. 1.

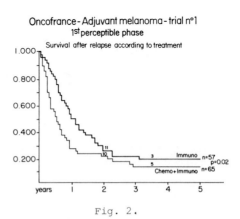

Fig. 2.

DISCUSSION

Several authors (Cunningham et al. 1979, Morton et al. 1982, Spitler & Sagebiel 1980) have reported that combined chemo-immunotherapy is valuable as adjuvant treatment for malignant melanoma. We observed in this trial that it may be less effective than immunotherapy alone. If immunotherapy is of any value in melanoma, it may be very important to give it soon after (or even before) surgical removal of the primary tumour and/or to avoid any chemotherapy which has not been effective in any trial (Beretta 1982) before immunotherapy.

REFERENCES

Beretta, G., 1982 Trial six : randomized study of prolonged chemotherapy, immunotherapy, and chemo-immunotherapy as an adjuvant to surgery for stage I and II melanoma. A progress report. In Recent Results in Cancer Research : "Adjuvant Therapy of Cancer" (G. Mathe, G. Bonadonna, S. Salmon, eds.). Springer Verlag p. 259.

Cunningham, J.T., Schoenfeld, D., Nathanson, L., Wolter, J., Patterson W., Cohen, M., Kuperminc, M., & Carbone, P.P., 1979. A controlled ECOG study of adjuvant therapy in patients with stage I and II melanoma. p. 507

In : "Adjuvant therapy of cancer II" (S.E. Salmon & S.E. Jones, eds).
New York, Grune & Stratton.

Eilber, F.R., Morton, D.L., Holmes, E.C., Sparks, F.C., & Ramming K.P., 1976.
Adjuvant immunotherapy with BCG in treatment of regional lymph node
metastasis from malignant melanoma. New England Journal of Medicine.
294, 237.

Mac Govern, V.J., Mihm, M.C., Bailly, C., Booth, J.C., Clark, J., Clark, W.H.,
Cochron, A.J., Hardy, E.G., Micks, J.D., Levene, A., Lewis, M., Little,
J.H., & Milton, G., 1973. The classification of malignant melanoma and
its histologic reporting. Cancer 32, 1446.

Mathe, G., Cancer active immunotherapy. Recent Results in Cancer Research.
Springer Verlag.

Morton, D.L., Holmes, E.C., Eilber, F.R., & Ramming, K.P., 1982. Adjuvant
immunotherapy of malignant melanoma : results of a randomized trial in
patients with lymph node metastasis. p. 245. In :"Immunotherapy of
Human Cancer" (W.D. Terry & S.A. Rosenberg, eds.) New York, Excerpta
Medica.

Spitler, L.E., & Sagebiel, R., 1980. A randomized trial of levamisole
versus placebo as adjuvant therpy in malignant melanoma. New England
Journal of Medicine. 303, 1143.

THE METASTASIZING PLEOMORPH ADENOMA OF THE SALIVARY GLAND

J.G.J. ROUSSEL[1], J.A. VAN DONGEN[2], and J.F.M. DELEMARRE[2]

[1]Department of Surgery, Lukas Ziekenhuis, Albert Schweitzerlaan 31,
7334 DZ Apeldoorn, The Netherlands
[2]The Netherland Cancer Institute, Plesmanlaan 121, 1066 CX Amsterdam,
The Netherlands

Keywords: pleomorph adenoma; satellitosis

ABSTRACT

A case of metastasizing pleomorph adenoma in which both the primary
tumor and metastasis were composed of benign pleomorphic structures is
reported, showing a peculiar type of metastasis-like satellitosis. Previously reported cases are reviewed. The metastasis commonly developed
many years after the excision of the primary tumor and was mostly preceded
by local recurrences. Mitotic activity and infiltrative growth pattern
are the histological features in the primary tumor important in predicting
the metastasizing potential.

INTRODUCTION

The pleomorphic adenoma of the salivary gland shows in clinical
behaviour three different patterns:

benign pleomorphic adenoma

carcinoma in pleomorphic adenoma

metastasizing pleomorphic adenoma

Benign pleomorphic adenoma is a circumscribed tumor, characterized
microscopically by its pleomorphic or 'mixed' appearance, clearly recogni-
zable epithelial tissue, being intermingled with a tissue of mucoid,
myxoid or chondroid appearance (WHO 1972).

Carcinoma in pleomorphic adenoma is a tumor showing definite evidence
of malignancy such as invasive growth and cytologic changes appropriate
to carcinoma and in which areas characteristic for pleomorphic adenoma
still can be found (Thackray and Lucas 1974).

Metastasizing pleomorphic adenoma is a tumor which shows the characteristic histological features of a pleomorphic adenoma in the primary tumor as well as in the metastases.

The respective definitions may establish order in the various clinicopathological features.

CASE REPORT

A 33 year old man presented with a two years existing lump in the left parotid area in 1970. The tumor was enucleated and histologic examination showed a pleomorphic adenoma in the salivary gland. In 1973 two recurrences were treated with excision. Finally a superficial parotid-ectomy was done. The patient subsequently received external radiation with a total dose of 3000 rads. In the following 5 years no evidence of disease was found until the patient experienced skin nodules in the face and scalp during a period of three years. In a first session in 1981 three skin nodules, localised near the left ear, eye and hair area, were removed (Figure 1).

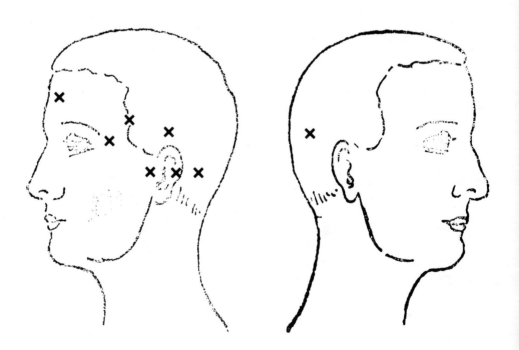

Figure 1. Sites of metastases in face and scalp.

Histological examination demonstrated a tumor type identical to the primary pleomorphic adenoma of the salivary gland. For this reason another 5 skin nodules, localised in the forehead on the left, the back of the head on the right, and near the left ear, were treated with simple surgical excision. Likewise the primary tumor and metastasis showed a similar histologic appearance and were composed of structures typical of benign pleomorphic adenoma. Up to now no further regional recurrences have arisen and distant metastasis has not occurred.

DISCUSSION

Pleomorphic adenoma, the most common tumor in the salivary glands, is generally considered a benign tumor, although it is recognised, that the tumor can become locally invasive. Non-radical rumor resection or peri-operative tumor spill may give rise to implantation in the operation site, resulting probably in local recurrence. Besides the more common pattern, a so-called 'malignant mixed tumor' occurring in a small number of all pleomorphic adenomas, may account for the potential to give distant metastasis.   The tumor in the metastatic sites is always composed of the carcinomatous component of the primary tumor. On the other hand a para-doxical feature of a 'benign' pleomorphic adenoma is the metastasizing sign, in which both the primary tumor and metastasis have a similar histologic appearance and are composed of structures typical of a benign pleomorphic adenoma.

Few similar cases have been reported in the literature and are listed in Table 1, including the present case.

Characteristics of metastasizing pleomorphic adenoma such as mitotic activity and the infiltrative growth pattern are indicated. Local re-currences preceding the metastasis frequently occur.   The sites of metastasis included bone, lung, lymphnode, liver and skin.

The pattern of metastasis in the present case history is distinct from other metastatic characteristics. The metastatic localisation outside the scar area raises the surmise that the satellitosis of skin nodules has its origin in purely skin metastasizing propensity.

Table 1.

Clinicopathologic Features of 11 Cases of Metastasizing Pleomorphic Adenoma.

Authors and references	No. of pts.	mitotic activity	infiltrative growth	No. of local recurrences preceding metastasis	interval between the detection of the primary and metastatic tumor (years)	metastatic sites	Outcome
Foote and Frazell 1954 Fascicle 11, Atlas of Tumor Pathology	1	-	-	5	19	lung	?
Thackray and Lucas 1957 Cancer 2, 154-167	1	-	-	1	22	Iliac bone	?
Fine and Marshall, 1961 Am. J. Surg. 102: 86-89	1	+	-	1	3	Femur, humerus ribs, lumbar vertebrae	Died in 3 years with multiple bony metastasis
Gerughty et al, 1969 Cancer 24: 471-486	3	-	+	?	?	Lung, bone, lymph nodes	?
Youngs and Scheuer, 1973 Journal Path. 109:171-173	1	+	-	0	11	Lung, bone, lymph nodes	Living with NED for 1 year
Chen, 1978 Cancer, 42, 2407-2411	1	+	-	5	12	Sacrum	Living with local recurrences and persistent sacral tumor for 4 years
Steffelaar, 1979 Ned. Tijdschr. Geneesk. 123. nr. 52 2209-2212	1	+	-	3	2	Thoracal vertebra VIII	Died some months after neurosurgery and radiotherapy
Morrison and Mc Mullin, 1984 Clinical Oncology,10, 173-176	1	-	-	4	51	Skull Nodule	?
Roussel et al, 1984 (present paper)	1	-	?	2	8	Satellitosis of face and scalp	Living with NED for 3 years

REFERENCES

Thackray, A.C. and Sobin, L.M., WHO 1972, Histologic typing of salivary gland tumors. International histologic classification of tumor no. 7.
Thackray, A.C. and Lucas, R.B. 1974, Tumors of the Major Salivary Glands. Fascicle 10, Second Series, Atlas of Tumor Pathology. Washington D.C. Armed Forces Institute of Pathology.

AN EXPERIMENTAL MODEL OF LIVER METASTASES FROM RAT COLORECTAL
ADENOCARCINOMA

P. van DALE, W. PENASSE, A POPOWSKI, D. JACOBOWITZ and P. GALAND
Laboratoire de Cytologie et de Cancerologie Experimentale de 1'U.L.B.,
Rue Heger Bordet, 1, 1000 Bruxelles

Keywords : liver, metastasis, experimental, colon carcinoma

INTRODUCTION

Following curative resection of colorectal cancer, of those patients
with recurrent disease at 5 years, 20 - 80% (depending on the Duke's
stage of disease) present with hepatic metastases. This relatively high
incidence of liver metastases makes it desirable to obtain an experimental
model of such lesions for fundamental and clinical investigations.

For this purpose we utilized DHD-K12-TR cells, a transplantable cell
line established from an intestinal carcinoma, induced in rats by 1,
2-dimethyl hydrazine (DMH) by Martin and Martin (1973) and generously
provided to us by them. The DMH-intestinal cancer model is remarkable for
its similarity to human colorectal adenocarcinoma (Martin & Martin, 1973).

MATERIAL AND METHODS

We used 27 BD IX rats (23 males and 3 females), provided by the
"Proefdieren Centrum" (KUL, Leuven, Belgium), weighing 250 to 350 g at the
time of intraportal injection. Culture medium for the DHD-K12-TR cells
contained HAM's F-10 medium, L-glutamine, 10% fetal calf serum and neomycin
(40 mg/ml). The cells (10^7 cells in 0.2 ml HAM's medium solution) were
prepared just prior to their injection. Laparatomy for intraportal injection
was performed under general anaesthesia with thalamonal (0.4 cc/100 g b.w.)
and atropine)0.1 to 0.2 mg/kg b.w.). When performed, partial hepatectomy
was accomplished immediately after cell injection according to Higgins and
Anderson (1931). This implies the removal of the median and left lobes
representing about 70% of the liver mass.

Four groups, corresponding to different experimental conditions were
constituted as follows : Group 1 or control group : 8 rats which received
tumour cell injection without prior treatment. Group 2 : 6 rats treated by
subcutaneous injection of cyclophosphamide (250 mg/kg b.w.) 2 days before
direct intraportal cell injection, according to Mendes da Costa (1978).
Group 3 : 6 rats treated by intraperitoneal injection of cyclophosphamide
(150 mg/kg b.w.) also 2 days before cell injection. Group 4 : 7 rats
submitted to a two-third partial hepatectomy 5 min. after portal injection.

RESULTS

   The results are summarized in Table 1. They show that treatment with
cyclophosphamide, either intraperitoneally or subcutaneously lead to a high
mortality rate, chiefly from generalized infection.

Table 1. Hepatic metastases formed after intraportal injection of 10^7
colorectal adenocarcinoma cells (DHD-K12 strain), under various conditions.

	CONTROLS	CYCLOPHOSPHAMIDE		PARTIAL HEPATECTOMY	
		I.P. (150 mg/kg)	S.C. (250 mg/kg)	1^d	2^d
Number of animals	8	6	4	3	4
Acute death (a) (at day)	3^b (3,4,7)	5 (6,7,10,11,13)	4 (0,1,3,3)	0 (e)	0 (e)
Animals with liver metastases	2	2^c	-	3	4
Animals with metastases	1 (Pu, Pe)	1 (Pe)	-	1 (Pe)	3 (1 Pe; 1 Pe-Pu; 1 Pu)

a. death occurring within less than 15 days. b. sepsis ? c. including
1 animal that died on day 13, scored among the "acute death" group.
d. experiment 1. and 2. were identical except for the animal age at the
time of injection (respectively 4 and 5 months). e. animals in these
groups survived at least 75 days and were killed on the basis of a drastic
loss of weight. This occurred between day 75 and day 111. f. abbreviations:
Pu : pulmonary; Pe : peritoneal.

All the animals in group 2 (cyclophosphamide, s.c.) died within 3 days,
without any detectable sign of liver invasion by adenocarcinoma cells.
In group 3, (cyclophosphamide i.p.) 4 animals died within 11 days without
liver metastases. The two others survived respectively 13 and 35 days; both

animals had developed multiple liver metastases and one also had pulmonary
involvement. In the control (group 1), 3 rats died within 7 days; among
the 6 others (that survived for at least 4 months), 2 developed well
defined liver metastases. Finally, as Fisher (1959) first demonstrated with
256 Walker carcinoma cells, partial hepatectomy performed immediately after
intraportal injection (group 4) resulted in a remarkably high incidence of
hepatic metastases. All the animals in this group survived more than 2
months following cell inoculation and were killed on the basis of their bad
condition and marked loss of body weight. All of them had developed
numerous liver metastases, (detectable macroscopically and confirmed by
anatomopathological examination).

DISCUSSION

   Our results indicate that the Fishers' model for liver metastasis seems
to be applicable to our system with colonic adenocarcinoma cells. To our
knowledge there are no clearcut experimental data to explain the mechanism
of this positive effect of partial hepatectomy on tumour cell take and
metastatic conversion. It will be noted that lethality of this procedure
is remarkably low. Our data seem to warrant the conclusion that our model
is a valid one for investigation of liver metastasis formation. The cells
in the metastases proliferate intensely, as shown by ^{3}H-thymidine autoradi-
ographic labelling and the cell mass seems to develop neovascularization,
as demonstrated by microangiographic studies. This, together with the fact
that metastases develop at a high incidence and within a relatively short
time, makes the model very promising.

REFERENCES

Druckrey, H., Preussmann, R., Matzkies, F. & Ivqnkovic, S., 1967,
   Naturwissenschaften, 54 (11), 285.
Fisher, B. & Fisher, E.R., 1959, Cancer, 12, 929.
Martin, M.S., Martin, F., Michiels, R., Bastien, H., Justrabo, E.,
   Bordes, M. & Viry, B., 1973, Digestion, 8, 22.
Mendes Da Costa, P., Defleur, V. & Lejeune, F.J., 1978, Acta Zoologica et
   Pathologica Antverpsia, 72, 65.

ACKNOWLEDGMENTS

   We thank Dr. P. Mendes Da Costa, Drs M.S. and F. Martin for their
generous help and advice at the start of this work. This work was
performed thanks to financial support from Belgium Research Foundation
for Medical Research and the Loterie Nationale.

TREATMENT OF A HYPERBILIRUBINEMIC PATIENT WITH DOXORUBICIN: CLINICAL AND PHARMACOKINETIC RESULTS

S. MARTINO, J.D. YOUNG, AND R.B. SCHILCHER

Wayne State University, Division of Medical Oncology, Detroit, Michigan, 48201 (USA)

Keywords: doxorubicin, hyperbilirubinemia

INTRODUCTION

Doxorubicin (DOX) remains a widely used agent in the treatment of human malignancies. Appropriate dosing in patients with impaired hepatic function remains unclear. Benjamin, et al (1974) observed increased toxicity with elevated and prolonged plasma levels of doxorubicin and its metabolites in such patients, and suggested dose reduction based on serum bilirubin and bromosulphalein (BSP) retention studies. In this report, we describe clinical and pharmacokinetic results in a patient with markedly elevated serum bilirubin treated with 3 courses of doxorubicin.

CASE PRESENTATION

The patient, a 55 year old caucasian female, was diagnosed in April 1982 with breast cancer ($T_2N_0M_0$, estrogen and progesterone receptor positive), and treated with a lumpectomy, axillary sampling, radiotherapy to the left breast, and radiation castration. Eleven months later, recurrent carcinoma was apparent in bilateral axillary lymph nodes, left supraclavicular lymph nodes, and the right breast. Systemic therapy with cyclophosphamide, 5-fluorouracil, methotrexate, prednisone, and vincristine (CMFVP) was begun, and a partial response obtained. Following four months of CMFVP, systemic therapy was interrupted, and radiotherapy to bilateral axillary, cervical, and supraclavicular lymph nodes, and the right breast, was carried out. Near completion of radiotherapy, liver and bone metastases were documented and CMFVP restarted, but without tumor response. In April 1984, the patient became febrile and dyspneic. Lung biopsy demonstrated fibrosis, lymphangitic metastases, and pneumocystis carinii. Antibiotic therapy ensued, with improvement in respiratory symptoms. Progressive tumor destruction of bone and liver continued with development of pronounced hyperbilirubinemia.

Treatment with doxorubicin at 21 day intervals was started with intra-venous bolus of DOX 20 mg/M^2 (course 1,2) and 27 mg/M^2 (course 3). On day 13 of course 1, after WBC nadir had been reached, the patient was placed on 40 mg/M^2 of prednisone as an effort to improve pulmonary symptoms. The dose was reduced to 33 mg/M^2 on day 2 of the second course, and to 26 mg/M^2 on day 12 of course 3. Examinations of blood counts, and liver function tests, were obtained at least weekly. Samples of blood for pharmacokinetic studies were obtained day 7,14, and 21 of the second course, and times 0,1, 15,30,45,60, and 90 minutes, and then daily on days 2,6,7,14,19 following the 3rd course.

METHODS

DOX and its primary metabolite,doxorubicinol(DOX-OL) were assayed in plasma by high-performance liquid chromatography (HPLC) using a method modified from Peng et al (1984). The HPLC system was composed of a Perkin-Elmer Model 650-10M fluorescence spectrophotometer (Perkin-Elmer Corp., Norwalk, Connecticut, USA), a Waters U6K injector (Waters Associates, Milford, Massachusetts, USA), a Waters u-Bondapak C$_{18}$ column (300 x 4.6 mm), a guard column containing about 400 mg of 40 micron corasil, and a Waters model M45 pump operated at 2.0 ml/min. The mobile phase was 65% 0.1M ammonium acetate buffer, pH 4.5, and 35% acetonitrile. The excitation and emission wave lengths were 470 and 588 nm, respectively, and both slit widths were 10nm. The analytical standards were a gift of Farmitalia Carlo Erba, Milan ,Italy. Samples of plasma were extracted with 10 volumes of ethyl acetate, the organic layer evaporated, the residue dissolved in the mobile phase, and an aliquot chromatographed. The retention time for DOX was 2.9 minutes and for DOX-OL was 2.2 minutes. The sensitivity of this method was 1-2 ng/ml plasma. Data were analyzed using the computer program AUTOAN to determine the most appropriate model and to determine values of the pharmacokinetic parameters.

RESULTS

In spite of the patient's low performance status (ECOG 3), treatment with 3 courses of DOX was well tolerated. Nausea and vomiting were minimal. Neither stomatitis nor infection occurred. No cardiac toxicity was ob-served. White blood cell nadir occurred on day 10,14, and 7 of course 1,2, 3, respectively, and promptly returned to normal, allowing each subsequent dose of DOX to be given on day 21 (Table 1). Though subjective improvement in the patient's clinical status was observed, and a lowering of serum SGOT and LDH occurred during treatment with DOX, an objective tumor response was not observed, and therapy discontinued after three courses.

TABLE 1. Hematological and hepatic parameters during DOX therapy.

Course	DOX mg/M^2	WBC (10^7/mm^3)	Hb (g/dl)	Platelets (10^3/mm^3)	Total[a] Bilirubin (mg/dl)	Alkaline Phos ((Iu/1))	LDH (Iu/1)	SGOT (I/ul)
1	20	6.4(0.9)[b]	9.8(7.0)	45(27)	15.0	3330	1185	561
2	20	5.6(2.2)	10.5(9.0)	91(78)	18.7	1435	696	425
3	27	4.8(0.2)	8.8(8.2)	115(110)	12.0	3170	558	250

a. normal value - 1.1 mg/dl b. (parenthesis) nadir per course.

    The plasma concentration time profile for course 3 is shown in Figure 1. The data were best fit to a 3-compartment model (R^2=0.9993) with half-life values of 5 min., 1.0 hr., and 10.1 hr. Other pharmacokinetic values were: area under the plasma curve, 1362 ng· ml·$^{-1}$hr; volume of the central compartment, 26 liters; total body volume of distribution, 2955 liters; and total body clearance, 29 liters/hour. On day 21 of course 2, both DOX and DOX-OL were detectable. However, in course 3, no levels were detectable beyond day 7.

DISCUSSION

    The importance of hepatic function in the metabolism of doxorubicin and its metabolites remains unclear. Liver extraction of 45-50 percent has been reported by Garnich et al (1979). Mucositis and severe pancytopenia were reported by Benjamin et al (1974) in eight patients with impaired liver functions when treated with 60 mg/M^2 DOX at 3-4 week intervals, re-sulting in three (38%) drug related deaths. Dose reduction based on serum bilirubin and BSP retention reduced toxicity in 9 subsequent patients. In contrast, Brenner et al (1984) reported that leukemic patients receiving full doses of doxorubicin with mild hepatic dysfunction as determined by bromosulphalin (BSP) retention and serum liver function studies had the same incidence of toxicity as those with normal liver function.

    In spite of marked abnormalities in all measured liver parameters, our patient tolerated treatment with minimal side effects. Though myelo-suppression was prominent, neither infection nor bleeding complications were encountered. Whether concomitant prednisone administered altered the level of myelosuppression or other toxicity cannot be determined.

    Robert et al (1982) have described pharmacokinetic parameters in 12

patients with locally advanced breast cancer treated with 50 mg/M^2 of doxorubicin plus vincristine and methotrexate. The successive half-lives were
4.75 min., 0.822 hr., and 18.9 hr. Our data demonstrate that pharmacokinetics of DOX differed in hyperbilirubinemia mainly in prolonging the third
phase of elimination. This was most pronounced in course 2 when the serum
bilirubin was 18 mg/dl, and both DOX and DOX-OL were still detectable on
day 21. In spite of an increased dose of DOX, when the serum bilirubin decreased to 12 mg/dl (course 3) neither parent compound nor its metabolite
were detectable beyond day seven, suggesting a close relationship between
bilirubin level and elimination of DOX.

Figure 1.

Plasma concentra-
tion time profile
following third
course of DOX at
27 mg/M^2.

(.) = measured
x=model predicted

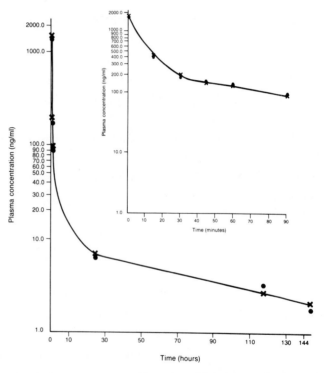

Benjamin, R.S.,et al, 1974, Adriamycin chemotherapy-efficacy, safety, and
    pharmacologic basis of an intermittent single high-dosage schedule,
    Cancer, 33, 19.
Brenner, D.E.,et al, 1984, Acute Doxorubicin toxicity, relationship to pre-
    treatment liver function, response, and pharmacokinetics in patients with
    acute nonlymphocytic leukemia, Cancer, 53, 1042.
Garnich, M.B., et al,1979, A clinical pharmacological evaluation of hepatic
    arterial infusion of Adriamycin, Cancer Research, 34, 4105.
Peng, Y.M.,et al, 1984, A method for the simultaneous measurement of the new
    anthracycline derivative 4' Deoxydoxorubicin and its metabolite by re-
    verse phase liquid chromatography,Investigational New Drugs,(in press).
Robert, J.,et al, 1982, Pharmacokinetics of Adriamycin in patients with
    breast cancer: Correlation between pharmacokinetic parameters and clin-
    ical short-term response,European Journal of Cancer Clinical Oncology,
    18, 739.

HETEROGENEITY OF HUMAN PRIMARY TUMORS AND METASTASES MEASURED BY
SOFT AGAR CLONING AND DNA-FLOWCYTOMETRY

D. FLENTJE[1], G.E. FEICHTER[2], M. FLENTJE[1], P. SCHLAG[1]
[1]Department of Surgery, Section Surgical Oncology,
[2]Department of Experimental and Comparative Pathology, University
of Heidelberg, FRG

Keywords: heterogeneity, human tumor colony assay, DNA-flowcytometry

INTRODUCTION

Heterogeneity in drug sensitivity is of major concern for the response
of malignant disease to chemotherapy and especially for the significance
of in vitro predictive drug tests that were developed to assess the tumor
response of individual patients to cytostatic drugs.   If such a
test system is to be of use for individual treatment planning in systemic
disease, the test results must be unequivocal and independent of biopsy
site. To address this question we report the results of soft-agar growth
and chemotherapy testing of patients with different lesions of the same
tumor and correlate these data with DNA-flow-cytometry to look for impact
of cell-cycle kinetics and possible deviations of DNA-stemlines.

MATERIAL AND METHODS

Surgically removed tumor material from different tumor lesions of 25
patients was immediately disaggregated mechanically and cultured using the
bilayer soft-agar method described by Hamburger et al 1978. Drug testing
was performed by a one hour preincubation at 1/10 of the clinically
achieved peak plasma level. Fixed day 0-control plates were checked for
the presence of artefacts. Colony growth was evaluated after a 14-21 day
incubation at 37°C and 5% CO_2 in air, 95% humidity. Experiments yielding
more than 25 colonies per control plate were considered evaluable for drug
sensitivity testing.

Tumor material from identical sites was available from 19 of these
patients for flow-cytometry analysis according to the method described by
Feichter et al 1982. Calculation of the cell cycle parameters was done
graphically using the integral of the DNA-histogram.

RESULTS AND DISCUSSION

In this study, in vitro colony growth and DNA-flow cytometry point to considerable differences between different tumor lesions of the same patient concerning both functional aspects like proliferative activity and clonal heterogeneity with regard to DNA-stemlines and chemosensitivity. Colony growth from more than one lesion was seen in 14/25 patients. The number of colonies was higher in the secondary lesion (either syn-or metachronous metastases) in 15/25 cases. This would mean, that cells from different lesions possess a varying potential for adaptive growth under altered physiologic circumstances. Technical reasons concerning sample viability and damage during culturing procedure cannot be ruled out entirely, although sample processing and culture conditions are widely standardized and there were no significant differences in trypan blue viability.

In vitro colony growth seems to be correlated with the proliferative activity of the tumor lesion. The median %-S-phase of lesions with positive colony growth was 8.7 compared to 3.8 in tumors without colony formation. We have previously analyzed the latter question in a greater set of tumors and found a statistically significant correlation between in vitro growth and DNA-parameters such as ploidy (Flentje et al 1984). Metastases showed a slightly higher %-S-phase (median 8.5) than the primary tumors (median 6.2). This effect seems to be more evident in metachronous lesions, but is not predictable as the contrary may also occur depending on the tumor type.

One aspect of tumor heterogeneity can be easily detected by differences in the DNA-content of the G_1-peak in different lesions. In 11 cases the distribution of ploidy was identical in primary and secondary lesions. In 5/5 cases with more than one DNA-stemline in the primary there was deletion of a subline in the metastasis. Three cases showed completely different DNA-content of the G_1-peak between the lesions analyzed (difference in DNA index⟩0.1). This points to a possible segregation of tumor cell subpopulations in metastases. This phenomenon may be due to varying DNA-characteristics in different sites of the primary tumor and inadequate representation in the biopsy sample or to mutation during tumor progression.

Variability between tumor lesions seems to concern in particular the in vitro chemosensitivity. In 14/25 patients in vitro drug testing was possible in more than one lesion. In these, an overall of 33 drug comparisons between the lesions was possible. In 14/33 cases (42%), considerable differences in in vitro chemosensitivity were seen, a difference being assumed when inhibition of colony growth of a particular drug was greater than   70% in one lesion and less than 50% in the other. There was no

correlation between in vitro drug sensitivity and the percentage of cells
within S-phase. A similar lack of correlation between chemosensitivity of
different tumor lesions has been reported in an earlier study from our own
group on 21 paired samples of primary tumors and their synchronous metastases
(Schlag & Schreml 1982), whereas in a recent publication by Tanigawa et al,
1984 a good correlation between different metastases, but not between
different sites of the same large primary tumor were observed.

The impact of an in vitro heterogenous response to cytostatic drugs
can be studied if in vitro/in vivo correlations are possible. In 11 of
our 25 patients an in vitro correlation could be obtained. Correct in vitro
predictions for response after at least two cycles of therapy were obtained
in 9/11 cases (7 S/S, 2 R/R). There were two false positive predictions.
However, due to differing growth in vitro, in only 6 of these, both lesions
have been evaluable for drug testing. In 2 of the remaining 6 patients
discordant test results of different lesions concerning the drugs used
for therapy were seen. In the first case, the test result of only one
of the 2 lesions predicted sensitivity and only a partial remission was
seen. In a second case, resistance was found in a metastasis of melanoma
that occurred after an initial remission of disease under cis-platinum and
actinomycin D which had shown an in vitro activity against a lesion assayed
before induction of therapy.

In our eyes, the significance of in vitro heterogeneity to drugs is
expressed by the fact that no complete remissions were seen. This is in
agreement with overall experience: while there was a higher response rate
in patients to drugs found sensitive in in vitro testing in prospective
studies (Von Hoff et al. 1983) and even an increase in survival to a
control on empirically chosen treatment (Alberts et al. 1982), no improve-
men with respect to cures seems to be obtained. This may well be caused
by selective killing of the sensitive cells and heterogeneity of advanced
tumors. Such a pattern is suggested in the case where in vitro sensitivity of one lesion was followed by in vitro resistance of a later
appearing metastasis after successful therapy with the respective drugs.
This problem is stressed by our in vitro findings, but apparently cannot
be settled even by using a presumably clonal in vitro assay.

REFERENCES

Alberts, D.S., Surwit, E.A., Leigh, S., Moon, T.E. and Salmon, S.E., 1982
    Stem Cells, 1, 294.
Feichter, G.E., Höffken, H., Heep, J., Haag, D., Heberling, D., Brandt, H.,
    Rummel, H., Goerttler, K., 1982, Virchows Archiv., 398, 53.
Flentje, D., Feichter, G.E., Krämer, K.L., Goerttler, K., Schlag, P., 1984

Langenbecks Archiv Chirurgie (suppl.).

Hamburger, A.W., Salmon, S.E., Kim, M.B., Trent, I.M., Soehnlen, B.S., Alberts, D.S., and Schmidt, H.J., 1978, Cancer Research, 38, 3438.

Schlag, P. and Schreml, W., 1982, Cancer Research, 42, 4086.

Tanigawa, N., Mizuno, Y., Hashimura, T., Honda, K., Satomura, K., Hikasa, Y., Niwa, O., Sugahara, T., Yoshida, O., Kern, D. and Morton, D.L., 1984 Cancer Research, 44, 2309.

Von Hoff, D.D., Clark, G.M., Stogdill, B.J., Sarosdy, M.F., O'Brien, I., Casper, J.T., Mattox, T.E., Page, G.P., Cruz, A.B. and Sandbach, J.F., 1983, Cancer Research, 43, 1926.

TUMOR PROXIMATE IMMUNE SUPPRESSION OF REGIONAL LYMPH NODES IN PATIENTS
WITH MALIGNANT MELANOMA

A.J. COCHRAN[1,2], D-R WEN[1], D.B. HOON[1], E.A. PIHL[3], M.V. FAIRHURST[1] and
E.L. KORN[1]
[1]Division of Surgical Oncology, Armand Hammer Laboratories, John Wayne
Clinic, Jonsson Comprehensive Cancer Center,
[2]Department of Pathology, UCLA School of Medicine, Los Angeles, CA.   90024
[3]Department of Pathology, Monash University School of Medicine, Melbourne,
AUSTRALIA   3181

Keywords: Melanoma; regional lymph nodes; immune suppression

INTRODUCTION

Spread of melanoma to the regional lymph nodes is an unfavorable event,
associated with a reduced survival. Patients with primary melanoma have
a five-year survival of 75-90% (Cochran 1969; Das Gupta 1977), while
after lymphadenectomy for melanomatous nodes five year survival is about
50% (Callery et al., 1982). Studies of factors related to survival after
lymphadenectomy indicate that the number of tumorous nodes correlates
with the survival of groups of patients (Cochran et al., 1977; Balch et al.,
1981; Day et al., 1981; Callery et al., 1982).

Placement of an individual in a favorable or unfavorable category
remains desirable but difficult. Assessment of node status has been
greatly facilitated by the utilization of anti-serum to S-100 protein,
an operationally useful marker for melanocyte-derived cells.

S-100 protein is an acidic protein of unknown function, named from its
solubility in saturated ammonium sulfate at neutral pH (Moore, 1965),
found in glial cells (Moore, 1965; Ludwin et al., 1976), Schwann cells,
and ganglion satellite cells (Eng et al., 1976). It exhibits strong
serological cross-reactivity among vertebrate species (Kessler et al.,
1968). S-100 protein was detected in cultured melanoma cells and biopsies
by Gaynor et al. (1980, 1981). Using an immunoperoxidase approach, S-100
protein was detected in most primary and metastatic cutaneous (Nakajima
et al., 1981; Cochran et al., 1982; Springall et al., 1983) and ocular
melanomas (Cochran et al., 1983). Despite the demonstration of S-100
protein in a range of cell types (lymphoid dendritic cells, Langerhans
cells, chondrocytes and adipocytes) it is, in defined situations, a useful
marker for melanocyte-derived cells.

In our study of 1273 nodes the detection rates of tumorous nodes using H&E and S-100 protein were 10% and 29% respectively (Cochran et al., 1984). The occult tumor cells were present singly or in small groups in the paracortex or lymph node sinuses. The difference was most marked in patients with Stage II disease. In 794 nodes from Stage II patients, the detection rate was improved from 16 to 46% by the use of anti-serum to S-100 protein. In 479 nodes from patients with high risk Stage I disease only one additional tumorous node was detected.

Penetration of nodes by small number of melanoma cells affected node groups with at least one node substantially replaced by melanoma. Once a node is colonized by melanoma, seeding of tumor to several adjacent nodes may occur. Even in thick, deep, high-risk melanomas, this event does not occur until at least one substantial tumor colony is established. This suggests that there is reduction in the capacity of nodes adjacent to tumor to resist penetration by single tumor cells.

This paper describes the distribution of lymph node hyperplasia in carefully oriented melanoma-draining nodes. We examined nodes from 87 patients with melanoma who underwent lymphadenectomy at UCLA for melanoma. Seventeen patients had "therapeutic" lymphadenectomy for node-spread melanoma and 69 a "prophylactic" lymphadenectomy for high risk primary melanoma.

Tissues were diagrammed and dissected fresh. Individual nodes were numbered on a grid drawn on the diagram and divided for routine histological assessment and in vitro studies. Each node was classified histologically by tumor status and by the strength of any reaction present. We assessed the reaction of the T-dependent paracortex, the B cell follicular areas and the nodal sinuses on a 0 to +++ scale.

Statistical analysis employed the Kruskall-Wallis test for differences between groups and Kendall's Tau Rank correlation test for trends (SAS Users' Guide, 1982).

RESULTS

The main reactions were in T-dependent areas and lymph node sinuses, with little follicular hyperplasia. The extent of paracortical hyperplasia was significantly different in nodes at varying distances from tumor. In the whole group, the maximum reaction was seen in nodes moderately removed from tumor ($.94 \pm .07$), a value significantly greater than that of nodes nearest to ($.72 \pm .08$, $P < 0.05$) and furthest from tumor ($.64 \pm .08$, $P < 0.001$). (Table 1.)

Table 1. Strength of reactions of melanoma patients' regional lymph nodes
oriented relative to nearest tumor. Comparing patients with* and without**
tumor in the node group. Hematoxylin and eosin stained sections, reactions
assessed on a 0 to +++ scale.

| | | Melanoma Patients | | | | | | |
| | | All Patients | | | Tumor Positive* | | | Tumor Negative** | | |
Type of Reaction	Position of Lymph Node	No.	Mean + SEM		No.	Mean + SEM		No.	Mean + SEM	
Paracortical (T-dependent)	Proximal	73	.72 + .08	}a	14	.48 + .11	}c	59	.78 + .10	}d
	Middle	81	.94 + .07		17	.96 + .11		64	.94 + .08	
	Distal	77	.64 + .08	}b	16	.83 + .16		61	.59 + .09	}b

a, $P < 0.05$; b, $P < 0.001$; c, $P < 0.025$; d, $P = 0.07$.

The proximal-middle difference (.48 + .11 and .96 + .11 respectively)
was greatest in patients with tumor in the node group ($P < 0.025$). In this
group middle and distal nodes showed similar (high) levels of reaction
(.96 + .11 and .83 + .16 respectively).

If the node group did not contain melanoma, the difference between
proximal and middle nodes (.78 + .10 and .94 + .08 respectively) approached
significance ($P = 0.07$), while the difference between middle and distal
nodes (.94 + .08 and .59 + .09 respectively) was highly significant
($P < 0.001$).

Substantial sinus histiocytosis was noted (data not shown), but showed
no zoned variations in strength.

DISCUSSION

These data indicate a non-random variation in node reactivity in nodes
regional to and draining or containing melanoma. This variation relates
to proximity to tumor, nodes nearest to tumor showing relatively low
reactivity while those more removed are strongly reactive. This, and the
fact that nodes nearest to tumor are least reactive suggest that the tumor
induces immune-suppression. The relatively strong reaction of nodes
further from tumor may indicate their exposure to less tumor-derived immune
suppressive material, or to a concentration that is immune stimulatory.
The relatively low reaction of the most distal nodes in the node negative
group may be due to lack of contact with a significant amount of tumor-
derived material. In the tumor positive group the amount of tumor-derived
material is likely to be higher and stimulatory of even distal nodes.

Studies in progress are designed to test the above hypothesis by counting interdigitating dendritic cells (as an index of paracortical hyperplasia) in accurately oriented nodes. We are also examining the response of lymphocytes from oriented nodes to phytomitogens, alloantigens and IL-2.

Preliminary data support our concept of tumor-proximal immune suppression in nodes draining primary melanoma or containing metastatic melanoma. Immune suppressed nodes are those which show early penetration by melanoma cells identifiable with anti-S-100 protein serum.

These studies are supported by DHHS grant CA 29938.

REFERENCES

Balch, C.M., Soong, S.J., Murad, T.M., Ingalls, A.L., Maddox, W.A., 1981 Annals of Surgery, 193 377.
Callery, C., Cochran, A.J., Roe, D.J., Rees, W., Nathanson, S.D., Benedetti, J.K., Elashoff, R.M., Morton, D.L., 1982, Annals of Surgery, 196, 69.
Cochran, A.J., 1969, Cancer (Philadelphia), 23, 1190.
Cochran, A.J., Wen, D-R, Herschman, H.R., Gaynor, R.B., 1982, International Journal of Cancer, 30, 295.
Cochran, A.J., Holland, G., Wen, D-R, Herschman, H.R., Lee, W.R., Foos, R.Y., Straatsma, B.R., 1983, Investigative Ophthalmology & Visual Science, 24, 1153.
Cochran, A.J., Wen, D-R, Herschman, H.R., 1984, International Journal of Cancer, 34, 159.
Cohen, M.H., Ketcham, A.S., Felix, E.L., Li, S-H, Tomaszewski, M.M., Costa, J., Rabson, A.S., Simin, R.M., Rosenberg, S.A., 1977, Annals of Surgery 186, 635.
Das Gupta, T.K., 1977, Annals of Surgery, 186, 201.
Day, C.L., Sober, A.J., Lew, R.A., Mihm, M.C., Fitzpatrick, T.B., 1981, Cancer (Philadelphia), 47, 955.
Eng, L.F., Kosek, J.C., Forno, L., Deck, J., Bigbee, J., 1976, Transactions American Society for Neurochemistry, 7, 211.
Gaynor, R., Irie, R.F., Morton, D.L., Herschman, H.R., 1980, Nature (London), 286, 400.
Gaynor, R., Herschman, H.R., Irie, R.F., Jones, P., Morton, D.L., Cochran, A.J., 1981, Lancet, 1, 869.
Kessler, D., Levine, L., Fassman, G., 1983, Biochemistry, 7, 758.
Kopf, A.W., Harris, M.N., Gumport, S.L., Raker, J.W., Malt, R.A., Golumb, F.M., Cosimi, A.B., Wood, W.C., Casson, P., Lopransi, S., Gorstein, F., Postel, A., Reichert, C.M., Rosenberg, S.A., Weber, B.L., Costa, J., 1981, Human Pathology, 12, 449.
Ludwin, S.K., Kosek, J.C., Engl, L.F., 1976, Journal of Comparative Neurology, 165, 197.
Moore, B.W., 1965, Research Communications, 19, 197.
Nakajima, T., Watanabe, S., Sato, Y., Kameya, T., Shimoshato, Y., 1981, Gann, 72,335.
SAS Users' Guide (1982).
Springall, D.R., Gu, J., Cocchia, D., Michetti, F., Levene, A., Levene, M.M., Marangos, P.J., Bloom, S.R., Polak, J.M., 1983, Virchows Archives (Pathol. Anat.), No. 697.

PREVENTION AND TREATMENT OF METASTATIC MELANOMA BY COUMARINS

R.D.Thornes

St. Laurence's Hospital, Dublin 7,Ireland

Keywords: Melanoma, Coumarin, Warfarin, Cimetidine

INTRODUCTION

The discovery of fibrin about human tumours by O'Meara and Jackson (1958) led to the use of anticoagulation to prevent spread of cancer (Thornes,1966 1969). In two controlled clinical trials anticoagulation with warfarin (3-(αAcetonylbenzyl)-4 hydroxy coumarin) was shown to double the survival of patients with breast cancer (D'Souza et al,1978) and small cell cancer of the lung (Zacharski,1983). A multicentre trial of urokinase and warfarin to prevent recurrence of large bowel cancer is in progress (Hilgard et al, 1981).

The role of anticoagulation in preventing cancer spread by coumarins was questioned (Thornes et al,1965) when warfarin therapy was found to inhibit locomotion of tumour cells in the rabbit ear chamber (Wood,1958). A vitamin K deficient diet was found by Hilgard (1981) to inhibit tumour growth and spread in a manner similar to warfarin type anticoagulation;while Maat (1980) showed that warfarin required macrophages to produce its effect on metastases. Pillar (1976) showed that coumarin also required macrophages to exert its action in preventing oedema following thermal injury. Coumarin has no anticoagulant action.

COUMARIN

Coumarin is widespread throughout nature,being present in plants and seeds. It is used in industry as a stabilizer in perfume and as a laser dye and was erroneously labelled as a carcinogen in rats by Bär and Griepentrog (1967). In fact coumarin is an anticarcinogen and when added to the diet of rats inhibits the carcinogenic effect of dimethylbenz(a)anthracene and benzo(a)- pyrene (Feuer,1976,Watterberg et al,1979). The erroneous assertion by Bar and Griepentrog led to the restriction of the use of coumarin in the

in the tobacco industry where it was used to stabilize aroma. This,with
hindsight,may be a mistake as it is an anticarcinogen.

   Coumarin was first used in Dublin(by Riordan) to treat human cancer
between 1947 and 1952,following his unpublished work on growth inhibition by
lactones (Thornes,1966). It is now mainly used clinically to prevent or
treat oedema (Pillar and Clodius,1980). Coumarin restores delayed hyper-
sensitivity and increases helper T.lymphocyte numbers (Thornes,1983). It
was the main treatment used in chronic brucellosis to correct the acquired
immune suppression associated with this disease (Thornes,1983). A recurrent
ulcerating Kaposi's sarcoma in a 65 year old heterosexual woman healed in
five days on treatment with coumarin 100 mg daily and all her lesions
completely regressed in five weeks (Thornes,1984). In Munich,Zänker et al
(1984) have shown that coumarin,like interferon,stimulates NK cell activity.

MELANOMA

   The use of cytotoxic therapy to prevent recurrence after surgical excision
of melanoma has been a failure. At the Colman K. Byrnes Research Centre in
Dublin between 1973 and 1979 we used B.C.G.,levamisole and DTIC (Dacarbazine)
in patients with Stage II and Ib melanoma. The recurrence rate within one
year of surgery was 8 out of 27 cases (30%). In 1980 we started using warfarin
anticoagulation alone after surgical excision and in 1981 we switched to
coumarin 50 mg daily as it had no anticoagulant action. The recurrence
rates within one year of surgery dropped to 2 in 28 cases (7%)

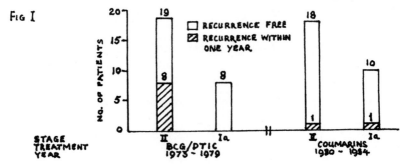

FIG I

   The recurrence of melanoma in both patients in the coumarin group was
treated by further surgery and the coumarin increased to 100 mg daily,then
when surgery was no longer possible cimetidine 1000 mg daily was started and
both patients responded within one week.

CIMETIDINE

   Cimetidine is an H_2(histamine) antagonist used in the therapy of peptic
ulceration. It was shown by Osband et al (1981) to inhibit tumour growth in

in mice and decrease suppressor T.lymphocyte levels.

Cimetidine 1000 mg daily given to the first patient with nonresectable recurrence on coumarin therapy decreased the suppressor T.lymphocytes from 30% to 18%. Cimetidine produces an initial inflammatory response in the area of the tumour and then within one week there is marked tumour reduction without any sign of toxicity. Five patients with nonresectable recurrent disease on long term coumarin responded to the addition of cimetidine (see Table I).

Table I.

EXTRAREGIONAL RECURRENT MELANOMA

RESPONDERS – CIMETIDINE 1000 mg. COUMARIN 100 mg.

No.	Sex	Age	Primary	Coumarins Months	A L C 10^9/L	Response Months
1	M	34	Leg	24	1.5	30
2	M	49	Eye	24	3.4	9
3	F	72	Foot	30	2.4	29+
5	F	69	Eye	72	3.8	22+
10	F	61	Thumb	36	1.7	3+

Five other patients with advanced melanoma on treatment with coumarin did not respond to cimetidine (Table II). One of the patients developed the inflammatory response when coumarin and cimetidine were started simultaneously but had rapid tumour progression leading to death in six weeks (Thornes et al,1982).Cimetidine given alone to 7 patients with advanced melanoma was without effect.

Table II.

EXTRAREGIONAL RECURRENT MELANOMA

NON-RESPONDERS – CIMETIDINE 1000 mg. COUMARIN 100 mg.

No.	Sex	Age	Primary	Coumarins Months	A L C 10^9/L
4	F	35	Back	0	0.7
6	F	39	?Brain	6	1.3
7	F	35	Arm	5	0.5
8	M	48	Face	1	0.7
9	M	77	Leg	7	0.4

All the responders were on coumarin for 2 years or more before cimetidine was started and they all had normal lymphocyte counts. It seems that the immune system needs to be primed by coumarin and be capable of response when suppressor T.lymphocyte levels are reduced by cimetidine.

CLINICAL TRIAL

A double blind randomised multicentre clinical trial has just started to assess the prevention of recurrence of melanoma by coumarin.

The trial is for patients with Stage II disease and Stage Ib with a

tumour thickness above 1.70 mm. Coumarin 50 mg daily or placebo is started
within one month of surgery and continued for 2 years. Patients are checked
every 3 months for 2 years and followed for 5 years in all. The trial is
organized by the National Foundation for Cancer Research in Bethesda,Maryland
U.S.A. and the coumarin and placebo tablets are made available free of charge
by Schaper & Brümmer,Salzgitter,West Germany. The trial secretariat is at
the Colman K. Byrnes Research Centre,Dublin.

ACKNOWLEDGEMENTS

This work is supported by the National Foundation for Cancer Research.

REFERENCES

Bär,Von F. and Griepentrog,F.,1967,Medizin und Ernahrung,11.244-251.
D'Souza,D.P., Daly,L.,Thornes,R.D.,1978,Journal of Irish Medical
    Association, 71. 605-608
Feuer,G.,Kellen,J.A. and Kovacs,K.,1976, Oncology, 33.35-39.
Hilgard,P.,White,H. and Turney,P., 1981,European Journal of Cancer and
    Clinical Oncology Supplement, 2.87-88.
Hilgard,P., 1981, The use of oral anticoagulants in tumour therapy in
    malignancy and the hemostatic system. Edited by M.B.Donati,J.F.Davidson
    and S.Garrattini. New York.Raven Press. p. 103-111.
Maat,B.,1980, British Journal of Cancer, 41. 313-316.
O'Meara,R.A.Q. and Jackson,R.D.,1958,Irish Journal of Medical Science,
    391.327-329.
Osband,M.E.,Hamilton, D.,Shen,T.J.,Cohen,E.,Shlesinger,M.,Lavin,P.,Brown,A.
    and McCaffrey,R., 1981. Lancet i, 636-638.
Pillar,N.B. The ineffectiveness of coumarin treatment on thermal oedema of
    macrophage free rats. British Journal Experimental Pathology,57.170-
    178.1976.
Pillar,N.B., & Clodius,   1980, Journal of Lymphology, 4.35-42.
Thornes,R.D., 1966,Irish Journal of Medical Science,6.265-276.
Thornes,R.D.,Edlow,D.W. and Wood,S.,Jr.,1968,Johns Hopkins Hospital
    Medical Journal,123. 306-316.
Thornes,R.D.,Lynch,G.,Sheehan,M.V., 1982,Lancet,ii, 328.
Thornes,R.D.,1983a, Coumarins,Melanoma and Cellular Immunity. In Protective
    Agents in Cancer. Edited by D.C.H.O'Brien & T.F.Slater, London
    Academic Press, p.43-56.
Thornes,R.D.1983b, Irish Medical Journal, 76.225.
Thornes,R.D.,1984, Irish Journal of Medical Science, 5.187.
Wattenberg,L.N.,Lam,L.K.T. and Flachmoe,A.V.,1979,Cancer Research,38.1651-165
Wood,S.,Jr.,1958. A.M.A. Archives of Pathology,66.550-568.
Zacharski,L.R., 1983, Warfarin anticoagulation in human malignancy. In
    Protective agents in cancer. Edited by D.C.H.O'Brien & T.F.Slater,
    London Academic Press, p.23-41.
Zänker,K.S., Blumel,G., Lange,J., Siewert,J.R., 1984. Submitted for
    publication.

THE COAGULATION HYPOTHESIS OF CANCER DISSEMINATION

L.R. ZACHARSKI
Dartmouth Medical School and the Veterans Administration Hospital, White River Junction, Vermont 05001

Keywords: Anticoagulants, warfarin, tumor procoagulant

Insight into mechanisms of malignant tumor dissemination has been obtained from studies of the interaction between neoplastic cells and the host coagulation mechanism. These studies, which have recently been reviewed (Zacharski 1982, Zacharski et al. 1979, 1982), reveal that the host coagulation mechanism is, in fact, activated in malignancy as determined by tests performed on peripheral blood; that elements of clots occur at tumor sites; that tumor cells themselves may be responsible for coagulation activation; and that administration of drugs with antithrombotic properties ameliorates the course of the disease. The complexity of this interaction is evidenced by the fact that the ability of tumor cells to influence fibrinolytic reactions, to initiate coagulation reactions that lead to fibrin formation, and to activate platelets varies both qualitatively and quantitatively between tumor cell types. Furthermore, work in a variety of experimental animal tumor systems has demonstrated different patterns of responsiveness to drugs which influence coagulation, platelet or fibrinolytic reactions by quite different mechanisms. It seems clear that various tumor types interact with the coagulation mechanism but by different pathways. Presumably such differences are the basis of the variability observed in responsiveness to different antithrombotic agents.

Based upon this evidence, a coagulation hypothesis of cancer dissemination has been formulated. According to this hypothesis, the interaction of neoplastic cells with the coagulation mechanism of the host constitutes a mechanism by which such cells modify their local environment permitting their growth and spread. Consideration of the beneficial effects of antithrombotic drugs in experimental animal tumor systems is essential to understanding the cause-effect relationships between host coagulation activation and neoplastic behavior.

In order to test the significance of the coagulation hypothesis for
human malignancy, a Cooperative Study Group was formed under the sponsor-
ship of the U.S. Veterans Administration Cooperative Studies Program to
investigate by means of prospective, randomized, controlled clinical trials
the effects of antithrombotic drugs in several types of advanced human
malignancy that are common within the VA Hospital system (Zacharski et al.
1979, 1982). The first study conducted by this group (designated CSP #75),
begun in 1976 and concluded in 1981, was of the anticoagulant, warfarin.
The second study, a double-blind trial (designated CSP #188) of the platelet antagonist RA-233, began in 1981 and currently has enrolled over 550
patients. It is scheduled for completion in 1986.

Warfarin was found in CSP #75 to provide a highly significant prolongation in survival but only in patients with small cell carcinoma of the lung
(SCCL) (Zacharski et al. 1981, 1984). This improvement could not be attributed to any other feature of the experimental versus control patient population. Survival for the control group was similar to that observed for VA
patients with SCCL who were not admitted to the study and also for patients
observed in other studies who were treated with the same standard combination chemotherapy regimen administered to all patients with SCCL admitted
to CSP #75. These favorable results, presented in the figure, support the
validity of the coagulation hypothesis and have apparently been independently confirmed in a recently completed study (Chahinian et al. 1984).

A major implication of the coagulation hypothesis is that it suggests
mechanisms of host-tumor interaction that promote tumor progression. For
example, tumor procoagulant may be responsible for the abundant fibrin that
is deposited locally in SCCL tumor masses (Zacharski et al. 1983) and this
fibrin may protect the tumor from host defenses (Dvorak et al. 1981) or
provide a local environment favorable to tumor cell growth. Platelets may
also cluster about certain types of tumor cells (Zacharski et al. 1982) increasing the opportunity for providing platelet granule constituents, such
as platelet-derived growth factor and other active peptides, that affect
neoplastic cell proliferation (Assoian et al. 1984). Thus, acquired properties that allow tissue cells to imitate the behavior of other cells designed for participation in hemostatic processes may allow malignant cells
to usurp normally quiescent coagulation reactions reserved for the self-
limited processes of hemostasis and wound healing. Such changes may be
fundamental to malignant behavior of cells.

A second implication of the coagulation hypothesis is that the suggested
mechanisms of interaction may be manipulated pharmacologically. This

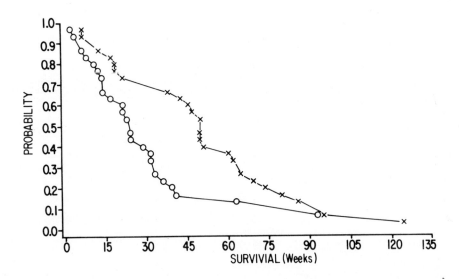

Figure 1. Comparison of survival for warfarin-treated (x) versus control (o) patients with small cell carcinoma of the lung entered to CSP #75. The median survival was 49.5 weeks for warfarin-treated and 23.0 weeks for control patients (p=0.018) (Zacharski et al. 1984, used by permission).

hypothesis is eminently testable now in human malignancy since a number of antithrombotic drugs are available for incorporation into controlled clinical trials. Such drugs are well studied, are relatively nontoxic and inexpensive, and have fairly well defined mechanisms of action. While the coagulation hypothesis is theoretically most applicable to prevention of subsequent distant recurrence in patients with localized disease treated for "cure" by surgery or radiation therapy, available evidence from CSP #75 indicates that gains may be realized in advance disease as well. This implies that biologic properties of the tumor may be as important as the stage of the disease in determining responsiveness. Studies of antithrombotic drugs may be timely in tumor types for which current therapy is inadequate or future planning stalemated.

REFERENCES

Assoian, R., Grotendorst, G., Miller, D., & Sporn, M., 1984, Nature, 309, 804.

Chahinian, A., Ware, J., Zimmer, B., Commis, R., Perry, M., Hirsh, V., Skarin, A., Raich, P., Weiss, R., & Carey, R., 1984, Proceeding of the American Society for Clinical Oncology, 3, 225.

Dvorak, H., Orenstein, N., & Dvorak, A., 1981, Lymphokines, 2, 203.

Zacharski, L., 1982, The biologic basis for anticoagulant treatment in cancer. In Interaction of Platelets with Tumor Cells, edited by G. Jamieson (Alan R. Liss, New York), P. 113.

Zacharski, L., Henderson, W., Rickles, F., Forman, W., Cornell, C., Forcier, R., Harrower, H., & Johnson, R., 1979, Cancer, 44, 732.

Zacharski, L., Henderson, W., Rickles, F., Forman, W., Cornell, C., Forcier, R., Edwards, R., Headley, E., Kim, S-H., O'Donnell, J., O'Dell, R., Tornyos, K., & Kwaan, H., 1981, Journal of the American Medical Association, 245, 831.

Zacharski, L., Henderson, W., Rickles, F., Forman, W., Van Eeckhout, J., Cornell, C., Forcier, R., & Martin, J., 1982, American Journal of Clinical Ongology, 5, 593.

Zacharski, L., Schned, A., & Sorenson, G., 1983, Cancer Research, 43, 3963.

Zacharski, L., Henderson, W., Rickles, F., Forman, W., Cornell, C., Forcier, R., Edwards, R., Headley, E., Kim, S-H., O'Donnell, J., O'Dell, R., Tornyos, K., & Kwaan, H., 1984, Cancer, 53, 2046.

MODELS FOR THE INTERACTION OF NEOPLASIA WITH BONES: MODULATION BY DIPHOSPHONATES

A. GUAITANI, G. TARABOLETTI, M. SABATINI, G. COCCIOLI[*], M.C. ANTONACCI[*],

S. FILIPPESCHI, S. GARATTINI and A. MANTOVANI

Istituto di Ricerche Farmacologiche "Mario Negri", v. Eritrea, 62, Milan,
[*]Ospedale L. Sacco, via G.B. Grassi, Milan

Key words: Bone metastases, hypercalcemia, bisphosphonates

INTRODUCTION

Neoplastic diseases frequently involve osseous tissues. Humoral mediators can cause bone resorption and hypercalcemia in the course of malignancy, as exemplified by multiple myeloma. In various tumors, such as prostate, colon and breast cancers, distant metastasis to bones occurs. Finally, in other malignant diseases (e.g. head and neck), tumors directly invade neighbouring bones. Little effort has been made to develop models for the heterogeneous interaction of neoplastic diseases with osseous tissues (reviewed in Garattini and Mantovani, 1984). The involvement (direct or indirect) of bones by neoplastic diseases poses specific problems related to the peculiarity of these anatomical sites. Such specificity of bone involvement in malignancy may offer opportunities for therapeutic strategies based on the particular properties of bone structure and metabolism.

Diphosphonates have been shown to enhance the resistance of osseous tissues to osteolysis.

Here we briefly report on our efforts to develop models for bone involvement in malignancy and to study the potential of diphosphonates to modulate the interaction of neoplastic diseases with osseous tissues.

Models for the interaction of malignancy with bone

As stated above the interaction of neoplasia with osseous tissue is multifaceted, including systemic resorption due to humoral mediators, local invasion and distant metastasis.

No available rodent tumor encompasses this wide range of phenomena, as discussed elsewhere in this book. A combination of two lines of Walker 256
carcinoma of rats offered us an opportunity to examine the three main aspects
of bone involvement in malignancy. As summarized in Table 1, the Walker
256 B line injected s.c. or i.m. and intra-arterially (i.a.) causes hypercalcemia and hypercalciuria, probably related to systemic bone resorption.

Table 1. Interaction with skeletal tissues of two sublines of Walker 256
          carcinoma.

LINE	Route of inoculation	Hypercalcemia and Hypercalciuria	Bone invasion	Bone metastasis
A	s.c.	−	−	−
	i.m.	−	+	−
	i.a.	−	−	−
B	s.c.	+	−	−
	i.m.	+	−	−
	i.a.	+	−	+

Tumor cells given subcutaneously (s.c.), intramusculary (i.m.) or into the
abdominal aorta (i.a.)

The same subline of Walker 256, inoculated into the abdominal aorta, results
in osteolytic bone lesions in both hind limbs. Areas of tumor-induced
osteolysis are particularly prominent in the distal femur and proximal tibia.
However, so far, we have been unable to obtain local invasion of bones by
contiguity using the B line of Walker 256 carcinoma.

In contrast to Walker 256 B, the A line inoculated i.m., s.c. or i.a. did
not cause appreciable hypercalcemia or hypercalciuria. When inoculated into
the abdominal aorta, Walker 256 A cells, unlike B cells, did not result in
osteolytic bone lesions, as detected by x-rays. However, when Walker 256 A
cells were injected i.m. in hind limbs, local bone swelling, zones of marginal erosion of bone cortex and diffuse rarefaction of osseous tissue were
observed radiologically. Local bone invasion by malignant cells was confirmed histologically. Light microscopy showed periostial growth and deep
invasion of the bone cortex starting from the tumor implanted in the

adjacent muscle. Further confirmation of bone lesions due to a contiguous
tumor mass is given by the increase in tibia weight.

Effect of EHDP on bone involvement by malignancy in rodents

Using the rat models described in the preceding section we performed a
series of experiments to assess the potential of diphosphonates in modulating
the interaction of neoplasia with bones. Among diphosphonates, our attention was focused mainly on sodium etidronate (EHDP), a compound already
available for clinical use in other conditions (Fleish and Felix, 1979).
The Walker 256 B line was used to assess the effect of EHDP on tumor-induced hypercalcemia and hypercalciuria. Treatment with EHDP (10-40 mg/day
from day 1 to day 15) inhibited the elevation of plasma levels and urinary
excretion of calcium observed in tumor-bearing rats (Guaitani et al., 1984).
The Walker 256 B line inoculated into the abdominal aorta was also used to
study the effect of EHDP on blood-borne bone metastasis. As reported elsewhere (Guaitani et al., 1984) treatment with this diphosphonate prevented
the formation of osteolytic bone lesions in hind limbs , as ascertained by
X-rays.

Finally, we investigated whether diphosphonates have the potential to interfere with local bone invasion by contiguity , using the Walker 256 A line.
EHDP appreciably inhibited bone invasion under these conditions (Table 2).

Table 2.   Inhibition of bone invasion by EHDP in rats implanted i.m. with
Walker 256/A.

TREATMENT [a]	BONE LESIONS IN RIGHT TIBIA [b]	
	BORDERLINE	SEVERE
Saline	–	7/9
EHDP 10 mg/kg	1/5	1/5
20 mg/kg	–	1/5
30 mg/kg	1/9	–

[a] EHDP was given s.c. from day 1 to day 13 after tumor implant. Walker
256/A line was inoculated i.m. in the right hind limb.

[b] Hind limbs were coded , fixed and examined by X-rays. Results are number
of rats with bone involvement over total number of tumor-bearing rats.

CONCLUDING REMARKS

While metastasis has been the subject of increasing interest in recent years, the biology of implantation and growth of tumors in bone has not received the same attention. Available models for bone invasion and metastasis have not been extensively characterized and those available suffer from serious limitations. For instance, the Walker 256 tumor used in the studies reported here, while providing a tool to probe the various aspects of the interaction of neoplasia with osseous tissues , has a long transplantation history, is maintained in outbred animals, and bone metastasis does not occur spontaneously but only after intraortic inoculation. These limitations emphasize the need to develop carefully characterized murine tumors of epithelial origin that represent the various possible aspects of the interaction of neoplasia with bones. Preliminary data along this line are encouraging. With these limitations inherent to the models , results reported here indicate that diphosphonates can modify the various aspects of the interaction of tumors with bones. These observations indicate the feasibility of pharmacological approaches to bone involvement in malignancy that take advantage of the peculiar properties of osseous tissues.

ACKNOWLEDGEMENTS

This work was supported by   special project "Oncology" from CNR, Rome, Italy , by a grant from Procter and Gamble, USA, and by a generous contribution of the Italian Association against Cancer.

REFERENCES

Fleisch, H. & Felix, R., 1979, Calcified Tissue International, 27, 91.

Garattini, S. & Mantovani, A. (Eds.), 1984, Bone Resorption Metastasis and Diphosphonates, (Raven Press, New York)(in press)

Guaitani, A., Polentarutti, N., Filippeschi, S., Marmonti, L., Corti, F., Italia, C., Coccioli, G., Donelli, M.G., Mantovani, A. & Garattini, S., 1984, European Journal of Cancer, 20, 685.

THE STABILISATION OF SKELETAL METASTASES

C.S.B. GALASKO, A.J. BANKS

Department of Orthopaedic Surgery, University of Manchester, Clinical Sciences Building, Hope Hospital, Eccles Old Road, Salford M6 8HD

Keywords: skeletal metastases; surgical stabilisation

INTRODUCTION

Evaluation of 175 patients with symptomatic skeletal metastases has shown that surgical stabilisation has an important role to play in the treatment of these patients, by relieving their symptoms and improving their quality of life. Surgical stabilisation of the metastasis does not affect the underlying malignancy.

LARGE LYTIC METASTASES

These usually present with pain. Radiographs reveal a large lytic metastasis often associated with much destruction of the cortex. Pathological fracture is a common complication, Fidler (1973) found that if more than 50% of the cortex of a long bone was involved there was a 50% chance of spontaneous fracture. Radiotherapy relieves pain, but temporarily weakens the bone, probably due to the associated transient osteoporosis and may increase the risk of fracture. Fourteen per cent of the pathological fractures in our series occurred through large lytic metastases which had been treated by irradiation.

Primary internal stabilisation of the weakened bone has certain advantages. It is easier to fix the bone whilst it is still intact, and the rehabilitation and convalescence are much shorter and easier. It is the authors' view that internal stabilisation should be the primary treatment followed by irradiation. Irradiation is essential to inhibit further tumour growth with progressive bone destruction and resultant loosening of the stabilisation with increased risk of fracture. It is also important that the stabilisation should be strong enough to allow unsupported weight bearing, and if the implant does not provide this, the stabilisation should be supplemented with methylmethacrylate.

PATHOLOGICAL FRACTURE

The femur is the commonest site, but virtually any long bone is at risk (Table 1). Although every malignant neoplasm can metastasize to bone and can be associated with a pathological fracture, the commonest cause is mammary carcinoma (Table 2).

Table 1. Sites of 122 pathological
fractures in 105 patients.

Femur	Transcervical	28
	Intertrochanteric	18
	Subtrochanteric	12
	Shaft	26
	Distal	4
Humerus	Proximal	7
	Shaft	24
	Distal	1
Tibia	Shaft	1
Radius	Shaft	1

Table 2. The primary tumour associated with
pathological fracture in 105 patients.

Primary Tumour	No.Patients	No.Fractures
Breast	57	71
Bronchus	12	13
Prostate	10	10
Kidney	4	4
Bladder	2	2
Melanoma	2	2
Stomach	2	2
Thyroid	1	1
Oesophagus	1	1
Bile duct	1	1
Uterus	1	1
Cervix	1	1
Penis	1	1
Squamous cell	1	1
Leukaemia	2	2
Myeloma	6	8
Site unknown	1	1
Total	105	122

The development of a pathological
fracture is not a terminal event, the mean
survival after fracture being 10.1 months.
(Galasko, 1974). Fifty four per cent of
patients survived for more than three
months and 23% for more than one year

following fracture (Table 3). The survival is
related to the primary tumour, none of our
patients with bronchial carcinoma surviving
for more than three months, but several of the
patients with carcinoma of the breast lived
for more than one year after developing a
pathological fracture.

There are three aspects to the treatment
of pathological fractures.

    (a) The orthopaedic management;

    (b) Localised irradiation; and

    (c) The treatment of the underlying
       tumours.

Evaluation of 28 patients with a trans-
cervical femoral fracture showed that no
fracture united, irrespective of the type
of orthopaedic management, probably due to
the effect of supra-added irradiation to an
area with impaired vascularity. Primary
replacement hemiarthroplasty gave optimum
results. All patients were mobilised within
a few days of surgery and had no further
problems from their proximal femur. Where
there was a metastasis affecting the acetabu-
lum a total hip arthroplasty was carried out.

The results obtained in the other 61
pathological fractures involving the femur or
tibia showed that the majority of fractures
united by bone in those patients who survived
for four months, irrespective of the type of
treatment. However, internal fixation provided definite advantages over external
support. It gave the patient much greater and
much more rapid relief of pain; it was
associated with easier nursing,more comfort-
able turning of the patient and prevention of
pressure sores; and it allowed much earlier
mobilisation of the patient and discharge
from hospital. It is essential to adequately
stabilise the bone, sufficient for weight

bearing, at the time of surgery. If necessary, the internal fixation must be supplemented
by methylmethacrylate (Harrington et al, 1972; Yablon and Paul, 1976), but had the dis-
advantage of interfering with callus formation. The method of internal fixation depended
on the site of the fracture. Intertrochanteric fractures were best stabilised with a Zickel
nail and fractures of the shaft by intramedullary nailing.

Local irradiation was essential. Only one pathological fracture, in our series, did not
receive post-operative radiotherapy. This was associated with progressive destruction of
bone, loosening and subsequent breakage of the plate used to stabilise a fracture of the
distal femur. The irradiation can be delayed until the wound has healed, but this is not
essential. The implant did not appear to affect the irradiation, providing megavoltage
was used.

Evaluation of the 32 pathological fractures of the humerus showed that internal fixation
was also of benefit in that it provided the patient with much greater mobility and earlier
use of the limb, although the advantages over conservative treatment were not as marked as
with pathological fractures of the lower limb.

There was no evidence that internal fixation disseminated tumour along the course of the
bone.

SPINAL INSTABILITY

Back pain is a frequent symptom in patients with disseminated carcinoma and in 10% is
due to spinal instability (Galasko and Sylvester, 1978). We have now treated 34 patients
with spinal instability secondary to spinal metastases. The primary tumours are shown in
Table 4 and the technique of stabilisation in Table 5. There have been three failures.
A Bank's rod had to be removed because of infection and one Harrington and one Bank's rod
loosened. In the other 31 patients there has been relief of their severe pain, which was
markedly worsened by movement and only partly improved by bracing. Pre-operatively, many
of the patients were confined to bed and found that turning was agonising even when carried
out by two or three trained nurses. There was an associated neurological deficit in 17.
The spinal cord or cauda equina was decompressed at the time of spinal stabilisation and
the results are shown in Table 6.

Like pathological fractures, spinal instability is not a terminal event. Twenty-five
of the 34 patients have died, the mean survival being 32.1 weeks and one patient living for
four years (Table 7).

CONCLUSIONS

The development of skeletal metastases and their major complications are not necessarily
terminal events. The aim of treatment is to provide maximum palliation and improve the
quality of life by relieving pain, providing early mobilisation and early discharge from
hospital. Major surgery may be required to achieve maximum palliation and internal
stabilisation of skeletal metastases has much to offer in the treatment of large lytic
lesions, pathological fractures and spinal instability.

Table 3.   Survival following pathological fracture in 69 patients.

Survival	No.
0 - 3 months	32
4 - 6 months	5
7 - 12 months	17
13+ months	15
Mean Survival	10.1 months

Table 4. The primary tumour associated with spinal instability.

Tumour	No. patients
Breast	15
Myeloma	5
Prostate	2
Melanoma	2
Bronchus	1
Parotid	1
Uterus	1
Cervix	1
Vaginal	1
Kidney	1
Colon	1
Chondrosarcoma	1
Histiocytoma	1
Cordoma	1
Total	34

Table 5. Method of spinal stabilisation.

Method	No. patients
Harrington rod	5
Harrington rod + sublaminal wiring	1
Bank's rod	26
Luque segmental stabilisation	2
	34

Table 6. Associated neurological deficit in patients with spinal instability.

No. patients	17
No. improved foll. surg.	12
No. late cord/cauda equina compression	1
No. recurrence	2

Table 7.   Survival following spinal stabilisation in 25 patients.

Length of survival	No. patients
0 - 8 weeks	5
8 - 16 weeks	7
17 - 24 weeks	2
25 - 36 weeks	6
9 - 12 months	0
13 - 24 months	4
2 - 5 years	1

REFERENCES
Fidler, M., 1973, British Medical Journal, 1, 341
Galasko, C.S.B., 1974, Journal Royal College Surgeons of Edinburgh, 19, 351
Galasko, C.S.B., Sylvester, B.S., 1978, Clinical Oncology,4, 273
Harrington, K.D., Johnston, J.O., Turner, R.H., Green, D.L., 1972, Journal of Bone and Joint Surgery, 54-A, 1665
Yablon, I.G., Paul, G.R., 1976,Surgery, Gynecology and Obstetrics, 143, 177

ADJUVANT CHEMOTHERAPY FOR NASOPHARYNGEAL CANCER CAUSES TUMOUR SHRINKAGE,
BUT FAILS TO PREVENT RECURRENCE OR METASTASES AFTER RADIATION TREATMENT

I. TANNOCK, K. HEWITT and D. PAYNE
Princess Margaret Hospital, 500 Sherbourne St., Toronto, Ontario M4X 1K9,
Canada

Keywords: nasopharyngeal carcinoma; adjuvant chemotherapy, radiotherapy

Radical radiation therapy to the nasopharynx and cervical nodes is
used world-wide as the standard treatment for nasopharyngeal cancer. A
recent review of 140 patients treated at this hospital between 1970 and
1975 (Payne 1983) gave results similar to those for other large series
with overall 5-year survival rates of about 30-40%. The study showed
that deaths from disease continued to occur beyond 5 years, and that there
was a high rate of tumour recurrence in both local and metastatic sites.
We decided to explore the use of adjuvant chemotherapy given prior to
radiation in an attempt to decrease recurrence and improve survival.

DESIGN OF STUDY
During the period April 1981 to December 1983, 50 of 52 consecutive
patients with locoregional nasopharyngeal cancer (T_{1-4}, N_{0-3}, M_0) were
treated with 2 courses of methotrexate, bleomycin and cisplatin given at
3-week intervals prior to radical radiation therapy. After overnight
hydration, methotrexate was given on Day 1 in 3 doses of $100/mg/^2$ i.v. over
6hr; folinic acid rescue (15 mg/m^2 every 6hr for 4 doses) was started
24hr after methotrexate. Bleomycin was given in a dose of $20U/m^2$ on
Day 1, and then as an infusion of $20U/m^2$/day for 3 days. Cisplatin
($60mg/m^2$) was given on Day 5. A preliminary study had demonstrated that
this schedule could be given to patients with head and neck cancer
without detectable increase in toxicity (Tannock et al, 1982), and seven
patients with nasopharyngeal cancer treated in the earlier study are
included in this analysis.
Patients were assessed with nasopharyngeal tomograms and CT scan,

bone scan, chest X-ray, standard biochemistry and measurement of neck nodes
at the start of the study.   Nasopharyngeal tomograms, CT scan and tumour
measurements were repeated for most patients at the start of radiation
therapy 6 weeks later.   Patients were seen weekly during radiotherapy and
at 2-3 month intervals thereafter.   Appropriate studies were undertaken
if the patient developed signs or symptoms suggestive of local recurrence
or metastases.   Neck dissection was performed if patients had persistent
or recurrent disease in neck nodes without other evidence of tumour.

Most patients had palpable neck nodes, and response to chemotherapy
was determined at the start of radiation therapy according to the
following criteria: Complete Response (CR) required complete disappearance
of neck nodes and normalization of nasopharyngeal tomograms and/or CT scan;
Partial Response (PR) required 50% shrinkage in cross section of all
palpable nodes and improvement in tomograms and/or CT scan.   Patients
without nodal disease were not assessed for response to chemotherapy
because of the difficulties associated with accurate radiologic assessment;   they were assessed for toxicity, recurrence and survival.

RESULTS

Forty-three of 57 patients receiving chemotherapy had measurable
disease in the neck: there were 3CR and 29PR giving a response rate to
chemotherapy of 74%.   Eight patients categorized as partial responders
had complete disappearance of nodal disease in the neck without complete
normalization of nasopharyngeal tomograms or CT scan. Of the 14 patients
without measurable disease in the neck, two had normalization of tomograms
and CT scans, and most had radiologic improvement. Chemotherapy caused no
life-threatening or irreversible toxicity in these patients, although most
of them experienced fever during bleomycin infusion, and nausea and
vomiting after cisplatin.   Thus chemotherapy can be given with acceptable
toxicity and is highly effective in causing tumour shrinkage.

All patients completed radical radiation therapy (50-60 Gy in 20-30
fractions) following their chemotherapy, except for one patient who
developed metastatic disease during the course of radiation therapy.

At a median follow-up of 27 months (range 9-53 months), the status of
patients is as shown in Table 1. Actuarial survival and recurrence-free
survival curves are shown in Fig. 2 for patients treated during the period
when it was our policy to give chemotherapy and are compared with those
for a historical control group of patients treated in this Institution with
radiotherapy alone (Payne, 1983).   Chemotherapy has not lead to improvement in patient survival, and has failed to prevent or delay either local

or metastatic relapse.

Table 1.   Current status of 57 patients treated with chemotherapy and radiation, and patterns of failures.

	Number of Patients	Failure Pattern		Historical Controls (N = 132)
Alive, no evidence of disease	25	Persistent disease	8 (14%)	13%
Dead, no evidence of disease	1	Locoregional recurrence	13 (23%)	35%
Alive with disease	10	Distant recurrence	8 (19%)	19%
Dead of disease	21	Local and distant recurrence	3	

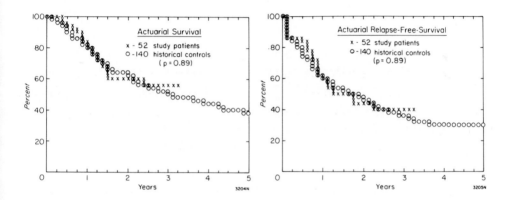

Figure 1. (a)   Actuarial survival curves and (b) recurrence-free survival curves for patients who were treated when our policy was to use chemotherapy and radiation and for historical controls receiving radiation alone.

DISCUSSION

Payne (1983) has analysed the survival and patterns of failure for patients with locoregional nasopharyngeal cancer who were treated with curative intent in this Institution using radiotherapy alone (Table 1). These patients had a similar distribution of stage to those in the present study, and all of them were followed for a minimum of 6 years.   In the current study 23% of patients have had locoregional failure and 19% have relapsed with distant metastases after median follow-up of only 27 months. With longer follow-up it seems inevitable that the rate of failure in meta-static sites will exceed that in historical controls.   Chemotherapy was effective in shrinking locoregional disease in the majority of patients; thus, failure to improve the rate of local control suggests that chemotherapy and radiation were effective against the same subpopulation of cells.

The rate of response to chemotherapy in patients who subsequently

relapsed in metastatic sites was similar to that of the whole group. It
is unexpected that chemotherapy which was effective in shrinking locoregional disease should not have had sufficient effect against microscopic
metastases to cause at least a delay in their overt appearance. One
explanation is that chemotherapy might cause damage to either normal
tissue or host defence mechanisms that could increase the retention of
circulating, potentially metastatic tumour cells. Several studies have
demonstrated an increase in lung colonies after intravenous injection of
tumour cells into mice that have been treated with anti-cancer drugs. This
effect is greatest for cyclophosphamide, where the efficiency of lung
colonization may be increased by more than 100-fold, but smaller increases
of up to 4-fold have been observed in some studies following treatment of
mice with methotrexate or bleomycin (e.g. Van Putten et al, 1975). If
such an effect were to exist in man, one would predict a possible increase
in metastases where adjuvant chemotherapy is given prior to local treatment of the primary, but not when adjuvant chemotherapy follows local
treatment as is usual for breast cancer.

   We conclude that chemotherapy which is effective in causing shrinkage
of nasopharyngeal cancer does not improve survival or relapse-free survival when given prior to radiation therapy; in particular, chemotherapy
does not prevent or delay the appearance of metastases. Chemotherapy
should be used as part of primary management of nasopharyngeal cancer only
in the context of a well-designed clinical trial.

REFERENCES

Payne, D.G., 1983, Carcinoma of the nasopharynx.   Journal of Otolaryng-
   ology, 12, 197.
Tannock, I., Cummings, B & Sorrenti, V, 1982, Combination chemotherapy
   used prior to radiation therapy for locally advanced squamous cell
   carcinoma of the head and neck.   Cancer Treatment Reports, 66, 1421.
Van Putten, L.M., et al, 1975, Enhancement by drugs of metastatic lung
   nodule formation after intravenous tumour cell injection.
   International Journal of Cancer, 15, 588.

AVCF COMPARED TO CMF IN PREMENOPAUSAL BREAST CARCINOMA ADJUVANT THERAPY :
LOSS OF BENEFIT FOR SURVIVAL

G. MATHÉ, J.L. MISSET, R. PLAGNE, D. BELPOMME, B. LE MEVEL, J. GUERRIN,
P. FUMOLEAU, R. METZ, M. DELGADO, F. de VASSAL, M. ERIGUCHI, M. SCHNEIDER
ONCOFRANCE, Service des Maladies Sanguines et Tumorales et ICIG, Hôpital
Paul-Brousse, VILLEJUIF

Keywords: Breast carcinoma; adjuvant chemotherapy premenopausal patients.

INTRODUCTION

When we published the preliminary result, at the third year, of
adjuvant AVCF (adriamycin, vincristine, cyclophosphamide and 5-fluoro-
uracil) compared to CMF (cyclophosphamide, methotrexate, 5-fluorouracil)
shown by Rossi et al. (1981) superior to abstention in premenopausal
patients but not in postmenopausal women, this quadruple combination,
shown efficient in advanced breast carcinoma (Gouveia et al. 1978),
appeared to give no significant difference after menopause, but a significant advantage before, for survival as well as for disease-free survival
(DFS) (Mathé et al. 1982).

At the fifth year analysis, the advantage persists for DFS, but not
for survival.

MATERIAL AND PATIENTS

The patients were stratified according to the following categories :
T2N-MP-, T2N-MP+, T1T2N+MP-, T3T4N-MP-, T3T4N+MP+, T3T4N+MP- and T3T4N+MP+.
They were eligible regardless of whether or not they had received post-
surgical radiotherapy which was performed in 50.8% of them according to
the center policy.

A total of 329 patients meeting the above criteria, recruited from
six French medical oncology services of cancer centers, entered the trial
until May 1981 when the study was closed to patient accrual.

After registration, patients were randomized within each stratification subgroup above described, to receive 12 monthly cycles of either CMF
according to Rossi's schedule (Rossi et al. 1981) (days 1 and 8 : MTX,
40mg/m2 IV and 5FU, 600mg/m2 IV ; days 1 to 14 : CPM, 100mg/m2 orally),

or 12 monthly cycles of the following combination : ADM, 30 mg/m² IV on
day 1 ; VCR, 1 mg/m² on day 2 ; CPM, 300 mg/m²/d and FU, 400 mg/m²/d,
both given on days 3 to 6 (AVCF) (Gouveia et al. 1978). The next cycle
was begun on day 29 if the patients hematologic recovery was satisfactory.
ADM was omitted in N-patients and in three N+ patients with medical
contra-indication : those patients will be later referred to as "VCF"
patients.

Four patients were lost to follow-up immediately after randomisation
leaving 325 women for analysis. The characteristics are listed in tables
I and II.

		CMF (154)			(A)VCF (171)		
	TOTAL	T	N+	N-	T	N+	N-
PREMENOPAUSAL	168	76	57	19	92	74	18
POST MENOPAUSAL	157	78	55	23	79	63	16
N+	249		112			137	
N-	76			42			34
N+ ≤ 3 NODES	101		49			52	
N+ > 3 NODES	125		49			76	
N+ NUMBER UNKNOWN	23						
PREVIOUS RADIOTHERAPY	166	82	64	18	84	73	11
NO PREVIOUS RADIOTHERAPY	159	72	48	24	87	64	23

Table I. Characteristics of the patients in the two groups.

N = 226

NODES	≤ 3			> 3		
	AVCF	CMF	P	AVCF	CMF	P
Mp-	33 (0.58)	24 (0.42)	0.26	35 (0.58)	25 (0.42)	0.25
Mp+	19 (0.43)	25 (0.57)	0.38	41 (0.63)	24 (0.37)	0.07
	52	49		76	49	
ROSSI'S PATIENTS	140				67	p < 0.01

Table II. Distribution of patients according to hormonal and node status
and treatment group.

RESULTS

The results will be described in detail in a later article (Mathé et
al. 1984). We have to mention the absence of any difference between the

irradiated and the non-irradiated subjects (Plagne et al. 1984), the absence of difference between the actions of AVCF and CMF after menopause and in N-patients (Mathé et al.   1984)   was   as observed at the third year (Mathé et al. 1982); the AVCF 100% alopecia versus the CMF 20% and the AVCF 100% amenorrhea versus the CMF 20%.

We shall only detail here three facts :

a) The significant difference for overall DFS, but the absence of signi-ficant difference for overall survival

When the entire group of patients is considered, a significant differ-ence appears in favor of the AVCF-VCF group over the CMF group with a p value adjusted for nodal status of 0.015 for DFS (fig. 1), but there is no significant difference (p = 0.37) for overall survival (fig. 2).

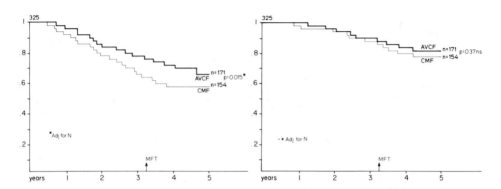

All patients (n=325) Disease free
survival according to treatment

Fig.1

All patients (n=325) Survival
according to treatment.

Fig.2

b) The significant difference for DFS and the absence of significant dif-ference for survival in overall node positive patients

For the 249 N+ patients, the difference is significant in favor of the AVCF group (the analysis includes three N+patients who received only VCF), with respect to DFS (p = 0.014). But, no significant difference (p = 0.39) appears for survival.

c) The significant difference for DFS, but the absence of difference for survival in premenopausal patients

The group of premenopausal N+ patients have a five year disease free survival of 77% after AVCF and 53% after CMF : according to the log-rank-test, the difference between the two curves is significant (p = 0.003) (fig. 3), but there is no significant difference in favor of AVCF for survival (p = 0.09) (fig. 4).

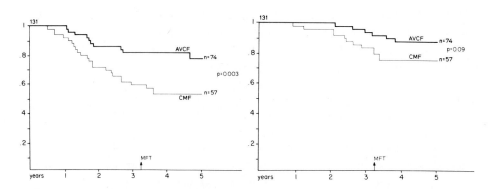

N+ Premenopausal patients (n=131)
Disease free survival according to
treatment.

N+ Premenopausal patients (n=131)
Survival according to treatment.

Fig. 3   Fig. 4

REFERENCES

Gouveia, J., Misset, J.L., Bayssas, M., Belpomme, D., De Vassal, F.,
Delgado, M., Gil, M., Hayat, M., Jasmin, C., Machover, D., Musset, M.,
Pico, J.L., Ribaud, P., Schwarzenberg, L.,   Mathé, G., 1978, Medical
Oncology, 4, 13 (abstract 49).

Mathé, G., Misset, J.L., Plagne, R., Belpomme, D., Guerrin, J., Fumoleau,
P., Metz, R. 1 Delgado, M. 1982 Superiority of AVCF (adriamycin, vincristin
cyclophosphamide, and 5-fluorouracil) as adjuvant chemotherapy for breast
cancer : International Symposium on Basic Mechanisms and Clinical Treatment of Cancer Metastasis, Fukuoka 6-8 December   (abstract book)
(in press).

Mathé, G., Misset, J.L., Plagne, R., Belpomme, D., Le Mevel, B., Guerrin,
J., Fumoleau, P., Metz, R., Delgado, M., De Vassal, F. , Eriguchi, M.,
Schneider, M., Controlled phase III trial of breast cancer adjuvant
chemotherapy comparing CMF and the combination of AVCF (adriamcyin,
vincristin, cyclophosphamide and 5-fluorouracil (submitted).

Plagne, R., Misset, J.L., Belpomme, D., Guerrin, J., Le Mevel, B., Metz,
R., Chollet, P., Delgado, M., Fargeot, P., Fumoleau, P., Jeanne, C.,
Ferriere, P., Schneider, M., De Vassal, F., Jasmin, C., Schwarzenberg, L.,
Hayat, M., Machover, D., Ribaud, P., Dorval, T. & Mathé, G.
Absence de différence avec la radiothérapie appliquée après la mastectomie
et avant la chimiothérapie adjuvante pour cancer du sein. In prepara-
tion.

Rossi, A., Bonadonna, G., Valagussa, P. & Veronesi, U., 1981 Multimodal
treatment in operable breast cancer: five year result of the CMF program.
British Medical Journal 282: 1427.

COMBINED TREATMENT OF MICRO-METASTASES OF SMALL CELL CARCINOMA OF THE LUNG

K. KARRER for the ISC-SMALL CELL LUNG CANCER STUDY GROUP
Institute for Epidemiology of Neoplasma of the University Vienna,
Borschkegasse 8a, A-1090 Vienna, Austria

Keyword : small cell carcinoma of the lung, adjuvant chemotherapy, surgery
for cure, combined modality treatment

INTRODUCTION

The system of the Lewis lung carcinoma implanted into BDF_1 mice possesses
the advantage of a solid tumour and, because of its spontaneous metastasis
early during the course of the disease, particularly to the lungs, it also
has the advantages of a disseminated malignant disease. It enables one to
estimate the number of tumour cells in the micrometastases by bioassaying
the lungs at different stages of tumour growth (Karrer et al. 1967).

Measurement of the effect of drugs on the survival of individual cells
has to include the function of time. At a given moment the effect of a drug
on one particular tumour cell cannot merely be described as positive or
negative. There exists also the possibility that this cell is sublethally
damaged and able to recover in time, or on the other hand, it could be
completely destroyed in time by the host (Humphreys et al. 1967).

Additionally, there always exists the possibility of the presence of so-
called "dormant" cells, which do not behave at this time as viable and
dividing tumour cells but which are able to do so at other times, perhaps
under different conditions, for reasons not yet known. This is also related
to the problem of differences in the uptake of drug by the tumour cells
under different kinds of metabolism, or with different utilization of the
drug, e.g., blood supply (Karrer et al. 1983).

METHODS

According to the results of their studies (Denk & Karrer 1956, Denk &
Karrer 1961) the Viennese cooperative group for lung cancer treatment began
in 1969 a further randomized cooperative trial using adjuvant polychemo-

therapy or radical surgery only for patients with bronchial carcinoma.
(Karrer & Denck 1971). The lifetable survival rate of patients with small
cell bronchial carcinoma treated by the combination of polychemotherapy and
surgery shows a rise in the survival rate 4 years after operation for stage
I or II diseases in comparison with patients treated with surgery only, and
also of the survival time for more advanced stages.

Therefore continuation of the trial was considered to be justified
(Karrer 1979). To improve the positive results of adjuvant chemotherapy
further new (designed alternating) polychemotherapy schedules were administered intermittently in a randomized two-arm cooperative study (Karrer
et al. 1982). This study was activated in 1979 and is still in progress.
(Karrer et al. 1983). For the first group the same polychemotherapy
protocol as before was administered intermittently as 13 courses of three
infusions, each containing: 12 mg/kg cyclophosphamide, 12 mg/kg 5-fluorour-
acil, 0.5 mg/kg methotrexate, 0.1 mg/kg vinblastine, 500 ml 5% laevulose
i.v. for 40 minutes. The first infusion of the first set starts 7 days
after operation, the second set one week later, followed by the third also
after one week interval. Three series, each of three infusions, should be
given within the first half year after operation. Two further series of
infusions are administered within every half year until three years after
operation.

The second group received three different drug combinations alternating
according to the following schedule : 7 days after radical operation the
combination A consisting of 1.500 mg/m^2 cyclophosphamide, 100 mg/m^2 CCNU and
15 mg/m^2 MTX given as infusion in 500 ml 5% laevulose intravenously for one
hour.

After an interval of 4 weeks combination A is given a second time,
followed after another interval of 4 weeks by combination B consisting of
1.000 mg/m^2 cyclophosphamide, 40 mg/m^2 adriamycin and 1 mg/m^2 vincristine.
4 weeks later the second infusion of combination B is administered, followed
by combination C consisting of 40 mg/kg ifosfamid and 200 mg VP-16 given
over 5 days after an interval of 4 weeks and a second time after another 4
weeks. Between the 21st week and the 33rd week after the operation chemotherapy is discontinued.

During this interval, from the 25th week to the 28th week, local radiation (30 Gy) is administered to the mediastinal area of the bronchial stump.
After a 5 week interval two further courses of scheme A,B and C each at 4
weeks interval are given. In this way each scheme would be intermittently
administered 4 times within the first year after operation.

Efforts have been made to increase the number of patients in this new
randomized trial by inviting several thoracic surgical departments for coop-
eration. So far 9 centres of thoracic surgery (from Austria 3, FRG 3,
Argentina 2, Yugoslavia 1) have entered 54 appropriate patients in this trial.

From the preliminary evaluation on August 1st, 1984, of this new current
trial, survival data in the form of life-table curves from 54 patients are
presented. Figure 1 shows the number of patients classified according to
pTNM based on the patho - histological examination of the operation
specimen, the numbers of patients at risk 1, 2, 3, and 4 years after operation and their life-table survival.

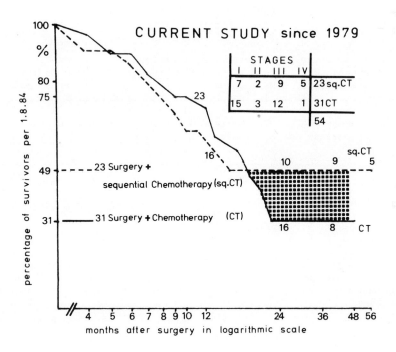

Based on observations of the 23 patients treated with the new alternating
sequential adjuvant chemotherapy during a median observation time of 17
months it can be stated that toxicity was in an acceptable range. So far the
administration seems to be clinically applicable. No unexpected side effects
occurred.

The histological classification of all long-term survivors (more than 2
years) was kindly confirmed by M.J. Matthews as small cell carcinomas.

In line with our decision to continue and further optimize this study a new treatment protocol for a two-arm randomized enlarged ISC-cooperative trial is proposed for October, 1984.

Preparations for this new protocol were initiated at the 13th International Congress of Chemotherapy in August, 1983 in Vienna. It was formulated together with the ISC-cooperating groups in consideration of comparability with ongoing trials of the NCI-lung Cancer Study in USA and the EORTC - Lung Cancer Study Group in Europe.

REFERENCES

Denk, W. & Karrer, K., 1955, Modellversuch einer Rezidivprophylaxe des Karzinoms. Wiener Klinische Wochenschrift 67, 986.

Denk, W. & Karrer, K., 1956, Chemotherapie zur Rezidivprophylaxe des Karzinoms. Wiener Klinische Woechenschrift 68, 977.

Denk, W. & Karrer, K., 1961, Combined Surgery and Chemotherapy in the Treatment of Malignant Tumors. Cancer 14, 1197.

Humphreys, S.R., Dewys, W.D. & Karrer, K., 1967, A Model System for the Selection of Drugs for Chemotherapy of Metastasis. Proceedings of the 5th International Congress of Chemotherapy, Vienna, June 26-July 1,B 9/17.

Karrer, K., Humphreys, S.R. & Goldin, A., 1967, An Experimental Model for Studying Factors which Influence Metastasis of Malignant Tumors. International Journal of Cancer 2, 213.

Karrer, K. & Denck, H., 1971, Weitere Vorschlage zur chemotherapeutischen Rezidivprophylaxe des Bronchuskarzinoms. Wiener Medizinische Wochenschrift 7, 112.

Karrer, K., 1979, Adjuvant Chemotherapy of Post-Surgical Minimal Residual Bronchial Carcinomas. Recent Results in Cancer Research 68, 246.

Karrer, K., Rella, W. & Goldin, A., 1979, Surgery Plus Corynebacterium Parvum Immunotherapy for Lewis Lung Carcinoma in Mice. European Journal of Cancer 15, 867.

Karrer, K., Denck, H., Pridun, N. & Zwintz, E., 1982, Zur Rezidivprophylaxe beim kleinzelligen Bronchuskarzinom mittels adjuvanter Polychemotherapie. Wiener Klinische Wochenschrift 94, 159.

Karrer, K., Denck, H., Pridun, N., Zwintz, E. & Cooperative Group, 1983, Combination of Early Surgery for Cure and Polychemotherapy in Small-Cell Bronchial Carcinoma. Proceedings of the 13th International Congress of Chemotherapy, Vienna, August 28 - September 2.

ISOLATION AND ANALYSIS OF A CELL SURFACE METASTASIS-ASSOCIATED SIALOGALACTOPROTEIN FROM RAT AND HUMAN MAMMARY ADENOCARCINOMA

PETER A. STECK[1,2] and GARTH L. NICOLSON[1]

Departments of [1]Tumor Biology, and [2]Neuro-Oncology, The University of Texas-M. D. Anderson Hospital and Tumor Institute, Houston, Texas 77030 USA

Keywords: mammary adenocarcinoma; sialogalactoprotein; gp580

INTRODUCTION

Breast cancer metastasis is responsible for more deaths of women in North America and Northern Europe than any other malignant disease. This has stimulated efforts in finding suitable biochemical markers that are associated with breast cancer metastasis. We have been investigating cell surface constituents of spontaneously metastasizing rat 13762NF mammary adenocarcinoma cells (Neri et al., 1982). These cells share several important characteristics with human breast cancer, including similar cell type and pathogenesis of metastasis. Cell clones derived from subcutaneously growing tumor and spontaneous pulmonary lesions have been characterized for a number of biological and biochemical properties, and have been shown to differ in metastatic behavior (Neri et al., 1982; Welch et al., 1983). The majority of these cell clones drift in their metastatic and biochemical properties upon prolonged cultivation in vitro (Neri and Nicolson, 1981; Neri et al., 1981). In particular, the expression of two cell surface glycoproteins correlated with metastatic potential (Steck and Nicolson, 1983). One, a sialoglycoprotein (gp80), was observed to decrease in expression with metastatic potential, whereas the other, a high molecular weight sialogalactoprotein (gp580), increased in expression with metastatic potential. Recently we described a procedure for purification and characterization of gp580 from the highly metastatic cell clone MTLn3 (Steck and Nicolson, 1984). In this report, we compare some biochemical characteristics of gp580 to a similar glycoprotein isolated from several human breast cancer lung metastases.

METHODS

Clone MTLn3 cells were grown in vivo or in vitro as previously described (Neri et al., 1982). Human breast carcinoma pulmonary metastases were obtained from autopsy specimens. Sialoglycoproteins from rat or human adenocarcinoma cells were purified according to Steck and Nicolson (1984). Briefly, 4M guanidine hydrochloride tissue extracts were subjected to cesium chloride density gradient centrifugation and fractions around p=1.48±0.05 g/ml were pooled and applied to a calibrated Sepharose CL-2B column. The void volume fractions were pooled, dialyzed and aliquots were radioactively labeled. Fractions were subjected to ion exchange chromatography on a DEAE column in 8M urea and eluted with a sodium chloride gradient. The individual labeled peaks were pooled, dialyzed and then analyzed for their sensitivities to various degradative enzymes and by SDS-polyacrylamide gel electrophoresis. Certain fractions were acid hydrolyzed for amino acid determination using a LKB model 4400 amino acid analyzer.

RESULTS AND DISCUSSION

Previously we found that rat gp580 could be isolated and partially purified by density gradient centrifugation (Steck and Nicolson, 1983). Extracts from rat or human lung metastases of similar buoyant density (p=1.48 g/ml) after cesium chloride gradient centrifugation were pooled individually and subjected to gel filtration chromatography on a calibrated Sepharose CL-2B column. Aliquots of the void volume fractions were radioactively labeled with periodate-$[^3H]$borohydride (for sialic and carboxyl acids) or Na ^{125}I (for protein) (Steck and Nicolson, 1984). The radiolabeled materials were applied to a Sephacel DEAE ion exchange column and eluted with a sodium chloride gradient (Figure 1). Four radioactive peaks (I-IV) were eluted from the column. The eluted material from rat and human origin yielded identical profiles. Either radiolabeling procedure gave similar results, except for the intensity of peak II, which was increased when the void volume fractions were labeled by the periodate-$[^3H]$borohydride method. The results indicated that DEAE peaks I, III, and IV contained the overwhelming majority of the protein material.

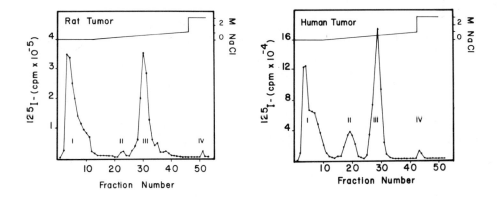

Figure 1. Left panel: The ion exchange chromatography of high density void volume fractions from rat MTLn3 metastasis extract radioactively labeled with [125]I. Right panel: Same as left panel except an extract from breast cancer lung metastasis was used columns were equilibrated with 8M urea, 20 mM Tris HCl pH 6.8, and eluted with a sodium chloride gradient.

When the different peaks from Sephacel DEAE chromatography were analyzed by SDS-polyacrylamide gel electrophoresis, the first peak contained free radiolabel or low molecular weight protein material (<10 kD). When labeled by the periodate-[^{3}H]borohydride protocol, the other three peaks contained high M_r glycoproteins that barely entered a 7.5% polyacrylamide gel. These gp migrated between the gel origin and M_r ~ 350 kD on a 2-17.5% DATD-crosslinked gradient acrylamide gel (Steck and Nicolson, 1984). Similar analyses with ^{125}I-labeled fractions demonstrated that only peaks III and IV could be radioactively labeled. Furthermore, peaks III and IV bound radiolabled peanut agglutinin after removal of their sialic acid residues, a technique used previously to identify gp580 (Steck and Nicolson, 1983).

Further characterization was accomplished by assaying the susceptibility of the various fractionated gp to a panel of degradative enzymes for 1 hour at 37°C. The ^{3}H-labeled peak II material was degraded by Streptomyces hyaluronidase, and together with the lack of detectable protein in this peak, suggested it is hyaluronic acid. [125]I- and ^{3}H- labeled materials from peaks III and IV were resistant to trypsin, chymotrypsin, hyaluronidase, chondroitinase ABC, and DNase, but were degraded by Pronase and Subtilopeptidase A. Fractions from human or rat extracts gave identical results.

Aliquots of peak III were hydrolyzed and subjected to amino acid analysis. The major amino acids present in each glycoprotein and their percentage of total amino acids are shown in Table 1.

Table 1.   Major Amino acids of isolated rat and human peak III sialogalactoproteins.

Amino Acid	Rat	Human
	(% of total amino acids)	
Aspartic acid	10	12
Threonine	6	6
Serine	15	18
Glutamic acid	13	15
Glycine	10	9

We have previously purified and characterized a high M_r glycoprotein (gp580) expressed on the cell surface and in the matrix of rat 13762NF mammary adenocarcinoma cells that correlates with sponataneous metastatic potential. A similar glycoprotein has now been identified in human breast cancer lung metastases. Both glycoproteins possess relatively high buoyant densities, are of high M_r (around 580 kD), bind peanut agglutinin after desialylation, are relatively resistant to proteases, and share similar ratios of major amino acids. Although high M_r glycoproteins have been observed on the cell surfaces of mammary epithelial cells, their functional roles remain obscure. They have been suggested as immunologic protective agents (Kim et al., 1975) or cell lubricants (Silberberg and Meyer, 1980). The increased expression of gp580 on rat cells of high metastatic potential and its identification in human metastatic lesions suggests that it might be useful as a marker for distinguishing metastatic cell subpopulations within primary breast adenocarcinomas.

ACKNOWLEDGMENTS

Supported by PHS grants RO1-CA-28844 (G.L.N.) and F32-CA-07224 (P.A.S.) from the U.S. National Cancer Institute. P.A.S. is currently supported by the John S. Dunn Research Foundation. Amino acid analyses were kindly performed by Dr. D. Ward of Biochemistry Department, M. D. Anderson Hospital and Tumor Institute.

REFERENCES

Kim, U., Baumler, A., Carruther, C., & Bielat, K., 1975, Proceedings of
   the National Academy of Sciences, U.S.A., 72, 1012.
Neri, A. & Nicolson, G.L., 1981, International Journal of Cancer, 28, 731.
Neri, A., Ruoslahti, E., & Nicolson, G.L., 1981, Cancer Research, 41, 5082.
Neri, A., Welch, D., Kawaguchi, T., & Nicolson, G.L., 1982, Journal of
   National Cancer Institute, 68, 507.
Silberberg, A. & Meyer, F.A., 1980, Advances in Experimental Medicine and
   Biology, 103, 53.
Steck, P.A. & Nicolson, G.L., 1983, Experimental Cell Research, 147, 255.
Steck, P.A. & Nicolson, G.L., 1983, Journal of Biological Chemistry (in
   preparation).
Welch, D., Neri, A., & Nicolson, G.L., 1983, Invasion and Metastasis, 3, 65.

A TRANSPLANTABLE OSTEOSARCOMA IN RATS WITH REGULAR OCCURRENCE OF LUNG METASTASES AS A MODEL FOR CHEMOTHERAPY

F. WINGEN and D. SCHMÄHL
Institute of Toxicology and Chemotherapy, German Cancer Research
Center, Im Neuenheimer Feld 280, 69 Heidelberg, F.R.G.

Keyword: Osteosarcoma

Osteosarcoma is the most frequent primary bone tumor in
childhood and is most dangerous because of its early metastases
in the lung and its chemoresistence. In recent years great
therapeutic progress has been made by adjuvant treatment with
high-dose methotrexate and leucovorin rescue (Jaffe et al. 1978).
The five-year survival time was considerably increased from 20%
to about 40% due to retardation of pulmonary metastases. The
hopes placed in this method, however, have not fully material-
ized during testing, even in combination therapy (Jaffe et al.
1981). Recent reports have described successful clinical trials
with intraarterial infusion of different cytostatics to be used
predominantly for preoperative chemotherapy of non-metastasized
osteosarcoma (Benjamin et al. 1984, Jaffe et al. 1984, Senn
1981). A standard therapy is not yet in sight because pulmonary
micrometastases are found in up to 80% of patients at the time
of resection of the primary tumor. Animal models suited for
chemotherapy of metastasizing osteosarcomas are therefore of
special relevance.

Xenografts in nude mice often do not metastasize (Masuda 1983).
The frequently used Ridgway osteosarcoma in mice is also inapt
to metastasize (Nelson 1982). Marked metastasis in the lung and
osteoid formation over several hundred passages characterize the
Dunn osteosarcoma (Hanamura and Urist 1978). For our investigations which were to include scintigraphic and surgical methods,
however, this mouse model is less appropriate than a rat model.
The beryllium-induced, slowly growing osteosarcoma in rabbits
(Komitowski 1974), which also metastasizes to the lung, is not
well suited for chemotherapy testing despite its good histo-

pathologic comparability with human osteosarcomas. In 1980 Delbrück et al. induced osteosarcomas in rats by administration of
^{144}Cer. The resulting tumor metastasized to the lung and formed
ample osteoid and alkaline phosphatase. In our laboratory, the
tumor is being maintained in passage 14 after transplantation of
tumor fragments into the medullary canal of the tibia in Sprague-
Dawley rats. The take rates reach about 90% within 30 days after
transplantation. Pulmonary metastases arise in 99% of these animals. Micrometastases can be seen histologically already after
14 days (Wingen et al. 1984) (Fig. 1).

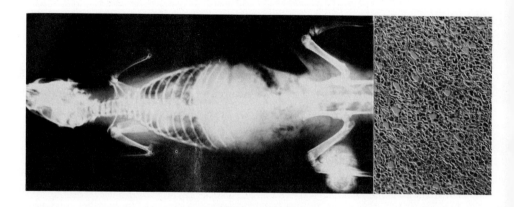

Fig. 1a. Radiograph of rat with large primary tumor and extensive pulmonary metastases on day 38 after transplantation
(corresponding approximately to the median survival time).
Fig. 1b. Histologic correlate to primary tumor shown in Fig. 1a
with polymorphous hyperchromic cells which are embedded in a
fine network of partly calcified osteoid and are very similar
to osteogenic osteosarcoma cells in man (Kissane et al. 1981).

Primary tumor and pulmonary metastases can be depicted by
X-ray and scintigraphy. Bone scintigrams taken two hours after
iv administration of ^{99m}Tc-methylene diphosphonate showed the
storage capacity of primary tumor and pulmonary metastases for
osteotropic compounds. This tumor model is therefore considered
suitable for diagnostic investigations (Wingen et al. 1984).

When the pulmonary metastases developed less rapidly, secondary metastases also occurred in the kidneys. Additional
metastases were found in regional lymph nodes of the lower ab-

dominal region at a rate of about 12%. In one case the lymph
node invasion originated from pulmonary metastases. The latter
mostly occurred as multiple metastases in both pulmonary lobes.
Occasionally, single giant metastatic nodes developed in the
hilus, but no preferred tumor site was seen for multiple metastases. Histologic examination revealed osteoid-forming, partly
confluent metastases with necrotic centers.

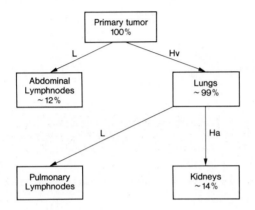

Fig. 2. Possible pathways of metastases of osteosarcomas after
intraosseous transplantation.

In chemotherapy experiments we tested new osteotropic cytostatic agents and diphosphonates beside cyclophosphamide and
dacarbazine (DTIC). 10 iv doses of 48 mg/kg DTIC resulted in a
median survival time of 84 days (78-87, p=0.003), and 2 iv doses
of 96 mg/kg DTIC increased the median survival time to 76 days
(63-80, p=0.005), this being twice the median survival time of
36 days in control animals (33-44). The present animal model is
only moderately chemosensitive, compared to other experimental
tumors, and thus resembles human osteosarcomas, because cures
cannot be achieved.

Only low-grade calcification is seen in small pulmonary metastasis (a), administration of the osteotropic compound BAD (b)
(4-(-/bis(2-chloroethyl)amino/phenyl)-1-hydroxybutane-1,1-
diphosphonic acid) induced clear pyknosis, karyolysis, necrosis,
and marked calcification with disaggregation of the cellular
structure. The primary tumor also reacted to BAD chemotherapy
by increased calcification.

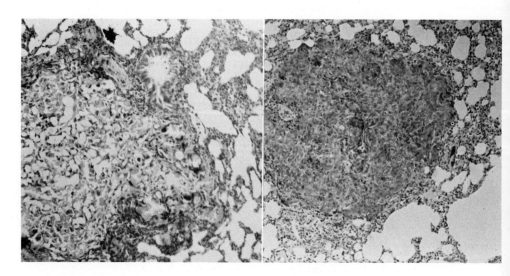

Fig. 3a. Pulmonary metastasis in untreated osteosarcoma-bearing rat. Fig. 3b. Pulmonary metastasis of BAD-treated osteosarcoma-bearing rat (X 300, staining: Masson Goldner).

Sutow et al (1981) demonstrated that especially the time of diagnosis of metastasis is a decisive factor for postmetastatic survival time of osteosarcoma-bearing patients. Chemotherapy was started 21 days after transplantation when the tumor was palpable and pulmonary metastases had already formed, thus simulating preoperative chemotherapy in patients with pulmonary metastases. Further experiments will have to investigate the influence of resection of the primary tumor on pulmonary metastasis under different therapeutic schemes.

Other modes of transplantation were also tested. Subcutaneous transplantation of fragments of the primary tumor and pulmonary metastases yielded a lower take rate (80%) and less frequent and irregular pulmonary metastases (70%). The model of subcutaneously growing tumors was therefore not followed up despite the easier handling. In summary, we consider the described osteosarcoma a suitable model for experimental adjuvant and primary chemotherapy because of its histologic structure, its transplantation-dependent metastasis formation, its relatively low chemosensitivity, and its being a rat tumor model, because it is easier to handle rats than mice for scintigraphic examinations and for surgical interventions, for instance, in experiments with tumor resection and limb perfusion.

REFERENCES

Benjamin, R.S., Murray, J.A., Wallace, S., Ayala, A., Chawla, S.
P., Raymond, A.K., Carrasco, C.H., Romsdahl, M.M., Papadopou-
los, N.E.J., & Plager, C., 1984, Intra-arterial preoperative
chemotherapy for osteosarcoma - a judicious approach to limb
salvage. The Cancer Bulletin, Vol. 36(1), p 32.

Delbrück, H.G., Allouche, M., Jasmin, C., Morin, M., Deml, F.,
Anghileri, L., Masse, R., & Lafuma, J., 1980, Bone tumours
induced in rats with radioactive cerium. British Journal of
Cancer, 41, 809.

Hanamura, H. & Urist, M., 1978, Osteogenesis and chondrogenesis
in transplants of DUNN and Ridgway osteosarcoma cell cultures.
American Journal of Pathology, 91, 227.

Jaffe, N., Frei, E. III, Watts, H., & Traggis, D., 1978, High
dose methotrexate in osteogenic sarcoma: a 5-year experience.
Cancer Treatment Reports, 62, 259.

Jaffe, N., Link, M.P., Cohen, D., Traggis, D., Frei, E.III,
Watts, H., Beardsley, G.P., & Abelson, H.T., 1981, High
dose methotrexate in osteogenic sarcoma. National Cancer
Institute Monographs, 56, 201.

Jaffe, N., Bowmann, R., Wang, Y.-M., Cangir, A., Ayala, A.,
Chuang, V.P., Wallace, S., & Murray, J., 1984, Chemotherapy
for primary osteosarcoma by intra-arterial infusion (review).
The Cancer Bulletin, Vol. 36(1), p. 37.

Kissane, J.M., et al., 1981, Sarcomas of bone in childhood:
Pathologic aspects. National Cancer Institute Monographs,
56, 29.

Komitowski, D., 1974, Experimentell durch Beryllium induzierte
Knochensarkome. Verhandlungen der Deutschen Gesellschaft für
Pathologie, 58, 438.

Masuda, S., Fukuma, H., & Beppu, Y., 1983, Antitumor effect of
human leucocyte interferon on human osteosarcoma transplanted
into nude mice. European Journal of Cancer and Clinical
Oncology, 19(11), 1521.

Nelson, J.A., Hokanson, J.A., & Jenkins, V.K., 1982, Role of the
host in the variable chemotherapeutic response of advanced
Ridgway osteogenic sarcoma. Cancer Chemotherapy and Pharmacology, 9, 148.

Senn, H.J., 1981, Chemotherapie von Knochentumoren. Röntgen-
Berichte, 10, 235.

Sutow, W.W., Herson, J., & Perez, C., 1981, Survival after
metastasis in oesteosarcoma. National Cancer Institute
Monographs, 56, 227.

Wingen, F., Schmähl, D., Berger, M.R., & Spring, H., 1984,
Itraosseously transplantable osteosarcoma with regularly
disseminating pulmonary metastases in rats. Cancer Letters,
23, 201.

OESTROGEN DEPENDENT RAT MAMMARY CARCINOMA AS A MODEL FOR DORMANT
METASTASES

P. V. SENIOR[1], P. MURPHY[2] and P. ALEXANDER[1]
[1]Dept. of Medical Oncology and [2]Dept. of Surgery, Southampton University,
Southampton General Hospital, Southampton SO9 4XY

Keywords: Dormant metastases, Carcinoma, Oestrogen dependence

INTRODUCTION

One of the reasons for the recurrence of primary and metastatic
cancer after therapy may be the existence of dormant, or non-cycling,
tumour cells which are refractory to cycle-specific agents and able to
repair damage inflicted by non-cycle specific drugs and radiotherapy,
(Alexander, 1982). To test this hypothesis we have evaluated a number of
in vivo models of tumour cell dormancy. In this paper we report on an
oestrogen-induced rat mammary carcinoma which when transplanted into virgin female animals will only grow if the animal is exposed to a continuous
supply of oestrogen. On transplantation into untreated rats the carcinoma
cells do not grow until the rats are oestrogenised. The response of
dormant carcinoma cells was studied both following subcutaneous inoculation and intra-cardiac injection into the left ventricle from where cells
are distributed to the capillary beds of all organs and tissues, providing
a model of metastatic growth from single cells.

METHODS

Tumours were induced in virgin female Lister hooded rats, using 80%
oestrogen and 20% cholesterol in a similar manner to that used by Noble
(Noble *et al.*, 1975). One pellet was implanted in the nape of the neck
of 10 rats. The first tumour arose after six months, by 12 months 9
animals had produced tumours. The six tumours that were tested all grew
when transplanted into oestrogenised recipients, but failed to grow in
untreated female rats. All six tumours remained dormant. If oestrogen
was administered two weeks following a subcutaneous implant, tumour growth
commenced. Five of these grew too slowly and produced necrotic

and haemorrhagic lesions rendering assessment of growth difficult. The
remaining tumour, OES 5, grew slowly in its earliest passages *in vivo* (1st
- 5th) taking 4-8 weeks to become palpable (0.5 - 1 cm.) following implantation in treated animals. In the passages used in these experiments (7th-
16th) the tumour showed consistent and more rapid growth, producing a solid
tumour mass until greater than 3-4 cms. diameter. The tumour can be
successfully stored in liquid N_2 in a serum rich medium i.e. 90% foetal
calf serum and 10% DMSO.

     Tumour cells were prepared by mechanical disaggregation in Hanks
salts containing 0.5 mg/ml. protease and 0.5 mg/ml. ribonuclease at
room temperature for 1½ hours. Some slight clumping of disaggregated
cells was noticed.

     Tumour cells (1 x 10^6) were injected s.c. into the flank of 30
animals. For left ventricular injection the right common carotid artery
was exposed under ether anaesthesia and a fine cannula passed through into
the left ventricle. In the initial experiments the animals were allowed
to recover, the cells being injected a day later in conscious but restrained rats. Subsequently the cells were injected immediately after cannulation, the cannula withdrawn and the vessel tied off. Tumour cells (1 x
10^6) were injected in 0.1 ml. Hanks salts. Groups of animals were
oestrogenised immediately, after 14 days, after 39 days or left unoestrogenised. Animals were killed when moribund or showing signs of tumour
growth and full post-mortem examinations performed.

RESULTS

     Ten animals were given oestrogen implants immediately after tumour
cell inoculation and all had palpable tumours (0.5 - 1 cm.) 14-20 days
later. In a second group of 10 rats oestrogen treatment was delayed for
14 days after tumour injection (day 0), 9 of these animals showed palpable
tumours, all within the period 28-34 days after inoculation (i.e. 14-20
days after oestrogenisation). The remaining animals were unoestrogenised
and were followed for 95 days after tumour injection, none developed
tumours. No difference in tumour incidence was noted between animals
inoculated under anaesthesia and those inoculated when conscious. The
table shows that if administration of oestrogen following intra-cardiac
injection of the carcinoma cells is delayed tumours grow in the same
organs and with the same frequency as when inoculated into oestrogenised
rats, except that their appearance is delayed. The time for appearance of
tumours after giving oestrogen is approximately the same in all groups.

This suggests that the carcinoma cells lie dormant and grow at the same rate after exposure to oestrogen. Adrenal and ovarian tumours were bilateral with the exception of one animal in the group oestrogenised after 39 days which had a single, right ovarian lesion. Apart from two animals in the simultaneous oestrogen group which developed intra-cardiac tumours, no tumour could be detected in any other organs.

Carcinoma cells remain dormant until administration of oestrogen in different organs; following inoculation into the left ventricle.

	Number of Animals with Tumours in:				
Treatment (Tumour given day 0)	Adrenals	Ovaries	Lung	Bone	Kidney
Oestrogen Day 0 Killed Day 27-37 (N=18)	17	14	9	14	0
Oestrogen Day 14 Killed Day 39 (N=5)	5	5	4	5	0
Oestrogen Day 39 Killed Day 76-79 (N=3)	3	3	1	1	0
No Oestrogen Still Alive Day 145+ (N=5)	—	—	—	—	—

DISCUSSION

This mammary tumour exhibits total dependence on exogenous oestrogen, the physiological levels of the hormones present in virgin female rats being insufficient to trigger growth. In the presence of oestrogen growth is rapid, a palpable tumour appearing from s.c. inoculation of 10^6 cells after 14-20 days. The actively growing tumour is sensitive to a number of cycle non-specific drugs, notably BCNU, Bleomycin, Cis-Platinum and Cyclophosphamide. In the absence of oestrogen, tumour cells will remain dormant but viable for at least two weeks when implanted s.c. We propose to use the s.c. dormancy model to examine whether cells in the dormant state are more resistant to chemotherapy than actively dividing cells.

When injected into the left ventricle cells are distributed to various organs and tissues via the arterial circulation. Experiments with other rat tumour cell types and studies of cardiac output to various organs using radiolabelled microspheres show that the proportion of an inoculum of tumour cells reaching any organ depends on the fraction of cardiac output it receives (Murphy *et al.*, this volume). As the table shows, the adrenals are the most common site of tumour growth, but together they received only 0.4% of cardiac output and hence only about 4×10^3 cells of the 1×10^6 injected. The kidneys receive about 12% of the cardiac output and hence 1.2×10^5 cells, yet no kidney tumours are encountered. This preference for the adrenals has been noted for a number of experimental and human tumours (Murphy *et al.*, this volume).

Similar experiments to those proposed for the s.c. model are planned in order to determine the response of dormant cells within organs to chemotherapy following intra-cardiac injection. Also, as the tumour grows in a number of locations in the body, the effects of site on pharmacodynamics and the influence of local metabolism on response to therapy may be investigated.

REFERENCES

Alexander, P., 1982 British Journal of Cancer, 46: 151.
Nobel, R. L., Honchachka, B. & King, D., 1975.   Cancer Research, 35:   766.

METASTATIC MODEL SYSTEMS

A. GOLDIN

Vincent T. Lombardi Cancer Research Center, Division of Medical Oncology,
Georgetown University School of Medicine, Washington, D. C. 20007, USA

Keyword: Leukemia, model, variants, metastasis

Classical tumor model systems may be useful for therapeutic investigations and the study of heterogeneity, including parameters such as tumor
growth rate, metastatic properties, the origin of tumor cell resistance, and
immunogenic potential. This has become possible with the advent of a number
of more effective antitumor agents, as indicted on re-examination of earlier
studies (Goldin et al. 1959; Humphreys & Goldin 1959). Two of the halogenated derivatives of amethopterin (MTX), namely, 3',5'-dichloroamethopterin
(DCM) and 3'-bromo-5'-chloroamethopterin (BCM) were capable of extensive
prolongation of the life span of mice carrying advanced systemic leukemia
L1210. At the time of initiation of treatment the animals had progressively
growing tumors at the site of inoculation and a remaining life span of only
a few days. With highly effective treatment of advanced disease the local
tumor at the site of inoculation as well as disseminated disease could be
eradicated, with the survival of a significant percentage of the animals.
These mice were quite resistant to reinoculation of the parental-sensitive
leukemia L1210 (Goldin & Humphreys 1960) and to MTX- or DCM-resistant sublines (Goldin et al. 1960). In most instances the reinoculated tumor either
failed to grow or grew slowly, with the animals showing increased survival
time. In the partially immune mice there was a positive correlation between
the tumor size achieved prior to death and the day of death.

However, despite total regression of the local tumor and apparent good
condition of the mice, the disease was not necessarily wholly eradicated.
A number of animals eventually developed tumors at various sites other than
at the initial site of inoculation. Tumors were found in the abdominal and
maxillary areas or internally in association with the kidney, liver, or other
organs. In some instances, intracranial disease was evidenced. Still other
animals, in apparently healthy condition, subsequently became moribund.

Autopsy frequently did not reveal an enlarged spleen or gross evidence of tumor, but transplantation of spleen mash or blood usually resulted in tumor growth.

These tumors, occurring in a single generation of treatment, comprise a spectrum of leukemic cell variants. Following daily treatment from the 7-8th day following leukemic inoculation to the 60-90th day, the median day of sacrifice of animals from which the tumor variants were obtained ranged from day 71 to 200. On transplant in untreated animals, there was a wide range in survival time and in tumor size prior to death (Table 1). Some of the tumor variants grew rapidly at the site of inoculation and were still small when the animal died at an early time, in comparability to the parental-sensitive tumor. Other tumor variants grew slowly, living for a more extended period of time with larger local tumors appearing at the site of inoculation. There was an approximately linear relationship between the average tumor diameter achieved prior to death and the survival time of the animals.

Table 1. Variants from mice treated for an extended period of time with halogenated derivatives of amethopterin. Comparison of survival time and tumor diameter.

Tumor[a] Variant	Generation Number	Median Survival Time, Days (range)	Tumor Diameter[b] Prior to Death (average mm)
J325 4C-2	20	7.0 (9-11)	12.5
S207 2-5	19	9.0 (8-12)	11.7
S207 2-4	17	9.0 (9-11)	13.0
J325 4A-2	19	10.0 (9-11)	11.7
J325 4A-9	6	17.0 (14-22)	15.5
J320 3A-7	15	26.0 (23-29)	22.2
J325 4A-4	6	26.0 (21-28)	27.7
J325 4B-5	7	30.5 (28-35)	25.6
J325 4C-9	7	30.5 (28-33)	25.9
J325 4B-10	7	40.5 (36-45)	30.6
Sensitive L1210 Z	232	9.0 (8-9)	12.5

[a]Trocar implants weighing approximately 20 mg each.
[b]Average of 2 dimensions.
Adapted from Humphreys & Goldin (1959).

The retarded growth characteristics of leukemic variants could not be attributed to a reduced inoculum. For the tumors listed in Table 1, trocar implants were employed. Also, serial dilution of the inoculum for the parent-sensitive leukemia resulted in some increase in survival time, but did not duplicate the extensive survival time or large tumors observed with the slow-growing tumor variants.

That retardation of metastatic growth accompanied the slow growth of the tumor variants is indicated by the increase in survival time of the animals and the increased difficulty in transmitting the disease by the transfer of blood from animals being treated for an extended period of time.

The growth characteristics and survival times elicited by the leukemic cell variants appeared heritable, persisting on serial transplant over a number of generations. The origin of the variants was not attributable to any carcinogenic action of the halogenated derivatives of MTX since no tumors appeared on prolonged treatment of normal mice. Whether the origin of the variants could reside in reinduction such as via possible association with a viral agent was not excluded. In any event, no histologic differences were observed between the tumor variants and the initial parent-sensitive line.

The tumor variants showed a wide range of sensitivity to therapy with MTX, ranging from definite sensitivity comparable to that of the parent-sensitive line to almost complete resistance (Table 2). But there was no clear relationship between the growth rate and metastatic potential and the degree of drug resistance. Varying degrees of resistance were obtained with both rapidly growing and slow-growing tumors. The resistance to antifolate therapy also appeared to be heritable without the need for additional treatment. One of the tumors (S207 2-5) still retained its acquired resistance after six generations. However, by the 16th generation it was only moderately more resistant to MTX than the parent-sensitive line.

Table 2. Sensitivity of variant sublines to treatment with methotrexate.

Exp. No.	Tumor Variant	Tumor Generation	Controls Med. S.T. Days	Methotrexate-Treated Optimal Dose mg/kg Daily	Median S.T. Days	ILS%
1	J325 4C-2	2	12.0	0.47	19.5	63
	J325 4H-5	3	12.5	1.30	34.0	175
	Sensitive	209	11.0	1.30	40.5	268
2	S207 2-4	3	14.0	1.30	19.0	36
	J325 4E-5	1	41.0	1.29	73.0	78
	Sensitive	211	10.0	1.29	39.0	290
3	S207 2-5	1	9.5	1.29	17.5	85
	J325 4A-2	2	10.0	1.29	34.0	240
	J325 4C-9	2	66.5	1.29	93.5	40
	Sensitive	212	13.0	1.29	64.5	396
4	J325 4A-3	3	37.5	1.0	63.0	69
	Sensitive	232	9.0	1.0	25.0	178
5	S207 2-5	6	10.5	0.8	20.0	90
6	S207 2-5	16	9.0	2.0	28.5	217
	Sensitive	228	9.0	2.0	35.0	282
7	J320 3A-7	8	36.0	1.0	37.0	3

[a]Treatment from day 2, exp. 1, 3; from day 3, exp. 2, 5, 6; from day 7, exp. 4; from day 17, exp. 7.

Adapted from Humphreys & Goldin (1959).

The resistant tumor variants tended to be somewhat more responsive to treatment with DCM than to MTX, apparently a reflection of the greater therapeutic effectiveness of the halogenated derivative.

Variant forms of tumor cell populations, appearing at a number of sites, have also been observed with a plasma-cell neoplasm (Potter 1958; Potter & Law 1957). Treatment of the plasma-cell neoplasm with the drugs azaserine (0-diazoacetyl-L-serine) or DON (6-diazo-5-oxo-L-norleucine) resulted in some instances in the origin of resistance in a single generation.

The origin of tumors at differing sites may provide additional models, as indicated by the example of a spontaneous mammary tumor model involving multiple tumor formation (Humphreys et al. 1966). In one experiment a comparison was made of surgery alone, cyclophosphamide alone, and surgery plus cyclophosphamide of spontaneous tumors of C3H/HeN at the time of their appearance. None of the treatments were effective in increasing the survival time of the animals. Interestingly, additional tumors appeared at various sites in the controls and in the animals undergoing therapy during the course of the experiment. The combination of surgery and therapy was instrumental in reducing the incidence of these new tumors to some extent.

Whether the new tumors that arose during the course of therapy with this spontaneous tumor model had an independent or common origin was not investigated.

Tumor variants occurring in a single generation of treatment may serve as experimental models for further therapeutic investigation, paralleling clinical relapse with appearance of tumors at distant sites and the recrudescence of generalized disease. They undoubtedly are of interest for investigation of tumor cell heterogeneity in relation to therapy.

REFERENCES

Goldin, A. & Humphreys, S.R., 1960, Journal of the National Cancer Institute 24, 283.
Goldin, A., Humphreys, S.R., Venditti, J.M. and Mantel, N., 1959, Journal of the National Cancer Institute 22, 811.
Goldin, A., Humphreys, S.R., Chapman, G.O., Chirigos, M. and Venditti, J.M., 1960, Nature 185, 219.
Humphreys, S.R. and Goldin, A., 1959, Journal of the National Cancer Institute 23, 633
Humphreys, S.R., Mantel, N. and Goldin, A., 1966, European Journal of Cancer 2, 1.
Potter, M., 1958, Annals of the New York Academy of Science 76, 630.
Potter, M. and Law, L.W., 1957, Journal of the National Cancer Institute 18, 413.

HORMONAL REGULATION OF B16 MELANOMA METASTASIS

RUSSELL G. GREIG, BRUCE LESTER, POUL SORENSEN, CHARLES BUSCARINO and
GEORGE POSTE
Department of Tumor Biology, Smith Kline and French Laboratories,
Philadelphia,
PA   19101, U.S.A.

Keyword: growth factors, pharmacology

A major objective in clinical oncology remains the need for
effective modalities for the therapy of established metastases.
Significant clinical benefits might also be gained, however, by
disrupting the metastatic cascade in patient populations recently
diagnosed as harboring malignant neoplasms or undergoing surgical
removal of their primary tumor. The objective of this approach would be
to pharmacologically manipulate circulating and/or arrested tumor cells
to render them incapable of forming secondary growths. Achieving this
goal requires a reasonably detailed knowledge of the molecular
mechanisms underlying tumor cell dissemination. Unfortunately, while
progress continues to be made in the cell biology of metastasis,
particularly in animal models, our understanding of this process at the
biochemical level is meager. Many attempts have been made to correlate
specific molecular events with the expression of metastatic properties
but causal relationships have yet to be defined and no biochemical
target has been identified for the design and development of novel
anti-metastatic drugs.

The pathogenesis of many diseases can be traced to aberrations in
hormonal regulation and/or responsiveness of major tissue/organ
functions. We reported recently that the ability of over 30 B16
melanoma clones to form experimental metastasis when injected into
syngeneic mice was positively correlated with their ability to
accumulate cAMP when challenged with activators of adenylate cyclase
(e.g. melanocyte stimulating hormone [MSH] and forskolin) (Sheppard et
al, 1984). Further biochemical investigations revealed that the
interclonal variation in cAMP accumulation could be attributed, at least
in part, to intrinsic differences in the catalytic component of the
adenylate cyclase complex. No significant differences were detected in

the activity of the regulatory components N_s or N_i. These results suggested that enhanced adenylate cyclase activity may partly account for increased metastatic potential in B16 melanoma clones and has lead to the working hypothesis that agents which antagonize adenylate cyclase in highly metastatic B16 melanoma clones might be expected to inhibit experimental metastasis; conversely, agonists of adenylate cyclase might be expected to enhance tumor cell dissemination by B16 melanoma clones of low metastatic potential.

To test this hypothesis and to identify endogenous mediators that might modulate the adenylate cyclase activity of tumor cells in situ we have begun to investigate a number of hormones and polypeptide growth factors for their effect on cyclic nucleotide metabolism in B16 melanoma cells. Two B16 melanoma clones, F1-C14 and F10-C23, exhibiting low and high metastatic capacities, respectively, were employed for these studies. Consistent with previous investigations, the highly metastatic clone F10-C23 accumulated high levels of cAMP following challenge with forskolin or MSH while under identical conditions the low metastatic clone, F1-C14, was only poorly responsive (Table 1).

In gaining entry into the circulation and during extravasation, metastatic tumor cells must penetrate the basement membrane and are thought to do so by secreting proteolytic enzymes including collagenase. Laminin, a major structural component of basement membrane, also binds specifically to receptors located on certain tumor cell surfaces including those of B16 melanoma. To evaluate whether laminin may also function as an important extracellular ligand that can modify tumor cell biochemistry, B16 melanoma clones were challenged with laminin in the presence and absence of either forskolin or MSH (Table 1). When treated with laminin alone (10^{-7} M), both F1-C14 and F10-C23 displayed a low, but reproducible increase in cAMP levels (Table 1). In contrast, laminin, at the same concentration, significantly potentiated the responsiveness of the high metastatic F10-C23 clone to challenge with MSH and to a lesser extent with forskolin. Under identical conditions, laminin augmented only slightly the responsiveness of the low metastatic F1-C14 clone to MSH, but failed to enhance sensitivity to forskolin. The results demonstrate that laminin, in addition to providing a mechanical support for invading tumor cells, can also sensitize them to hormones that stimulate adenylate cyclase, thus directly influencing a biochemical pathway that may be necessary for expression of B16 metastatic capacity.

Platelet-derived growth factor (PDGF) is a mitogenic hormone released by platelets at the site of vascular injury (Stiles, 1983). The effect of PDGF on metastatic tumor cells has not been studied to date, although there is considerable evidence from in vitro investigations that certain tumor cells can induce the platelet release reaction and that tumor cell-platelet interactions can influence tumor cell dissemination in vivo. As a single agent, PDGF (10^{-7} M) induced a 28-fold increase in cAMP accumulation in the low metastatic F1-C14 clone (Table 1). In contrast, challenge of the high metastatic F10-C23 clone under similar conditions, failed to increase cAMP levels. While PDGF potentiated the responsiveness of F1-C14 to both MSH and forskolin challenge, this mitogen antagonized cAMP accumulation in F10-C23 provoked by both of these agents. These preliminary studies provide a basis for detailed molecular investigations on the influence of platelet release-products on tumor cell biochemistry, dissemination and proliferation.

Vasopressin, a small peptide with known mitogenic properties (Rozengurt et al, 1979) produced only marginal elevations of intracellular B16 melanoma cAMP levels. However, vasopressin significantly potentiated responsiveness of both clones to MSH challenge and to a lesser extent to forskolin (Table 1).

The differential responsiveness of the two B16 clones to challenge with laminin, PDGF and vasopressin invites speculation that sensitivity to these agents mirrors metastatic performance. However, we consider that basing such an association on the investigation of only two clones is premature and could simply reflect a biochemical phenotype that exhibits interclonal variation with no causal correlation with metastatic potential. Further studies are in progress to examine these relationships in a larger panel of clones of defined metastatic potential. Whether PDGF and vasopressin are mitogenic for B16 melanoma cells in general or only for the clones examined here remains to be established and the physiological significance of the current data has yet to be determined. However, these observations reinforce the belief that regulation of cellular cyclic nucleotide metabolism by specific extracellular signals may be a key element in controlling the biochemical events that underlie the expression of the B16 metastatic phenotype.

Table 1.

Modulation of cAMP metabolism in B16 melanoma clones of low (F1-C14) and high (F10-C23) lung colonizing properties.

Fold-stimulation of intracellular cAMP levels[a]

	F1-C14			F10-C23		
	Single agent	MSH (1 µM)	Forskolin (50 µM)	Single agent	MSH (1 µM)	Forskolin (50 µM)
	-	1.3	1.9	-	54.3	45.2
Laminin (10^{-7}M)	1.7	2.2	1.5	2.4	80.2	56.3
PDGF (10^{-7}M)	27.9	3.1	13.4	0.9	17.0	1.0
Vasopressin (10^{-7}M)	1.7	7.0	2.7	1.4	120.1	76.7

[a]   Monolayer cultures were challenged with test agents in the presence or absence of either MSH or forskolin for 10 min. at 37^{0}C. Intracellular cAMP levels were assayed as described (Sheppard et al, 1984).

ACKNOWLEDGMENTS

We thank Dr. Lance Liotta for laminin preparations and Nancy Signora for typing the manuscript.

REFERENCES

Rozengurt, E., Legg, A. and Pettican, P., 1979, Proceedings National Academy Science (USA) 76, 1284.

Sheppard, J.R., Koestler, T.P., Corwin, S.P., Buscarino, C., Doll, J., Lester, B., Greig, R.G., and Poste, G., 1984, Nature, 308, 544.

Stiles, C.D., 1983, Cell, 33, 693.

Terranova, V.P., Rao, C.N., Kalebic, T., Margulies, I.M., and Liotta, L.A. 1983, Proceedings National Academy Science (USA), 80, 444.

REPAIR OF DNA STRAND BREAKS IN METASTATIC VARIANTS OF MURINE B16 MELANOMA

G.V. SHERBET, S. JACKSON and A.L. HARRIS

Cancer Research Unit [North of England Cancer Research Campaign], University of Newcastle upon Tyne, Royal Victoria Infirmary, Newcastle upon Tyne

Keywords: DNA; strand breaks; repair; 3-aminobenzamide

INTRODUCTION

Metastatic dissemination of cancer is a major cause of cancer deaths. Success of chemotherapeutic regimes will therefore be determined by the ability of anticancer agents to control metastatic growth. DNA is the major cellular target of a majority of anticancer agents. Alkylating agents and antibiotics produce DNA lesions of various types. Their cytotoxic potential is, however, reduced because mammalian cells can repair the damage. We have therefore examined if tumour cells differing in metastasizing ability have different DNA repair capacity. Here we present evidence that the metastasizing variant BL6 of the B16 melanoma and the F1 variant, which has virtually no ability to form natural metastases (Sherbet, 1982), differ considerably in their DNA repair properties.

MATERIALS AND METHODS

Mouse melanoma B16 BL6 and F1 cells were grown in culture (Sherbet, 1983). 24 hours after seeding, the cells were grown for $1\frac{1}{2}$ generations in the presence of 1 µg/ml (methyl-^{3}H) thymidine (Amersham).

The labelled cells were harvested using 0.25% trypsin in 0.02% EDTA, resuspended in PBS (5×10^5 cells/ml) and exposed to γ-radiation (20 Gy) from a ^{60}Co source. They were allowed to recover in fresh medium at 37°C for varying periods and resuspended in PBS at a density of 5×10^5 cells/ml. $1 - 2 \times 10^4$ cells were gently layered onto a lysing layer on top of 4.8 ml linear alkaline sucrose gradients, prepared as described by McGrath and Williams (1966). The gradients were centrifuged at 25,000 r.p.m. at 20°C in a SW50.1 rotor in a Kontron Centrikon T-2055 centrifuge. Four-drop fractions were collected on filter strips (Whatman 3MM), and the TCA-insoluble radioactivity estimated by scintillation spectrometry.

Cell monolayers were exposed to bleomycin (BLM) (50 µg/ml) for 30 minutes. They were then washed 3x with PBS, covered with fresh medium and allowed to recover as previously. After recovery, the cells were scraped off in 0.02% EDTA, spun down, resuspended in PBS and subjected to alkaline sedimentation.

In parallel experiments, cells were treated with 3 mM 3-aminobenza-mide (3AB) 30 minutes prior to exposure to drug/radiation, during exposure and during recovery.

RESULTS

Method of analysis of DNA repair

The analysis of the DNA repair process using the alkaline sedimenta-tion method is based on the principle that when cellular DNA is exposed to radiation or BLM, single strand breaks are produced and that rejoining of these strand breaks increases the effective size of the frag-ments, which causes them to sediment more rapidly. An assessment of the increase in the high molecular weight components (HMW DNA) is used here as a basis for semi-quantitation of the repair process. The percentage of radioactivity recovered from fractions 1 - 8 of the sucrose gradient is determined in each experiment.

DNA repair in cells exposed to γ-radiation and bleomycin

The metastatic variants of B16 melanoma which were exposed to γ-radiation and then allowed to recover over a period of 3.5 hrs showed in-creases in the percentage of radioactivity recoverable in the HMW DNA. Figs. 1 and 2 represent data obtained from three experiments each with F1 and BL6 cells. There was considerable variation between the experiments, but a linear regression analysis revealed that the points were distributed along the regression line, and the regression coefficients were statistic-ally significant in both F1 and BL6 (F1 $r = 0.8802$, $p < 0.001$; BL6 $r = 0.7982$, $p < 0.01$). But the difference in the slopes of the regression lines was considerable with the slope, which reflects the degree of DNA strand rejoining, being 5.9 for F1 and 10.1 for BL6 cells.

Fig. 3 represents the repair of strand breaks in BL6 and F1 cells which had been exposed to BLM. In 2/3 experiments with BL6 cells, the scission of DNA strands continued to occur for up to 1 hr after BLM was withdrawn. This was then followed by the repair process. In F1, on the other hand, the repair process began as soon as BLM was removed from the culture medium. However, unlike γ-irradiation-induced damage, BLM-induced damage was repaired at the same rate in both BL6 and F1 cells.

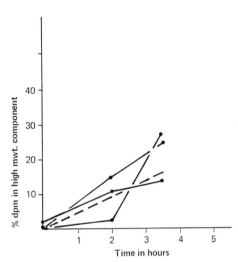

Fig. 1

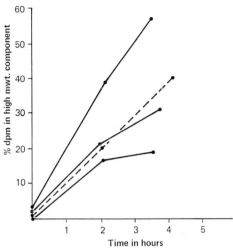

Fig. 2

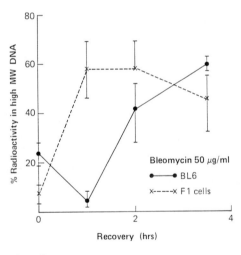

Fig. 3

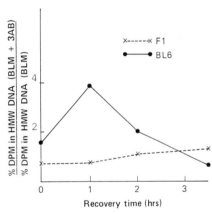

Fig. 4

Figs. 1 & 2.   Repair of strand breaks induced by ϒ-radiation in F1 and
              BL6 cells respectively.
Fig. 3.   Repair of strand breaks caused by BLM.   x---x F1, ●——● BL6.
Fig. 4.   Effect of 3AB on repair of BLM-induced strand breaks.   x——x F1,
          ●——● BL6.

Effect of 3AB on the repair process

3AB did not affect the repair process occurring in F1 cells exposed to BLM. However, in BL6 cells repair was augmented, especially in the first 2 hrs of recovery (Fig. 4). F1 cells were twice as sensitive to BLM as BL6. But 3AB did not affect the cytotoxicity of BLM.

DISCUSSION

The experiments described here demonstrate that there are differences between the metastatic variants in their ability to repair DNA lesions, but this is dependent upon the agent causing the lesion. BL6 is able to repair radiation-induced damage nearly twice as efficiently as F1, but BLM-induced damage appears to be repaired at similar rates. This could be due to the differences in the type of damage induced by these agents. In BL6 cells, the DNA strand scission continued for an hour after removal of BLM, when the repair process became evident. In contrast, in F1 this occurred immediately upon removal of BLM. This could be due to differential sensitivity of part of the DNA of the BL6 cells or to differences in the sensitivity within the cell population. Such differential effects have, in fact, been described by Iqbal et al. (1976).

The two metastatic variants also differed with respect to the effects of 3AB on the repair process. 3AB is said to inhibit the activity of ADP-ribosyl transferase which has been implicated in the repair of DNA strand breakage (Durkacz et al., 1980). In our experiments, 3AB had no effect on F1. In BL6 it had a pronounced effect on the repair of strand breaks in the first 2 hrs of the recovery phase, but repair was augmented rather than inhibited. Such stimulation of repair by 3AB has been reported by others (Waters et al., 1982; Berger and Sikorski, 1980; Bohr and Klenow, 1981). It would seem, therefore, that the metastatic variants may differ in their repair mechanisms as well.

REFERENCES

Berger, N.A. & Sikorski, G.W., 1980, Biochemical and Biophysical Research Communications, 95, 67.
Bohr, V. & Klenow, H., 1981, Biochemical and Biophysical Research Communications, 102, 1254.
Durkacz, B.W., Omidiji, O., Gray, D.A. & Shall, S., 1980, Nature, 283, 593.
Iqbal, Z.M., Kohn, K.W., Ewig, R.A.G. & Fornace, A.J., 1976, Cancer Research, 36, 3834.
McGrath, R.A. & Williams, R.W., 1966, Nature, 212, 534.
Sherbet, G.V., 1982, The Biology of Tumour Malignancy (Academic Press, London).
Sherbet, G.V., 1983, Experimental Cell Biology, 51, 140.
Waters, R., Ramsay, F. & Barrett, I., 1982, Carcinogenesis, 3, 1463.

PREVENTION OF LEUKEMIC SPREAD IN MICE BY ANTIMETASTATIC AGENTS

T. GIRALDI, G. SAVA, L. PERISSIN*and G. DECORTI*

Istituto di Farmacologia, Universita' di Trieste, I-34100 Trieste, Italy.

*Clinica Podiatrica, Università di Trieste, Istituto per l'Infanzia,

 I-34100 Trieste, Italy

Keyword: leukemia, metastasis, antimetastatic drugs

INTRODUCTION

Therapeutic interventions aiming to prevent the metastatic spread of solid tumors rather than attempting neoplastic eradication by killing tumor cells with cytotoxic drugs have been increasingly developed with success in experimental animal systems (Giraldi 1981). Leukemic metastases, whose establishment offers therapeutic problems as difficult to be solved as those encountered with solid tumor metastases (Woodruff 1978), appear largely less investigated in animal systems, either in terms of pathogenetic mechanism or of pharmacological treatment. The aim of the present investigation has been therefore that of determining the effects of the antimetastatic drug p-(3,3-dimethyl-1-triazeno)benzoic acid potassium salt (DM-COOK) (Giraldi 1984), in comparison with the antiinvasive drug vinblastine (VBL) (Atassi et al. 1982), and with the cytotoxic drug cyclophosphamide (CY), on tumor cell replication and spread in mice bearing transplantable leukemias.

MATERIALS AND METHODS

The transplantation of P388 leukemia was performed by i.p. inoculation of 10^6 tumor cells obtained from donors bearing 8 days old tumors; TLX5 lymphoma was similarly transplanted using inocula of 10^5 tumor cells. P388 and TLX5 lymphoma were inoculated into syngeneic DBA/2 or CBA/Lac mice, respectively. I.c. inoculations were made using the same inoculum size. The total number of peritoneal tumor cells was measured at the end of treatment after their careful collection by repeated washing of the peritoneal cavity using a Coulter counter mod. ZF. The presence of clonogenic tumor cells in the brain was determined by transplanting the whole brains in syngeneic normal mice s.c. in the case of TLX5 lymphoma, or i.p. for P388 leukemia. The survival time of the recipient mice was recorded, providing an indirect indication of the viability and number of tumor cells present (Sentjurc et al. 1979).

RESULTS AND DISCUSSION

After daily i.p. administration for 7 days following i.p. tumor implantation, the tested drugs increase the survival time of leukemic mice. DM-COOK and CY are active on P388, L1210 and TLX5 leukemias, whereas the effects of VBL are limited to P388 leukemia. TLX5 lymphoma exibits the greatest responsiveness to the effects of DM-COOK, and P338 leukemia is more responsive to CY and VBL (unreported results). Consequently the tumor lines used in the following reported experiments are TLX5 for DM-COOK and P388 for CY and VBL. The dosages used are chosen as equieffective, causing an increase in life span of 50% as compared with untreated controls after daily i.p. treatment for 7 days following i.p. tumor implantation.

Table 1. Number of peritoneal tumor cells and bioassay of the brains of mice bearing i.p. leukemias, treated i.p. with the tested drugs.

Tumor line	Drug	Dose (mg/Kg/day)	Number of peritoneal tumor cells (%T/C)	Brain bioassay %ILS	cured
TLX5	DM-COOK	25	57.6+10.9	95.0+44.1	4/10
P388	VBL	74*	0.0	60.0	4/5
P388	CY	9.8	0.0	20.0	4/5

*: ug/Kg/day
Groups of 5 mice (10 controls) were implanted i.p. with the tumor indicated on day 0, and were treated i.p. daily on days 1-7. After sacrifice on day 8, peritoneal tumor cells were collected and counted, and the brains were transplanted into normal recipients whose survival time was recorded.

Data reported in Table 1 show the absence of detectable peritoneal tumor cells after treatment with CY and VBL, which is consistent with the increase of life span observed and with the growth kinetic of the tumors (Sentjurc et al. 1979). On the other hand, DM-COOK causes a marginal reduction of the number of peritoneal tumor cells, which can not account for an increase of life span of 50%. At the same time, the bioassay of the brains of the treated animals indicates a marked reduction of the presence of clonogenic tumor cells. These findings might be interpreted considering the occurrence of cytotoxic effects for CY and VBL, and of antimetastic effects for DM-COOK, and data in Table 2 support this view.

Table 2. Survival time of mice bearing i.c. leukemias, treated i.p. with the tested drugs.

Tumor line	Drug	Dose (mg/Kg/day)	%ILS
TLX5	DM-COOK	25	31.8+6.8
P388	VBL	74*	10.8+9.9
P388	CY	9.8	83.8+24.5

*: ug/Kg/day
   Groups of 5 mice were implanted with the tumor indicated on day 0, and were treated i.p. daily on days 1-7. The dosages used for each compound cause an ILS of 50% in mice bearing tumors implanted i.p..

   Indeed, CY markedly increases the survival time of mice implanted i.c. with the tumor, thus showing a marked cytotoxic action of this drug also on tumor cells localized cerebrally. VBL is inactive, suggesting the possible occurrence of antimetastatic effects in addition to cytotoxic ones. The marginal cytotoxic effects of DM-COOK on peritoneal tumor cells, together with its similarly marginal effects on intracerebrally implanted tumor cells, indicate that the increase of survival time caused by this drug in mice implanted i.p. with the tumor has to substantially ascribed to its antimetastatic action. Similar unreported results are obtained also on P388 leukemia (Sava et al. 1983), and are confirmed by the histological analysis of the brain and liver of the treated animals (Sava et al. 1984).

   It thus appears that antimetastatic drugs might be employed for preventing leukemic metastases, as already suggested for solid tumor metastases, and that the considerations made on the implications of the extrapolation of experimental work on metastasis prevention to human treatment (Hellmann 1984) should be extended to include also leukemias.

ACKNOWLEDGEMENTS: This work was supported by Italian National Research Council, Special Project 'Oncology', contract n. 83.00838.96, and by grants from the Italian Ministry of Education (MPI). Including contract n.2831.

REFERENCES

Atassi, G., Dumont, P. & Vandendris, M., 1982, Invasion and Metastasis, 2, 217.

Giraldi, T. & Sava, G., 1981, Anticancer Research, 1, 163.

Giraldi, T., 1984, Drugs of the Future, 9, 503.

Hellmann, K., 1984, Clinical and Experimental Metastasis, 2, 1.

Sava, G., Giraldi, T., Lassiani, L. & Nisi, C., 1983, Mechanism of the antileukemic action of DTIC and its benzenoid analog DM-COOK in mice. In The Control of tumor growth and its biological bases, edited by W. Davis, C. Maltoni & St. Tannenberg (Akademie-Verlag, Berlin), p. 309.

Sava, G., Giraldi. T., Bartoli-Klugmann, F., Decorti, G. & Mallardi, F., 1984, European Journal of Cancer and Clinical Oncology, 20, 287.

Sentjurc, M., Shara, M., Nemec, M., Cotic, V., Pecar, S., Sava, G. & Giraldi, T., 1979, 75, 13.

STUDIES OF THE EFFICACY OF BACTERIOCIN (COLICIN) TREATMENT ON LUNG METASTASES OF A MURINE FIBROSARCOMA

R.P. HILL[1] and H. FARKAS-HIMSLEY[2]

[1]Department of Medical Biophysics, and

[2]Department of Microbiology, University of Toronto, Toronto, Ontario, Canada

Keyword: Micrometastases, KHT Sarcoma, Colicin Treatment

INTRODUCTION

Bacteriocins are polypeptide antibiotics produced by various bacteria. Previous work with a number of different bacteriocins has indicated that these polypeptides can act as growth inhibitors of neoplastic cells both in vitro and in vivo (Farkas-Himsley and Kuzniak, 1978). In the present study, purified bacteriocin extracted from E. coli has been tested for its efficacy in inhibiting the growth of small experimentally induced or naturally arising, metastatic foci of murine KHT fibrosarcoma cells, growing in the lungs of C3H/Jax mice. The results are compared with the effect of the bacteriocin on normal mouse bone marrow stem cells and on KHT sarcomas growing intramuscularly.

METHODS

The bacteriocin was prepared from cultures of E. coli HSC10 and purified by ammonium sulphate precipitation and chromatography using a Sephadex-ion exchange column. The active fractions were identified by their ability to kill sensitive bacteria and to inhibit ^{3}HTdR uptake by mouse L60T malignant fibroblast cells (Jaywardene and Farkas-Himsley, 1969). The protein content of these fractions was determined (Lowry et al, 1951). Appropriate dilutions were made in TRIS buffer so that the mice were injected intraperitoneally with 0.5 ml each.

The metastatic foci were induced by intravenous (i.v.) injection of KHT sarcoma cells admixed with plastic microspheres or arose spontaneously from

Supported by the National Cancer Institute of Canada and The Ontario Cancer Treatment and Research Foundation.

KHT sarcomas growing in the leg. The efficacy of the bacteriocin treatment
was assessed by counting the number of metastatic lung nodules which had
formed 21 days later or by determining the number of mice which survived to
63 days after the cell injections.

Local tumours were induced by injecting 2×10^5 KHT sarcoma cells
intramuscularly into the left hind leg of the mice and the effect of
bacteriocin treatment was determined by measuring tumour growth as a
function of time.

RESULTS AND DISCUSSION

Small metastatic tumours, induced by ι.v. injection of tumour cells,
were treated one day later with various doses of bacteriocin. Previous
studies (Hill and Bush, 1969) have demonstrated that, under the conditions
used, a linear relationship between the number of lung metastases formed
and number of tumour cells injected would be expected. Thus it was
possible to determine a survival curve for the small metastatic foci
(Figure 1). The results are derived from groups of 7 mice each and
indicate that the metastatic foci are very sensitive to the bacteriocin
treatment. Also shown in figure 1 (insert) are the results of an
experiment to examine the effect of bacteriocin treatment on mouse bone
marrow stem cells using a spleen colony assay (Till and McCulloch, 1968).
Doses up to 10 μg protein/mouse, had no effect on these normal cells.

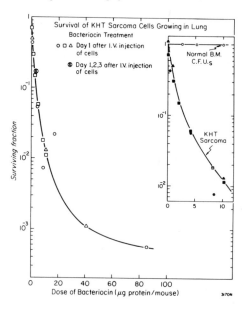

To investigate whether the
bacteriocin treatment might be
inhibiting or reducing the growth
rate of the tumour cells rather
than killing them, groups of mice,
were treated with bacteriocin 24
hours after tumour cell injection
and held for 63 days. The results
(Table 1) indicate that the
bacteriocin was indeed able to
cure a significant fraction of the
mice, with 3 doses of 10.4 μg
protein/mouse being more effective
than a single dose of this size.
It is also seen, however, from the
table that single large doses of

Figure 1.

bacteriocin, though highly effective, were toxic to the mice, resulting in death between 2 and 8 days after treatment. Further studies have indicated that the LD_{50} is about 70 µg protein/mouse for C3H/HeJ mice.

TABLE I   SURVIVAL OF ANIMALS WITH TUMOURS (KHT SARCOMA) TREATED WITH BACTERIOCIN

Treatment	Cells injected I-V	Expected no. of tumours in lung	Fraction of mice surviving to day 63	% of mice cured of tumour (excluding toxicity)
10.4 µg/mouse Day 1	2.5×10^2	25	4/7	57% (3/7)
41.6 µg/mouse Day 1	2.5×10^3	250	6/7 (1 died of toxicity)	100% (6/6)
83 µg/mouse Day 1	2.5×10^3	250	1/7 (6 died of toxicity)	100% (1/1)
10.4 µg/mouse Day 1, 2, 3	2.5×10^2	25	7/7	100% (7/7)

KHT sarcomas growing intramuscularly were treated with up to 4 doses of bacteriocin (10.4 µg protein/mouse) given daily starting 4 days after the injection of tumour cells. There was minimal effect on the growth of the tumour due to these injections of bacteriocin (see Figure 2). However these mice were also examined for spontaneous metastases, and it was found that the number of observable lung metastases (Table 2a) was significantly reduced in mice given multiple bacteriocin treatments. A second experiment of similar design was then performed in which the primary tumour growing in the leg was irradiated (Siemann *et al* 1977) with a dose of 50 Gray on day 8 when it had reached about 0.5 g. This irradiation caused regression of the primary tumour allowing the animals to be held until day 25, sufficiently long for previously seeded metastases to grow to detectable size. All

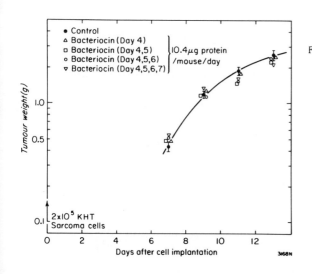

Figure 2. Growth of KHT sarcomas as a function of time after intramuscular injection of tumour cells. Mean values (7 mice) are shown with S.E. (control).

TABLE II   EFFECT OF BACTERIOCIN ON SPONTANEOUS METASTASES FROM KHT SARCOMA GROWING IN LEG

a)	No. of mice	No. of Metastases Median	(Range)
Control (No Treatment)	7	50	(25-59)
10.4 μg/mouse Day 4	7	31	(16-41)
10.4 μg/mouse Day 4 & 5	7	18	(9-66)
10.4 μg/mouse Day 4, 5, 6	6	12.5	(1-23)*
10.4 μg/mouse Day 4, 5, 6, 7	6	1.5	(8-23)*
b) Control (No Treatment)	7	69	(35-100)
Primary Irradiated Day 8			
Control	7	44	(20-66)
2 x 10.4 μg/mouse Day 4, 5	6	1.5	(0-32)*
4 x 10.4 μg/mouse Day 4, 5, 6, 7	5	2	(0-11)*

* Significantly different from control

metastases observed were in the lung, and the number is shown in Table 2b. Again, the bacteriocin treatment resulted in a reduction in metastases, with the multiple treatments giving a significant difference from control. It is to be noted that in some animals, there were no observable metastases.

In conclusion the results clearly indicate that the purified bacteriocin isolated from E. coli is very effective in preventing the growth of small metastatic deposits in the lung. Nontoxic doses of the bacteriocin can give greater than 99% killing of tumour cells under such conditions. These findings are noteworthy in that treatment of tumours growing intramuscularly show little evidence of growth inhibition, even though the treatment was initiated prior to the tumour becoming palpable, suggesting that the bacteriocin has some specificity for small micrometastases. One possible explanation for this observation is that, since the bacteriocin interacts primarily with the cell membrane (Farkas-Himsley, 1980), it may be most accessible to cells which are in the vascular system. Thus, its action against the metastatic KHT sarcoma cells may be greatest during the time prior to their extravasation into the interstitial space. The relatively large size of the bacteriocin (80,000 daltons) (Farkas-Himsley and Yu, 1984) may reduce its effective diffusion to attack the tumour cells. Further studies will be necessary to investigate whether the bacteriocin can demonstrate activity against larger micrometastases.

REFERENCES

Farkas-Himsley, H., 1980. Journal of Antibiotics and Chemotherapy, 6, 424.

Farkas-Himsley, H. & Kuzniak, R., 1978, Bacteriocins as inhibitors of neoplasia, In Current Chemotherapy Vol. II, Ed. Siegenthaler, W. & Luthy R., (American Society of Microbiology, Washington, D.C.), p.1188.

Farkas-Himsley, H. & Yu, H., 1984, Cytobios in press.

Hill, R.P. & Bush, R.S., 1969, International Journal of Radiation Biology, 15, 435.

Jaywardene, A. and Farkas-Himsley, H., 1969, Microbios, 1B, 87.

Lowry, O.H., Rosebrough, N.J., Farr, A.L. & Randall, R.J., 1951, Journal of Biological Chemistry, 193, 265.

Siemann, D.S., Hill, R.P. & Bush, R.S., 1977, International Journal of Radiation Oncology, Biology, Physics, 2, 903.

Till, J.E. & McCulloch, E.A., 1968, Radiation Research, 14, 213.

RADIO- AND CHEMOPROTECTION AS A MEANS OF INCREASING THERAPEUTIC RATIO IN THE TREATMENT OF TUMORS AND THEIR METASTASES

L. MILAS, N. HUNTER, H. ITO, T. BASTC, P.J. TOFTION & L.J. PETERS
Department of Experimental Radiotherapy, M. D. Anderson Hospital and Tumor Institute, Houston, TX

Keywords: radioprotectors; chemoprotectors; therapeutic gain

INTRODUCTION

Since normal tissue damage is often a dose-limiting factor in tumor radio- and chemotherapy, prevention of normal tissue injury without affecting the response of tumor cells should result in a therapeutic improvement for the treatment of both primary tumors and metastatic disease. Agents capable of "scavenging" free radicals caused by ionizing radiation or certain chemotherapeutic agents appear as good candidates for this purpose. The rationale for their use is based primarily on the assumptions that these agents concentrate less in tumors than in normal tissues due to compromised tumor blood circulation and because severe hypoxia, commonly existing only in tumors, limits radioprotection (Phillips et al. 1973; Denekamp et al. 1981; Milas et al. 1982). Also, tumor cells may be intrinsically less capable of absorption of radioprotective agents than normal cells (Yuhas 1980). Here, we briefly describe some of our studies on the potential of two radioprotective agents, S-2-(3-aminopropylamino)-ethylphosphorothioic acid (WR-2721) and diethyldithio-carbamate (DDC) for increasing therapeutic gain.

MATERIALS AND METHODS

The following assays were used to assess normal tissue damage induced by ionizing radiation, cyclophosphamide (CY), and cis-platinum: the LD50/30 and spleen colony assay for bone marrow; crypt epithelial cell survival for jejunum and colon; LD50/42 for esophagus; hair loss for hair follicles; seminiferous tubule stem cell survival for testis; NK-cell chromium release assay for the immune system; and leg contractures for leg damage. The TCD50 and growth delay assays were used to study the response of leg tumors to irradiation and chemotherapeutic agents, respectively.   The lung micrometastasis assay was used to study response of metastatic lesions to both chemotherapy and irradiation.   WR-2721, usually 400 mg/kg, was given i.p.   30 min. before irradiation.   DDC, either 600 or 1000 mg/kg, was given 30 min. before irradiation or CY, and 30 min. after cis-platinum.   Graded doses of irradiation and chemotherapeutic agents were used.   A detailed description of most of the above assays can be found in Milas et al. 1982, 1984a, and 1984b.

RESULTS

Table 1 contains a summary of protection factors (PFs) obtained when WR-2721 or DDC were combined with single doses of ionizing radiation.   Both agents protected most normal tissues studied against acute and late radiation injury, although the extent of protection varied greatly.   For WR-2721, PFs ranged from 1.24 to > 2, and for DDC, from 1.2 to 1.59.   In general, WR-2721 was more radioprotective than DDC.   Compared to the majority of normal tissues, tumors were protected to a lesser extent, implying that in many of our experimental settings a substantial therapeutic gain was achieved.   WR-2721 was less protective of solitary FSA leg tumors than of lung micrometastases, but the opposite was observed for DDC.

DDC was investigated for its ability to increase the therapeutic ratio of cis-platinum and CY.   DDC given 30 min. after (but not before) graded doses of cis-platinum protected bone marrow cells by a PF of about 4, as assessed by the spleen colony assay.   In the LD50/9 assay (which assays intestinal damage), the PF was 2.5. In an initial study with 4-day old FSA micrometastases, the PF was approximately 2, which is high but still smaller than PFs for normal tissues.   In studies with CY, DDC enhanced normal tissue damage and the response of FSA leg tumors and micro-metastases to a similar degree, thus providing no therapeutic gain.

DDC was effective in preventing BCNU-induced enhancement of spontaneous metastasis formation of a murine hepatocarcinoma (HCA). Mice bearing 5 mm HCA were treated with BCNU (16.5 mg/kg), DDC (600 mg/kg) or with both drugs.   None of the treatments significantly affected the growth of the primary tumor.   Tumor-bearing legs were amputated 6-8 days after treatment when tumors were approxi-mately 12 mm.   Sixteen days later, the lungs of mice were checked for the presence of metastases.   BCNU treatment increased the number of metastasis from 3.9 ± 1.2 in control (amputation only) mice to 9.7 ± 1.4 (P < 0.005).   DDC alone was ineffective (4.8 ± 0.5), but reduced the BCNU-induced enhancement of metastasis (6.4 ± 0.9).

Table 1. Radioprotection by WR-2721 of different normal tissues, solitary tumors in the leg, and lung micrometastases in C3Hf/Kam mice. The extent of radioprotection was expressed in PFs. PF of 1 designates no change in radioresponse.

	Protection Factors with WR-2721 for		Protection Factors with DDC for	
	Acute Damage	Late Damage	Acute Damage	Late Damage
Normal Tissues				
Bone marrow	>2		1.59	
Esophagus	1.58			
Jejunum	1.64		1.2	
Colon	1.72	1.58		
Hair follicles	1.24		1.44	
Testis	1.54		1.2	
Leg (contractures)		1.51		1.38-1.51
Immune system	1.6			
Tumors in the leg				
FSA tumor	0.96-1.13		1.24	
MCA-4 tumor	1.23-1.3			
Lung Micrometastases				
FSA tumor	1.24		1.1	
NFSA tumor	1.22			

DISCUSSION

Our data presented show both WR-2721 and DDC protected most normal tissue against radiation-induced injury to a significant degree, but the extent of protection varied considerably. Reasons for this variability might include variations in absorption of radioprotective agents among tissues, the levels of endogeneous thiols, and metabolism of the agents. Compared to most normal tissues, tumors were less radioprotected, either when grown as solitary tumors or as micrometastases. There is an indication that micrometastases are more amenable to radioprotection with WR-2721 than solitary tumors, probably because delivery of the drug is less compromised in micrometastases as compared to solid tumors and because they are not severely hypoxic. Overall, the results show that in many instances, therapeutic gain can be achieved by WR-2721 and DDC treatment.

DDC was a very potent protector of normal tissue damage by cis-platinum. It also protected FSA and micrometastases but to lesser degree thus providing some increase in the therapeutic ratio. On the other hand, DDC potentiated CY damage of both normal tissues and tumors, thus providing no benefit. It is likely that the protective activity of DDC against cis-platinum could be attributed to its thiol properties and to its potent chelating ability. The reason for its sensitizing effect when combined with CY is not known.

Inhibition of BCNU-induced enhancement of spontaneous metastasis was a further important activity of DDC. The enhancement of metastasis formation by chemotherapeutic agents is a potential problem in chemotherapy, especially when the agents administered are ineffective in tumor cell destruction. They induce metastasis enhancement due to direct damage of tissues in which tumor cells lodge and due to immunosuppression of host resistance mechanisms (Milas and Peters 1984).

Thus, the use of radioprotective agents can, in certain experimental settings, increase the therapeutic ratio of the therapy of solid tumors and metastases and, as such, these agents are of potential clinical use.

REFERENCES

Denekamp, J. et al., 1981, British Journal of Radiology, 54, 1112.
Milas, L. & Peters, L.J., 1984, In Cancer Invasion and Metastasis: Biologic and
    Therapeutic Aspects, edited by G.L. Nicolson and L. Milas (Raven Press), p. 321.
Milas, L., et al., 1982, Cancer Research, 42, 1888.
Milas, L., et al., 1984a, Int. J. Rad. Onc. Biol. Phys., 10, 41.
Milas L., et al., 1984b, Cancer Research, 44, 2382.
Phillips, T.L., et al., Cancer, 32, 528.
Yuhas, J.M., 1980, Cancer Research, 40, 1980.

MECHANISMS OF ABDOMINAL IRRADIATION-INDUCED INHIBITION OF LUNG METASTASES

K.ANDO, S.KOIKE and T.MATSUMOTO
1.Division of Clinical Research
2.Section of Animals and Plants
National Institute of Radiological Sciences, Chiba, Japan 260

key words: enteric bacteria, macrophage, natural killer cell

INTRODUCTION

We(Ando et al 1980) previously reported that irradiation of abdomen of mice prior to i.v. challenge of syngeneic fibrosarcoma cells reduced metastases in lung, and designated the phenomenon as AIRIM. Transmigration of enteric bacteria across the radiation-damaged mucous membrane of the cecum was proposed as the mechanism underlying the inhibition of metastases (Ando et al 1983). In this communication, we describe further investigations into the mechanisms of AIRIM.

MATERIALS AND METHODS

Animal tumor

Animals used here were 8-to-10 week old C3Hf/Kam and C3Hf/HeMsNrs male mice, produced in specific pathogen free (SPF) facilities. For some experiments, germ-free mice of the MsNrs substrain were used. A fibrosarcoma of spontaneous origin(NFSa), which arose in a C3Hf/Bu female mouse, was kept in liquid nitrogen, of which 18th generation transplants were used throughout these experiments. The procedure to make single cell suspensions from this tumor has been described elsewhere (Ando et al 1980).

Radiation

We used a ^{137}Cs γ ray unit with a dose rate of 0.9Gy min^{-1} and a 250Kvp x ray machine(HVL 1.2mm Cu, FSD 60cm) with a dose rate of 0.7Gy min^{-1}. For shielding the head, chest and legs,

50mm and 3mm lead were used in γ ray and x ray irradiations, respectively.

Antibody and silica

    Anti-asialo GM1 antibody (Wako Pure Chemical, Osaka) was dissoved in Dulbecco solution, and 250μg protein was administered. Silica (2-10μm, BIO-RAD) was suspended in 0.85% NaCl solution and 3mg was administered.

Enteric bacteria

    Ent. cloacae and Lactobacilli were used. Ent.cloacae possess endotoxin or lipopolysaccharide (LPS), and cannot attach to mucous membranes. On the other hand, Lactobacilli lack LPS and can attach to mucous membranes. These bacteria were cultured at 37°C in DHL agar and blood agar. For detecting plasma endotoxin, Toxicolor test (Seikaguka Kogyo, Tokyo) which can detect endotoxin as low as 1 picogram was employed.

Lung colony assay

    Mice were injected i.v. with $0.5-1x10^5$ NFSa tumor cells, and killed 11 days later. Their lungs were removed and fixed in Bouins solution, and tne numbers of tumor nodules on the surface of the lungs were counted macroscopically.

RESULTS AND DISCUSSION

    Kinetics of cecal bacteria in SPF mice that received 12Gy of abdominal irradiation were investigated. Ent.cloacae increased at day 3 of irradiation and remained at high levels until day 7. By day 14, Ent.cloacae decreased to unirradiated levels. On the other hand, Lactobacilli decreased at day 3 and remained low level until day 7. By day 14, Lactobacilli increased to reach unirradiated levels. Kinetics of AIRIM was parallel to that of Lactobacilli, but opposite to that of Ent.cloacae. This suggested that either Ent.cloacae or Lactobacilli were significant in AIRIM. The following experiments were therefore performed to identify bacteria responsible for AIRIM. Germ-free mice were monocontaminated with either Ent.cloacae or Lactobacilli one month before experiments (Table 1). AIRIM was clearly observable in Ent.cloacae-monocontaminated mice but not in Lactobacilli-monocontaminated ones. Mesenteric lymph nodes contained large numbers

of <u>Ent. cloacae</u> at day 5 and day 7 of irradiation, a
timing which coincided with maximum reduction of metastases.
Plasma endotoxin level was significantly high at Day 1 of
irradiation and remained high till Day 5.

Table 1. Identification of microorganisms responsible for
          abdominal irradiation-induced inhibition of lung
          metastases.

monocontamination	Number of lung colonies ((mean and s.e.(# of mice))	p value
1. none	117.6 ± 17.7 (5)	p<0.001
2. <u>Ent.cloacae</u>	17.2 ± 6.5 (5)	
3. none	159.4 ± 16.8 (5)	N.S.
4. Lactobacilli	125.8 ± 17.8 (6)	

1×10^{5} NFSa cells were i.v. challenged 7 days after
abdominal irradiation with 10.2Gy x ray.

Working hypothesis

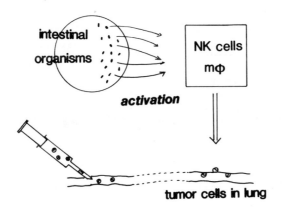

tumor cells in lung

As PARR et al(1973) suggested that endotoxin-activated macrophages could protect mice from tumor challenge, we hypothetized that transmigrated Ent.cloacae across the radiation-damaged mucous membrane into mesenteric lymph nodes could have stimulated macrophages that, in turn, attacked i.v. injected tumor cells(Fig.1). We tested our hypothesis in the following experiments. Administrating either silica or anti-asialo GM1 antibody prior to tumor cell challenge profoundly increased lung metastases, indicating that macrophages and NK cells might be inhibiting lung metastases in normal mice (Table 2). Abdominal irradiation failed to inhibit lung metastases in mice that were pretreated with the 2 agents, results supporting our hypotesis.

Table 2. Significance of natural killer cells and
          macrophages in abdominal irradiation-induced
          inhibition of metastases.

treatment	Number of lung colonies[a] abdominal irradiation		p value
	no	yes	
1. none	$19.3 \pm 4.3(8)$	$5.3 \pm 1.2(8)$	$p < 0.001$
2. anti-asialo GM1 antibody[b]	$119.5 \pm 15.1(8)$	$104.3 \pm 12.1(8)$	N.S.
3. silica[c]	$137.5 \pm 39.7(8)$	$122.1 \pm 33.6(8)$	N.S.

a) 1×10^5 NFSa cells were i.v. challenged 7 days after 12Gy
   irradiation to the abdomen.
b) 250µg of antibody was i.v. administered 1 day before
   tumor cell challenge.
c) 3.0mg silica was i.v. administered 1 day before tumor
   cell challenge.

REFFERENCES

Ando,K., Hunter, N. & Peters, L.J., 1980, British Journal of
    Cancer, 41, 250.

Ando,K., Peters,L.J., Hunter,N., Jinnouchi,K. & Matsumoto, T.,
    1983, British Journal of Cancer, 47, 73.

PARR,I., Wheeler, E. & Alexander,P., 1973, British Journal of
    Cancer, 1973, 23,370.

INHIBITION OF EXPERIMENTAL METASTASES BY DS-POLYNUCLEOTIDES

D. NOLIBÉ[1] and M.N. THANG[2]

1) C.E.A - IPSN - DPS - Laboratoire de Toxicologie des Transuraniens -
BP 12 - 91680 Bruyères le Châtel - France

2) INSERM U 245 and CNRS ER 238 - Institut de Biologie Physico-Chimique -
13, rue Pierre et Marie Curie - 75005 Paris - France

Keywords : metastases - natural killer - ds-polynucleotides - rat

INTRODUCTION

An increase in the Natural Killer (NK) cell cytotoxicity displayed by lung intracapillary lymphocytes (LIC) as compared to blood lymphocytes was observed by Nolibé et al. (1981). This observation correlates well with previous findings of Fidler (1970). Concomitantly, it was demonstrated in mice by Hanna & Fidler (1980) and in rats by Nolibé et al. (1982) that interferon inducers (r I_n. r C_n) are able to stimulate NK activity and markedly inhibit the lung metastatic process. Taken together these results provide a way of immunotherapeutic treatment of metastasis in cancer patients. However, many adverse effects of r I_n. r C_n have been observed whereas a mismatched polynucleotide duplexe, the r I_n. r$(C_{12},U)_n$, has been shown by Ts'o et al (1976) to be devoid of immediate secondary effects. The purpose of the present study was therefore to assess the in vivo effects of this mismatched polynucleotide duplexe on lung NK cell activity and the incidence of artificial metastasis using the same syngeneic lung tumor cells (P 77) for the two tests.

MATERIALS AND METHODS

Animals and treatments

Inbred Wistar AG rats (CNRS, Orleans la Source, France) were injected intratracheally (IT) with r I_n. r C_n (Sigma) or r I_n. r$(C_{12},U)_n$ provided by P.O.P. Ts'o (Johns Hopkins University School of Hygiene and Public Health, Baltimore, USA). Each rat received 400 µg/kg in 0.2 ml of saline.

In vitro assay for natural cell mediated cytotoxicity

Cell suspensions of LIC effector cells were obtained from lung capillaries as previously described by Nolibé et al. (1981). In vitro natural killer cell

cytotoxicity against YAC-1 mouse lymphoma cells or syngeneic P 77 rat lung
fibrohistiocytoma cells was evaluated by a standard 4hr ^{51}Cr assay according
to Herberman (1975). Cells from rats were tested at four effector to target
ratios, and the percentage of killing was calculated as followed : experimental release-spontaneous release/maximum release - spontaneous release x 100.

In vivo tumor cell clearance

   P 77 tumor cells prelabelled in vitro with (^{125}I)-Iododeoxyuridine (IdUrd)
according to Fidler (1970) were injected (10^6/rat) into syngeneic rats. Groups
of 10 rats were killed 24 hr post injection and lung radioactivity was assessed by γ scintillation counting. The number of viable labelled tumor cells
present in the lungs was calculated.

Assay for experimental pulmonary metastasis

   P 77 tumor cell were inoculated IV (10^5/rat) into syngeneic rats. Recipient rats were killed 27 days later and the number of visible lung metastases counted.

RESULTS

   The cells removed from lung capillaries (LIC) were tested for NK activity
one day after IT injection of 400 µg/kg of the two double-stranded (ds)-poly-
nucleotides. The treatment with r I_n. r C_n resulted in a minimal two fold increase of NK cytotoxicity against YAC-1 tumor cells whatever the effector to
target ratio used. The enhancement produced by r I_n. r(C_{12},U) was of the same
magnitude. Syngeneic lung tumor cells (P 77) displayed similar sensitivity
to LIC cytotoxicity as YAC-1 target cells (figure 1).

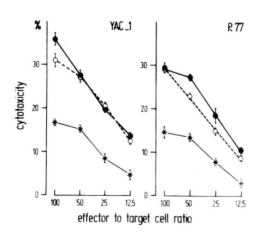

Figure 1.   Augmentation of rat LIC
NK activity 24 hrs after treatment
by interferon inducers.

●——● : r I_n. r C_n 400 µg/kg

○--○ : r I_n. r$(C_{12},U)_n$ 400 µg/kg

— : controls

Four days after ds-polynucleotide injection a significant augmentation was observed, after which, LIC NK activity returned to the control level in one week. Attempts to stimulate NK cytotoxicity in tumor bearing animals was also successful : however, the stimulatory effect seems less important than in controls. The pattern of arrest and survival of (^{125}I) IdUrd labelled syngeneic P 77 tumor cells was studied in rats given the interferon inducers IT one day before tumor cell injection. The initial tumor cell arrest in the pulmonary capillary bed was not significantly different in control and treated groups. However, in all treated animals the number of viable tumor cells in lungs was 60 fold lower than in control rats (Table 1). In addition, no significant difference was observed as regards the ds-polynucleotides injected. To substantiate this result, the development of lung tumor colonies was examined four weeks after IV injection of 10^5 P 77 tumor cells. The animals had a significantly lower number of tumor nodules on the lung surface when they were treated with ds-polynucleotides 24 hr before tumor cell injection (Table 1). The importance of the timing on the treatment should be emphasized : when ds-polynucleotides were administered 7 days or even 1 day after tumor cell injection, no inhibitory effect on lung tumor nodules was observed.

Table 1. Effect of *in vivo* ds-polynucleotide treatment on lung survival and development of IV injected syngeneic P 77 tumor cells.

IT treatment day - 1	N° of viable P 77 tumor cells (+ SD) retained in lungs at day + 1	N° of P 77 lung tumor nodules (+ SD) at day + 27
O	64500 + 15200	186 + 94
r I_n. r C_n	1220 + 430	14 + 9
r I_n. r$(C_{12},U)_n$	1280 + 370	22 + 7

Day o : day of IV injection of P 77 tumor cells.

DISCUSSION

As a way of stimulating NK cytotoxicity of lung intracapillary cells, applied to treatment of lung metastases, the present results show firstly that r I_n. r$(C_{12},U)_n$ is as effective as r I_n. r C_n. These observations are in agreement with those of Zarling et al. (1980) obtained *in vitro*. The magnitude of stimulation when the agent is delivered locally by IT injection may be directly related to the *in vitro* results of Djeu et al. (1979) showing the need for macrophages in the induction of the NK cytotoxicity enhancement. It seems that *in vivo* the alveolar macrophage could play a similar role to others macrophages.

Secondly, it is demonstrated that higher NK activity found in LIC of treated animals correlates well with an increased capacity for eliminating tumor
cells injected intravenously or to inhibit their development in tumor nodules. However, these beneficial effects are only observed when ds-polynucleotides are injected one day before tumor cell injection, although the NK stimulation of LIC is observed four days after stimulation. This short duration of
the in vivo effect could be explained by a rapid extravasation of tumor cells
in lung parenchyma, a compartment probably devoid of NK cells or inacessible
to NK cells from the capillaries.

Since the NK activity is known to be enhanced by interferon, one might correlate its increase to the production of interferon induced by ds-polynucleotides. However, the possibility that the inhibition of metastasis might result jointly from other effects of ds-polynucleotides cannot be excluded.
Although a single treatment by interferon inducers has a beneficial effect on
the development of experimental metastases, one should keep in mind that this
model represents an artificial situation in which a large number of tumor
cells are injected into the blood stream of a non cancerous animal. Moreover,
the beneficial effect occurred during a short period after polynucleotide injection, probably because tumor cells rapidly escape the lung intracapillary
NK cells. This last observation leads to the suggestion that efficient therapeutic treatment would require the induction of a chronic NK cytotoxicity
stimulation. The non toxic ds-polynucleotide r I_n. r$(C_{12},U)_n$ presents an advantage in such therapeutic treatments. Experiments are in progress to test
the efficiency of repeated ds-polynucleotide stimulation in a model based on
spontaneously metastasising tumors.

REFERENCES

Djeu, J.Y., Heinbaugh, J.A., Holden, H.T. & Herberman, R.B., 1979, Journal of
     Immunology, 122, 182.

Fidler, I.J., 1970, Journal National Cancer Institute, 45, 773.

Hanna, N. & Fidler, I.J., 1980, Journal National Cancer Institute, 65, 801.

Herberman, R.B., Nunn, M.E. & Lanvrin, D.H., 1975, International Journal of
     Cancer, 16, 216.

Nolibé, D., Bérel, E., Masse, R. & Lafuma, J., 1981, Biomedicine, 35, 230.

Nolibé, D., Bérel, E., Masse, R. & Lafuma, J., 1982, International Journal
     of Immunopharmacology, 4, 252.

Ts'o, P.O.P., Alderfer, J.L., Levy, J., Marshall, L.W., O'Malley, J.,
Horoszewicz, J.S., Carter, W.A., 1976, Molecular Pharmacology, 12, 299.

Zarling, J.M., Schlais, J., Eskra, L., Greene, J.J., Ts'o, P.O.P. & Carter,
W.A., 1980, Journal of Immunology, 124, 1852.

POTENTIAL VALUE OF LIPOSOMES AS CARRIERS OF LIPOPHILIC MURAMYL DIPEPTIDE
DERIVATIVE FOR RENDERING HUMAN MONOCYTE-MACROPHAGES TUMORICIDAL

S. SONE

3rd Department of Internal Medicine, The University of Tokushima
School of Medicine, Kuramoto-cho, Tokushima 770, Japan

Keywords: Liposomes; muramyl dipeptide; human mononuclear phagocytes

INTRODUCTION

There is increasing evidence that activated macrophages are important
in host defense against primary and/or metastatic tumors. At least in
vitro, macrophages can distinguish tumorigenic from nontumorigenic cells
by a mechanism that is independent of such phenotypic diversity as
metastatic potential, drug sensitivity, and antigenicity (Poste & Fidler
1980). These findings have resulted in the discovery of new biological
response modifiers (BRMs) that can enhance macrophage-mediated tumor cell
killing. For example, muramyl dipeptide (MDP), which is synthesized, is
the principle unit of the active component from Mycobacterium responsible
for the immunopotentiating activity of Freund's complete adjuvant (Adam &
Lederer 1984). We demonstrated that the efficacy of MDP encapsulated
within the aqueous space of phospholipid vesicles (liposomes) greatly
enhanced its potential to render murine macrophages tumoricidal in vitro
(Sone & Fidler 1981) and in vivo (Fidler et al.1981). Moreover, systemic
administration of liposome-entrapped MDP into tumor-bearing mice eradicated
disseminated metastatic diseases (Fidler et al.1981). We examined whether
these findings in animals could be applied to humans. Recent studies in
this laboratory have shown that liposomes containing MDP or its lipophilic
derivative (MTP-PE) potentiate the tumoricidal activity of human monocyte-
macrophages in vitro (Sone & Tsubura 1982, Sone et al. 1984a, Sone et al.
1984b). This paper provides a brief review of our in vitro studies which
provide a rationale for the clinical use of MTP-PE encapsulated in
liposomes for potentiating the host's defense against metastatic tumors.

MATERIALS AND METHODS

The origin, properties and cultivation of A375 melanoma cells, the
methods used for isolation and separated by adherence of alveolar

macrophages (AM) and peripheral blood monocytes (PBM) from normal human
volunteers, the preparation of large multilamellar (MLV) liposomes
composed of phosphatidylserine (PS) and phosphatidylcholine (PC) in a
molar ratio of 3 to 7 or 5 to 5, the activation of monocyte-macrophages by
hydrophilic muramyl dipeptide (MDP) or lipophilic muramyl tripeptide
phosphatidylethanolamine (MTP-PE) (Ciba-Geigy) encapsulated in MLV
liposomes, and the quantitative assay of the cytotoxicity of treated and
control monocyte-macrophages against ^{125}I-IUdR-labeled target cells, have
been described in detail elsewhere (Sone & Tsubura 1982, Sone et al.
1984b).

RESULTS AND DISCUSSION

We previously showed that systemic administration of liposomes
containing soluble MDP resulted in eradication of established pulmonary
metastasis (Fidler et al.1981).   Encapsulation of the lipophilic MDP
analog, MTP-PE in the bilayer membrane is interesting for several reasons.
First, lipophilic MTP-PE can be directly inserted into the lipid bilayer
of MLV liposomes. Second, for significant activation of murine AM *in vitro*
and *in vivo*, MTP-PE in liposomes was found to be effective at a much lower
concentration than free MDP (Fidler et al.1982).   Third, liposome-MTP-PE
can activate rat AM for a longer period than free MDP.   To extend these
observations obtained in mice to humans, we examine activation of human
alveolar macrophages (AM) by liposomes containing MTP-PE.   Treatment of
human AM with 5 µg/umol of MTP-
PE encapsulated in liposomes
induced maximal cytotoxicity
against human A375 melanoma
cells (Table 1). This amount of
entrapped MTP-PE was lower than
the effective amount of free
MDP.

Phagocytic uptake of
liposomes by macrophages seems
to be the most important factor
for their effectiveness in
activation. Murine macrophages are known to phagocytize negatively-charged
liposomes composed of PS and PC more rapidly than neutral liposomes
(Schroit & Fidler 1982). We also observed that addition of PS to PC
liposomes resulted in significant increase in both their phagocytosis and
their enhancement of the tumoricidal activity of human AM (Sone et al. 1984).

Table 1. *In vitro* activation of human AM by liposomes containing MTP-PE.

AM treatment[a] (per well)	AM-mediated cytotoxicity against A375 cells	
Tumor cells alone	2140 + 35[b]	
Untreated AM	1384 + 104	
Free MDP 1 µg	1011 + 52	(27 %)[c]
MTP-PE 0.5 µg/10 nmol	924 + 89	(33 %)[c]
0.05 µg/10 nmol	840 + 77	(38 %)[c]
0.005 µg/10 nmol	909 + 101	(34 %)[c]
0.0005 µg/10 nmol	1393 + 54	

[a] AM were treated for 24 hr with 10 nmol of liposome-MTP-PE. [b] Cpm ± SD
[c] % cytotoxicity by treated AM (p < 0.05).

The finding that iv injection of liposomes containing MDP or MTP-PE
resulted in eradication of established spontaneous pulmonary metastasis
suggests that the first step in in situ activation of tissue macrophages
such as AM or macrophages infiltrating tumors may require the direct
interaction of circulating peripheral blood monocytes with MLV liposomes
injected intravenously. As shown in Fig. 1, human monocytes (named
monocyte-derived macrophages) that had been incubated for 4 days in
medium, were activated and rendered tumoricidal by liposome-entrapped MTP-
PE at much lower concentrations than the effective concentration of free
MDP. Moreover, freshly isolated monocytes treated for 24 hr with 25 nmol
of liposomes containing MTP-PE (5 µg/umol) maintained their tumoricidal
potential for a longer period than those treated with free MDP (Fig. 2),
suggesting that monocytes circulating in the blood could be activated by
liposome-entrapped MTP-PE administered intravenously.

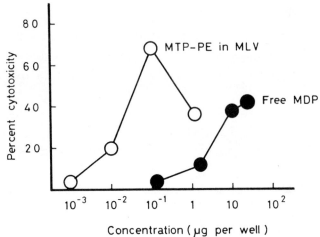

Fig. 1. Activation of
human PBM by free MDP
or MLV liposomes
containing MTP-PE at
the indicated doses
before cytotoxicity
assay.

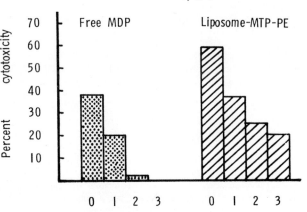

Fig. 2. Maintenance
of tumoricidal
activity of human PBM
treated for 24 hr with
10 µg of MDP or 10
nmol of MTP-PE (0.05
µg) per well.

Duration of incubation in medium after
monocyte activation (days)

It will be very interesting to see whether liposomes containing MTP-PE
are effective in cancer patients for treatment of disseminated diseases.
There is promising evidence for their clinical use. Recently, Lopez-
Berestein et al. (1984) reported that systemic injection of MLV liposomes
is safe, without undesirable side effects, and that 24 hr after iv
injection of negatively charged MLV liposomes, they become localized in
organs rich in reticuloendothelial cells. These observations, together
with our findings that liposome-entrapped MTP-PE can activate human
monocyte-macrophages to the tumoricidal state, and has a therapeutic
effect on murine cancer metastasis, indicate that systemic administration
of liposome-entrapped MTP-PE should be useful for treatment of disseminated metastatic diseases in humans.

CONCLUSION

Human AM and PBM can be activated and rendered tumoricidal in vitro by
incubation with liposomes containing the lipophilic MDP derivative,
muramyl tripeptide-phosphatidylethanolamine (MTP-PE). Negatively-charged
liposomes are preferentially incorporated into monocyte-macrophages by
phagocytosis. Liposome-encapsulated MTP-PE is effective at much lower
concentrations than free MDP and causes more prolonged activation than the
latter of human monocyte-macrophages. These results indicate that
systemic administration of liposomes containing MDP or MTP-PE may be
useful clinically for activation of macrophages responsible for eradication of cancer metastasis.

ACKNOWLEDGEMENT
   This research was supported by a Grant-in-Aid for Cancer Research and a
Grant-in-Aid for Scientific Research from the Ministry of Education,
Science and Culture of Japan.

REFERENCES
Adam, A. & Lederer, E. 1984, Medicinal Research Review, 4, 111.
Fidler, I.J., Sone, S., Fogler, W.E. & Barnes, Z.L. 1981,
    Proceedings of National Academy of Science, U.S.A., 78, 1680.
Fidler, I.J., Sone, S., Fogler, W.E., Smith, D., Braun, D.G.,
    Tarcsay, V., Gisler, R.H. & Schroit, A.J. 1982,
    Journal of Biological Response Modifiers, 1, 43.
Poste, G. & Fidler, I.J. 1980, Nature (Lond.), 283, 139.
Schroit, A.J. & Fidler, I.J. 1982, Cancer Research, 42, 161.
Sone, S. & Fidler, I.J. 1981, Cellular Immunology, 57, 42.
Sone, S. & Tsubura, E. 1982, Journal of Immunology, 129, 1313.
Sone, S., Tachibana, K., Shono, M., Ogushi, M. & Tsubura, E.
    1984a, Journal of Biological Response Modifiers, 3, 185.
Sone, S., Mutsuura, S., Ogawara, M. & Tsubura, E. 1984b,
    Journal of Immunology, 132, 2105.

IMMUNOTHERAPY OF METASTASIS: COMPARATIVE EFFICACY OF BRM'S FOR PROPHYLAXIS AND THERAPY OF SPONTANEOUS METASTASES AND AUTOCHTHONOUS TUMORS

J.E. TALMADGE[1], I.J. FIDLER[2], B.F. LENZ[1], D.M. LITTON[1], C.W. RIGGS[3], S. GUO[3], R. SIMMON[4], and R.K. OLDHAM[5]

[1]Program Resources Incorporated, NCI-FCRF, P.O. Box B, Frederick, Maryland 21701

[2]Cell Biology M.D. Anderson, Hospital and Tumor Institute, Houston, Texas 77030

[3]IMS, NCI-FCRF, Frederick, Maryland 21701

[4]Biometrics Research Branch NCI, Bethesda, Maryland 20205

[5]Biological Therapy Institute, Franklin, Tennessee 37064

Keywords: biological response modifiers; autochthonous tumors

Immunomodulation as a clinical therapeutic modality has in general been disappointing with results that are inferior to those obtained with transplantable tumor models (Oldham & Smalley 1983). The positive results observed with experimental tumor systems appear to be due in part to the initiation of therapy in "normal" animals with minimal tumor burdens. Indeed, many models of immunotherapy use a prophylactic approach in which the BRM is administered prior to tumor challenge. In contrast, patients present with established disease. Therefore, we must develop and utilize relevant therapeutic models which may predict clinical efficacy, rather than using experimental models of immunoprophylaxis or the treatment of animals with minimal tumor burden (Talmadge et al. 1984a). Routine tumor therapy models should be directed against preexistant metastatic disease in a tumor "conditioned" host. Ultimately, the most rigorous test of immunotherapy will be derived from studies utilizing induced or spontaneously arising autochthonous tumors.

Because metastasis is the major threat to the cancer patient, tumor therapy models that also effect the cure of secondary lesions are most desirable. Immunotherapy may be directed against metastatic foci from a primary tumor (spontaneous metastasis) or against tumor cells introduced into the host systematically by i.v. injection (experimental metastasis). The spontaneous metastasis model utilizes a host "conditioned" by tumor growth (rather than a "normal" host) if therapy is initiated following the surgical resection of the primary tumor. Therapeutic models directed against metastatic disease, in which therapy is initiated one or two days following primary tumor transplant represent a form of prophylaxis since therapy is started prior to metastatic tumor cell seeding. Furthermore, in such a model the primary tumor volume in

the treated animals is often smaller than that in saline treated hosts
thereby reducing metastatic disease and preventing a comparison of metastatic burden to control animals with a more extensive primary tumor burden.   This does not suggest that useful information cannot be obtained
from studies of nonspecific immunoprophylaxis or the treatment of primary
tumors (Herberman 1983) but rather that such approaches may not be predictive of systemic therapeutic efficacy in the clinical setting (Hewitt
1982).

It is apparent that as one progresses from models of immunoprophylaxis
to more stringent and rigorous models of immunotherapy only those BRM's
with increased therapeutic efficacy will have activity.   Thus, a BRM with
prophylactic activity may not have striking therapeutic activity against
established systemic disease in a relatively normal host (experimental
metastases), or in a host conditioned by the growth of an established primary tumor with preexistent spontaneous metastases which are treated following surgical resection of the primary tumor.   Even the spontaneous
metastasis model utilizes young, healthy hosts, bearing transplantable
tumors; a model which is disparate from cancer patients who may have
been exposed to "carcinogenic" insult and have progressive primary and
metastatic tumor growth.   The development of a clinically analogous model
is complex and optimally should include primary, autochthonous tumors
that metastasize.   These studies are more difficult and tedious than experiments with transplantable tumors but provide a rigorous test of therapeutic efficacy.   The difficulties associated with these studies are
similar to those routinely encountered in clinical trials; including tumor
accrual, randomization, statistical evaluation, and duration of the studies.

One of the metastatic autochthonous tumor models which we have developed utilizes UV induced skin tumors, including squamous cell carcinomas,
fibrosarcomas, hemangiosarcomas, rhabdomyosarcomas, and other less well
differentiated sarcomas.   The tumors are induced 22 to 50 weeks following
the onset of UV radiation (2.8 J/M^2/sec for 2 hr, 3 times per week) which
is maintained for eight months.   The animals are randomly assigned to one
of several arms of a protocol as palpable tumors accrue and treatment is
initiated when the initial lesion is noted.   The therapeutic efficacy is
determined based on the survival of the animals, tumor growth, as well
as development of systemic disease.

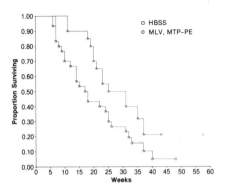

Kaplan Meyer survival curve of mice bearing autochthonous, UV induced
skin tumors, treated with saline (N=30) or liposomes incorporating MTP-PE
(N=20). The treatment with liposomes significantly prolonged survival
(p = 0.01) as determined by the Krauskal-Wallace analysis. Animals were
treated twice a week for 4 weeks.

It is apparent from the above figure that autochthonous UV induced tumors
presents a stringent challenge for testing a therapeutic protocol. In this
study, animals treated with liposomes incorporating MTP-PE have a significantly prolonged survival as compared to the saline treated controls.
Furthermore, such a treatment significantly reduced the tumor burden as
compared to the saline treated group (multivariant distribution free test)
from week 5 to week 42 of the protocol. Based on this and other studies
of the immunotherapy of autochthonous tumors we suggest that a BRM, such
as liposomes incorporating MTP-PE, that has a moderate efficacy against
autochthonous tumors holds promise for clinical trials.

Clearly, the development of successful immunotherapy protocols requires
additional strategies for the development of clinically predictive tumor
models and protocols (Fidler et al. 1982, Talmadge et al. 1984b). In addition to the determination of a maximum tolerated dose (MTD) it is also important to determine the optimal immunomodulatory dose (OID) not only in
animal models but also clinically. However, both of these levels of activity (MTD and OID) may not represent the optimal therapeutic dose (OTD).
The OTD appears to be dependent not only on the augmentation of effector
cell activity but also on the number and sequestering (tumor) of effector
cells. Furthermore, the determination of an optimal therapeutic protocol
requires additional information on therapeutic schedule and duration.
Studies of scheduling parameters have revealed that toxicity will be noted
if an immunomodulator is delivered frequently at high levels. However,
if the BRM is administered at either a lower level or less frequently there
is a decrease in toxicity which is often paralleled by a greater therapeu-

tic activity. The studies with the autochthonous tumor models have stressed the importance of maintaining the therapeutic schedule for prolonged
periods to obtain maximum therapeutic benefits. This is in contrast to
phase I trials in which patients are treated for a short time period to
determine the MTD. We suggest that the demonstration of clinical immunotherapeutic activity may require the prolonged administration of a BRM in
the phase I-II treatment schedule. This may involve an initial loading
dose followed by maintenance therapy or the consistant administration of
an OID in conjunction with an optimal therapeutic schedule.

   In summary, we suggest that the ultimate test of therapeutic efficacy
will come from the use of autochthonous tumor models, which should provide the greatest predictive value of a treatment protocol or BRM for
clinical trials. In addition animal models should be utilized to determine the optimal therapeutic schedule and dose required to provide
therapeutic activity. Because host effector mechanisms following BRM
activation are capable of controlling only a limited number of tumor
cells while the treatment of more extensive tumor burden generally results in progressive disease (Fidler et al. 1981), immunotherapy may
have its greatest role as an adjunct against clinically inapparent secondary disease or in conjunction with debulking treatment modalities. In
summary, immunomodulation as a fourth therapeutic modality has considerable potential and will ultimately provide an important therapeutic
adjunct for the treatment of systemic disease.

Fidler, I., Sone, S., Fogler, W. & Barnes, Z., 1981, Proceedings of the
    National Academy of Sciences of the United States of America Vol.78,
    p.1680-1684.
Fidler, I., Berendt, M. & Oldham, R., 1982, Journal of Biological Re-
    sponse Modifiers Vol.1, p.15-26.
Herberman, R., 1983, Journal of Biological Response Modifiers Vol.2,
    p.39-46.
Hewitt, H., 1982, Journal of Biological Response Modifiers Vol.1, p.107-
    119.
Oldham, R. & Smalley, R., 1983, Journal of Biological Response Modifiers
    Vol.2, p.1-37.
Talmadge, J., Lenz, B., Collins, M., Uithoven, K., Schneider, M., Adams,
    J., Pearson, J., Agee, W., Fox, R. & Oldham, R., 1984a, Behring Insti-
    tute Mitteilungen Vol.74, p.219-229.
Talmadge, J., Oldham, R. & Fidler, I., 1984b, Journal of Biological Re-
    sponse Modifiers Vol.3, p.88-109.

Research sponsored by the National Cancer Institute, DHHS, under contract
No. N01-23910 with Program Resources, Inc.

IMMUNOSTIMULANT DRUG TARGETED BY MONOCLONAL ANTIBODIES AND NEOGLYCOPROTEINS

A.C. ROCHE and M. MONSIGNY

Centre de Biophysique Moléculaire, CNRS, 1, rue Haute, 45045 Orléans Cédex (France)

Keywords : MDP, Macrophage activation, Metastasis regression

INTRODUCTION

Macrophages may be rendered tumoricidal upon activation with different agents such as lymphokines (Piessens et al., 1971) or bacterial products (Juy and Chedid, 1975). In vitro, $\underline{N}$-acetyl muramyl dipeptide (MDP), the minimal structure of mycobacteria able to induce stimulation (Adam et al., 1981) may activate macrophages. Unfortunately, MDP is very rapidly cleared from the body (Parant et al., 1979) and so has a low in vivo activity in tumor growth inhibition (Chedid et al., 1982). The in vivo efficiency of MDP is highly improved when is carried by liposomes (Fidler et al., 1981). In this paper, we report that murine alveolar and peritoneal macrophages are activated both in vitro and in vivo by MDP bound to mannosylated serum albumin (Monsigny et al., 1984b) and to IgM monoclonal antibodies specific for L1210 leukemic cells, and for Lewis lung carcinoma cells.

MATERIAL AND METHODS

Lewis rats were obtained from CSEAL, CNRS, Orléans, France. DBA/2 and C57/Bl 6 mice were purchased from IFFA CREDO, Lyon, France. DBA/2 lymphoma L1210 cells (kindly given by Dr. I. Gresser, Villejuif, France) and Lewis lung carcinoma cells (3LL) (kindly provided by Dr. F. Lavelle, Rhône-Poulenc Recherches, Vitry-sur-Seine, France) were adapted to grow in culture. $\underline{N}$-acetyl muramyl dipeptide was synthetized according to Merser et al. (1975). Neoglycoproteins such as mannosylated bovine serum albumin were obtained by allowing phenylisothiocyanate-α-$\underline{D}$-mannopyranoside to react with bovine serum albumin (Monsigny et al., 1984b), leading to a neoglycoprotein containing 20 mannosyl residues. $\underline{N}$-acetyl muramyl dipeptide was converted into its hydroxysuccinimide ester (MDP-ester), then the MDP-ester

was added to either a solution of immunoglobulins (IgM) or of serum albumin as previously described (Monsigny et al., 1984a) leading to MDP-bound
IgM and MDP-bound BSA containing 10 and 45 MDP units per molecule, respectively. The absence of lipopolysaccharide was checked as previously described (Monsigny et al., 1982). Monoclonal antibodies against L1210 lymphoma cells and 3LL Lewis lung carcinoma cells were selected and cloned as
previously described (Roche and Monsigny, 1982, and Midoux et al., 1984b,
respectively). The selected IgM monoclonal antibodies $F_{2.10.23}$ which bind
L1210 cells and 6B6 which bind 3LL cells were shown to be specific enough
to allow a selective visualization of L1210 tumors and 3LL tumors respectively, by γ-scintigraphy (Maillet et al., 1984, and Midoux et al., 1984a, respectively).

The cytostaticity activity of rat alveolar macrophages (obtained according to Holt, 1975) and of thioglycolate elicited mouse peritoneal macrophages was assessed by radioactive incorporation assay using ^{3}H-thymidine ;
the determination of in vivo activation of macrophages was checked by using
alveolar macrophages harvested one to four day(s) upon injection of a MDP-
bound carrier (Monsigny et al., 1984a). The therapeutic effects of MDP-
bound neoglycoproteins were estimated by direct examination of the lung metastases and by determining the radioactivity incorporated into the lungs 24
hr after injection of ^{125}I-IUdR (Bonmassar et al., 1975). C57 Bl/6 mice
were injected subcutaneously in the thigh with 10^5 viable 3LL cells. When the
tumor reached about 10 mm in diameter, the tumor bearing leg was amputated. The treatment began two days later by injection in the tail vein of 10
µg MDP-bound to neoglycoproteins (or monoclonal antibodies) and was repeated every third day.

RESULTS AND DISCUSSION
Rat alveolar macrophages from healthy and untreated animals were not
able to significantly inhibit the incorporation of ^{3}H-thymidine into L1210
lymphoma cells or into 3LL carcinoma cells. Conversely when rat alveolar macrophages were preincubated with MDP-bound Man-BSA, their cytostaticity
was quite high (Table 1). Because free MDP or MDP-bound BSA were much
less effective and because macrophages are known (Stahl et al., 1978) to
actively endocytose glycoconjugates containing mannose residues, it may be
concluded that rat alveolar macrophages are activated by MDP-bound mannosylated serum albumin through a specific adsorptive endocytotic process.
Similar results were obtained when mouse peritoneal macrophages were
assayed (Table 1). Mouse peritoneal macrophages are known to be devoid of

Table 1. Macrophage activation. Cytostaticity[a] of mouse peritoneal and rat alveolar macrophages in vitro activated by free and carrier substituted MDP.

Activator	Target cells	Rat alveolar macrophages		Mouse peritoneal macrophages	
		1^b	10^b	1^b	10^b
MDP	3LL	0	8	5	10
	L1210	0	8	5	10
MDP-BSA	3LL	0	20	15	15
	L1210	0	20	15	20
Man-MDP-BSA	3LL	40	75	80	90
	L1210	45	75	60	70
MDP-IgM-6B6	3LL	n.d	n.d	30	75
α 3LL	L1210	n.d	n.d	5	25
MDP-IgM F-2.10.23					
α L1210	L1210	n.d	n.d	50	80

a Cytostatic activity is expressed as growth inhibition (GI):GI % = (R–S/R) 100, where R is the radioactivity incorporated in tumor cells cultivated on unstimulated macrophages and S is the radioactivity incorporated in tumor cells cultivated on stimulated macrophages
b MDP (free or bound) concentration : µg/ml

plasma membrane receptors able to bind MDP or MDP-bound serum albumin but to have a membrane lectin able to induce the endocytosis of mannose-containing glycoconjugates (Tenu et al., 1982). So, the MDP-bound neogly-coprotein acts as a specific carrier forcing the internalization of MDP.

MDP-bound monoclonal antibodies were not able to activate macrophages when macrophages were preincubated in the presence of MDP-bound IgM and in the absence of the target tumor cells. When tumor cells were preincubated with the specific MDP-bound IgM or when tumor cells were preincubated with both the specific MDP-bound IgM and macrophages, the activation of macrophages was very efficient (Table 1). MDP-bound Man-BSA was found to render mouse and rat alveolar macrophages tumoricidal, two to three days after intravenous or intraperitoneal injection of 10 to 30 µg carrier-bound MDP (Monsigny et al., 1984a). According to the above data, MDP-bound Man-BSA are efficient activators of macrophages both in vitro and in vivo and would be suitable drugs to induce metastasis regression by systemic activation of macrophages as liposome-encapsulated MDP does (Fidler et al., 1981). Indeed, injection of MDP-bound Man-BSA led to the regression of spontaneous 3LL metastases developed upon excision of the primary tumor. All the untreated mice died with a high number of large metastases, but 40 % of mice which received MDP conjugates had no trace of lung metastases, 40 % had small lung metastases and only 20 % had as many lung metastases as untreated mice (Roche et al., 1984b). Injection of MDP-bound monoclonal antibodies under similar conditions leads to metastasis regression in more than 50 % of the treated mice.

In conclusion, it appears that MDP-bound neoglycoproteins and MDP-bound specific monoclonal antibodies are suitable macrophage activators and that such MDP-bound specific carriers could be used as anticancer drugs in animal therapy.

Adam, A., Petit, J.F., Le Francier, P. & Lederer, E., 1981, Molecular and Cellular Biochemistry, 41, 27.

Bonmassar, E., Houchens, D. Fioretti, M. & Goldin, A., 1975, Chemotherapy 21, 321.

Chedid, L., Morin, A. & Phillips, N., 1982, In Bacteria & Cancer, edited J. Jeljaszewicz, G. Pulverer & W. Roszkowski, p. 49 Academic Press.

Fidler, I.J., Sone, S., Fogler, W.E. & Barnes, Z., 1981, Proceedings of the National Academy of Science, USA, 78, 1680.

Holt, P.C., 1919, Journal of Immunological Methods, 27, 189.

Juy, D. & Chedid, L., 1975, Proceedings of the National Academy of Science, USA, 72, 4105.

Maillet, T., Roche, A.C., Thérain, F. & Monsigny, M., 1984, Cancer Research (submitted).

Merser, C., Sinaÿ, P. & Adam, A., 1975, Biochemical and Biophysical Research Communications, 66, 1316.

Midoux, P., Maillet, T., Thérain, F., Monsigny, M. & Roche, A.C., 1984a, Cancer Immunology and Immunotherapy (in the press).

Midoux, P., Roche, A.C. & Monsigny, M., 1984b, Immunology Letters, 8, 131.

Monsigny, M., Kiéda, C. & Maillet, T., 1982, The European Molecular Biology Organization Journal, 73, 127.

Monsigny, M., Roche, A.C. & Bailly, P., 1984a, Biochemical Biophysical and Research Communications, 121, 579.

Monsigny, M., Roche, A.C. & Midoux, P., 1984b, Biology of the Cell, 51 187.

Parant, M., Parant, F., Chedid, L., Yapo, A., Petit, J.F. & Lederer, E., 1979, International Journal of Pharmacology, 1, 35.

Piessens, W.F., Churchill, W.H.Jr & David, J.R., 1975, Journal of Immunology, 114, 293.

Roche, A.C., Bailly, P., Midoux, P. & Monsigny, M., 1984, Cancer Immunology and Immunotherapy (in the press).

Roche, A.C., Bailly, P. and Monsigny, M., 1984b, Invasion and Metastasis (submitted).

Roche, A.C. & Monsigny, M., 1982, Cell Biology International Reports, 6, 557.

Stahl, P.D., Rodman, J.S., Miller, M.J. & Schlesinger, P.H., 1978, Proceedings of the National Academy of Science, USA, 75, 1399.

Tenu, J.P., Roche, A.C., Yapo, A., Kiéda, C., Monsigny, M. & Petit, J.F., 1982, Biology of the Cell, 44, 157.

HIGH METASTATIC MURINE T-LYMPHOMA CELLS SHOW DECREASED SENSITIVITY TO THE CYTOSTATIC AND CYTOLYTIC EFFECTS OF AN ANTI-TUMOR LYMPHOTOXIN PRODUCED BY ACTIVATED PORCINE PERIPHERAL BLOOD LEUKOCYTES

E. RUSSMANN[1], M. D. KRAMER[1], J. H. WISSLER[2] and V. SCHIRRMACHER[1]

[1] Institut für Immunologie und Genetik, Deutsches Krebsforschungszentrum, D-6900 Heidelberg, FRG

[2] Arbeitsgruppe Biochemie, Max-Planck-Institut für Physiologische und Klinische Forschung, D-6350 Bad Nauheim, FRG

Keyword: metastasis, lymphotoxin, lymphoma

INTRODUCTION

Several cytolytic mediators which are produced by either activated macrophages or stimulated lymphoid cells have formerly been described. Their anti-tumor cytostatic and/or cytolytic activity has been demonstrated in different in vivo and in vitro test systems. McCabe and Evans (1982) found that an increase in tumorigenicity of transformed fibroblasts coincides with increased sensitivity to lymphotoxin (LT). However, little is known about the correlation of tumor cell's sensitivity to cytotoxins in vitro and their metastatic capacity in vivo. Furthermore, the biochemical nature and the exact mechanism of action of tumor cytotoxic mediators has so far not been elucidated. This is mainly due to the relatively small quantities of cytokines obtained after stimulation of lymphocytes on a normal scale in conventional cell culture systems.

In a collaborative venture we thus examined the effects of cytotoxic mediators that had been produced on a biotechnological scale (Wissler et al. 1980). Highly active supernatant solutions were tested for their cytostatic/cytotoxic effect using a well characterized experimental tumor system. This system consists of a low-metastatic murine T-lymphoma (Eb) with a high metastatic spontaneous variant (ESb) (Schirrmacher et al. 1982). In addition, we included normal peripheral T-lymphocytes and thymocytes into our studies.

MATERIAL AND METHODS
The Eb/ESb-tumor model system

The tumor model used was the chemically induced DBA/2 lymphoma L5178Y

with the two sublines Eb and ESb. Detailed descriptions have been published elsewhere (Schirrmacher et al. 1982).

Production of supernatant solutions

    The leukocyte culture supernatant was prepared as previously described
(Wissler et al. 1980). Briefly, preparations of at least 200 l porcine
blood were treated with methylcellulose to eliminate platelets and erythrocytes. The remaining leukocytes were cultured for 40 hrs in a modified
serum-free medium and stimulated by 50 nMol/l ConA.

    Porcine cytotoxin (PCT) used in this study was prepared from crude
supernatant by fractionated ammonium-sulphate precipitation and extensive
dialysis against phosphate-buffered saline containing 10^{-3}M L-cysteine.

Assays for cytostatic and cytolytic activities of PCT

    To test the cytostatic activity of PCT we determined the ^{3}H-thymidine
incorporation of ConA-activated spleen-cells, of thymocytes stimulated by
Il-2 and ConA and of autonomously growing transformed T-lymphocytes (Kramer
& Koszinowski 1982). To measure and characterize the PCT-induced cytolysis
we used a conventional 4 hrs ^{51}Cr-release assay (CRA).

RESULTS AND DISCUSSION

    In agreement with data published by McCabe and Evans (1982), we demon-
strate that sensitivity to PCT-mediated cytostasis is considerably increased in T-lymphomas as compared to activated peripheral T-cell blasts
(Fig. 1). Moreover, in all T-lymphoma variants of our tumor system we found
a strong correlation between high metastatic potential in vivo and low
sensitivity to PCT-induced growth inhibition in vitro (Fig. 1, Tab. 1).
Resistance of ESb-type cells to the cytolytic activity of PCT was not
affected by inhibitors of protein synthesis. Furthermore, we could not find
a difference in the absorption of PCT by either Eb or ESb cells.

    Further characterization of the lytic event allowed a preliminary
comparison to the established cytolytic factors lymphotoxin (LT) and tumor
necrosis factor (TNF).
i) Whereas LT-and TNF-mediated lysis is reduced by about 90% at 27° C the
    PCT-induced effect is only reduced by about 50% at 24° C (Fig. 2A).
ii) The cytolytic event of LT and TNF is preceeded by a lag phase of about
    4 hrs; in contrast, the PCT-mediated lysis starts immediately after
    coincubation of the mediator with the appropriate target cell (Fig.2B).

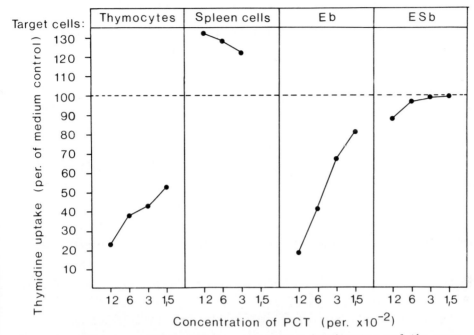

Fig. 1. PCT acts preferentially on immature T-lymphocytes and the non-metastatic T-lymphoma Eb.

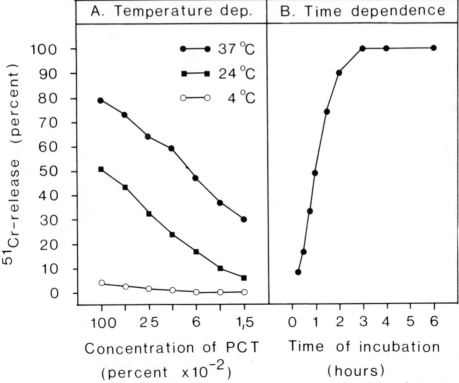

Fig. 2 The lytic event of PCT is temperature dependent (A) and starts immediately after coincubation of PCT and target cells (B).

iii)In contrast to LT and TNF, the PCT-induced cytolysis is not enhanced by
  inhibitors of protein synthesis.

iv) In contrast to TNF, PCT is absorbed to the cell surface and the
  cytolytic effect is not destroyed by pretreatment of the target cell
  with colchicin or cytocholasin B. The absorption of PCT to the target
  cell is not affected by pretreatment of the target cell´s membrane with
  trypsin - this is different to LT.

Taken together, we describe a cytotoxic cytokine which is distinguish-
able from LT or TNF by its mechanism of cytodestruction.

As was shown for lysis by cytotoxic T-cells, macrophages, NK-cells
and LT, tumor cell´s sensitivity to lytic events may decrease during
progression towards higher malignancy. In addition to these observations,
we found in our system that sensitivity to PCT decreases in the course of
tumor progression towards metastasis.

Table 1. Sensitivity of related T-lymphoma lines to PCT mediated lysis
         negatively correlates with their metastatic potential.

Tumor variant	Reduction of maximal ^{3}H-thymidine uptake (%)	Metastasizing capacity	TATA Eb	ESb
Eb 288	69	-	+	-
ESb 289	0	+ +	-	+
Eb Cl 34.2	65	-	+	-
ESb Cl 18.1	0	+++	-	+
ESb Cl 809.1	11	++	-	+
ESb Cl 809.4	6	+++	neg.	
ESb 08 TG^R	0	+	-	+
EB Cl 34.1 (pre)	65	-	+	-
Eb Cl 34.1 (post)	9	+	-	+
ESb-M (prim.)	44	-	-	+
ESb-M (rev.)	0	+ +	-	+
Eb-F1	1	+ +	-	+
Eb-F2	0	+ +	-	+

REFERENCES

Kramer, M. & Koszinowski U., 1982, Journal of Immunology, 128, 784.
McCabe, R. P. & Evans, C. H., 1982, Journal of the National Cancer Insti-
    tute, 68, 329.
Schirrmacher, V., Fogel, M., Rußmann, E., Bosslet, K., Altevogt, P. & Beck,
    L., 1982, Cancer Metastasis Reviews, 1, 241.
Wissler, J. H., 1982, Inflammatory mediators and wound hormones: Chemical
    signals for differentiation and morphogenesis in tissue regeneration and
    healing. In Biochemistry of Differentiation and Morphogenesis, ed. by L.
    Jaenicke, Springer-Verlag, Heidelberg, p.257.

SUCCESSFUL IMMUNOTHERAPY OF A HIGHLY METASTATIC MURINE LYMPHOMA BY MEANS OF VIRALLY XENOGENIZED AUTOLOGOUS TUMOUR CELLS

R. HEICAPPELL, P. v. HOEGEN, B. APPELHANS, V. SCHIRRMACHER
Institut für Immunologie und Genetik, Deutsches Krebsforschungszentrum,
D-6900 Heidelberg, FRG

Keyword: metastasis, xenogenization, lymphoma

INTRODUCTION

Modification of tumour cells with viruses could be shown to enhance the immunogenicity of several experimental tumours by making the tumour 'foreign' to the host ('xenogenization'). This concept has been success- fully applied to relatively slow growing experimental tumours (for review see Kobayshi 1979). In man, clinical responses were seen in patients bearing melanomas (Wallack et al. 1983) and ovarian cancers (Lotzova et al. 1984). We will demonstrate that also fast growing and highly metastatic mouse lymphoma ESb 289 can be curatively treated with viral xenogenization. ESb 289 (Schirrmacher et al. 1982) metastasizes preferentially into spleen and liver even if the primary tumour is removed surgically at an early stage of growth. No curative chemo- or immunotherapy existed so far for this tumour. Now we report that with a combination or surgery and immuno- therapy using irradiated autologous tumour cells infected by Newcastle Disease Virus (NDV) we were able to prevent the establishment of metastases in 50-70% of the animals. By in vitro analysis it could be shown that on the clonal level viral xenogenization leads to a significant increase of tumour specific precursor cytotoxic T-lymphocytes (p-CTL).

MATERIALS AND METHODS

Virus propagation

Newcastle Disease Virus (NDV) of the avirulent strain Ulster was grown in 10-days-old chicken eggs. Allantoic fluid was collected after 48 hours and partially purified and concentrated by differential centrifugation. Virions were finally suspended in Phosphate Buffered Saline (PBS) to give a standard batch with a hemagglutination titer of 1:2048.

Tumour cell lines

Details of chemically induced T-lymphoma Eb 288 and its highly metastatic variant ESb 289 have been published previously (Schirrmacher et al. 1982). For in vivo experiments, the cells were grown as ascites. In vitro, the cells were grown in suspension cultures as described (Schirrmacher & Jacobs 1979).

Therapy

On day 0 the mice were inoculated with 5×10^4 ESb 289 cells i. d. in their right flanks. On day 2 the animals received 1ml live NDV 1:500 s. c. and i. m. The primary tumour was removed surgically at a size of 5-7 mm. Immediately after surgery each animal was injected s. c. + i. m. with 2.5×10^7 irradiated (7000 rad) ESb 289 cells in 1 ml of live NDV at 1:500 dilution.

Limiting dilution analysis

DBA/2 mice were injected with 5×10^4 ESb 289 cells into the ear on day -7. For immunization with xenogenized tumour cells 1×10^7 ESb cells were infected with 160 hemagglutinating units (HU) of NDV. Limiting dilution analysis was performed as described (Lefkovits 1979, Langhorne & Fischer-Lindahl 1981). Briefly, limiting numbers of immune spleen cells (responders) were incubated with 1×10^6 irradiated syngeneic spleen cells and 3×10^4 mitomycin C-inactivated tumour cells (according to the cells used for priming) in round bottom culture plates containing IL-2-enriched complete RPMI 1640 medium. After 8 days, the cultures were split into two aliquots and analysed on ESb 289 and Eb 288 target cells in a 4h ^{51}Cr-release assay.

RESULTS AND DISCUSSION

Surgical removal of the primary tumour alone had no curative effect in the highly metastatic ESb 289 system: within 30 days after tumour transplant 100% of the animals died of disseminated visceral metastases (Table 1). However, under optimal post-operative immunotherapy conditions 55% of the animals survived at least 60 days after tumour transplant (group 6). Furthermore, the overall survival depended on the time of surgery during tumour progression and on the concentration of virus given (data not shown).

Table 1. Antimetastatic therapy by xenogenization with Newcastle Disease Virus (NDV); data of two independent experiments.

Group	day 0	day 7	therapy	survivors
1	ESb i. d.	–	–	0/16
2	"	surgery	–	0/16
3	"	"	ESb ⇃	0/14
4	"	"	– NDV	3/14
5	"	"	ESb ⇃ + NDV	6/18
6	"+NDV Day 2	"	ESb ⇃ + NDV	16/30

Animals which had survived ESb/NDV therapy were divided into two groups: one received 5 x 10^4 ESb 289 cells, the other one was inoculated with 5 x 10^4 SL-2 lymphoma cells i. d.. Two groups of normal DBA/2 mice were inoculated in the same way and served as controls. There was not a single ESb tumour take in the ESb-´immune´ animals whereas DBA/2 derived SL-2 lymphoma grew out in all of the animals inoculated with it. Furthermore, all ESb-immune animals survived ESb 289 challenge for at least 120 days whereas nearly all of the control animals died. Thus, the animals which had survived ESb/NDV therapy were in fact immune to a second ESb 289 challenge. There was no curative effect of this therapy protocol in T-cell deficient nu/nu mice and not when using a tumour antigen (TATA) negative variant of ESb (data not shown).

After in vivo immunization of DBA/2 mice with ESb 289 cells the frequency of TATA-specific p-CTL was estimated to be about 1/15,000 after 7 days. By in vivo immunization with NDV-coupled ESb cells and in vitro restimulation with the analogous cells the frequency of ESb-specific p-CTL could be significantly increased to 1/6,500, whereas no clone could be detected, which was specific for NDV antigens. Xenogenization of the antigen-presenting tumour cells did not lead to a loss of specificity.

These in vitro findings suggest an important role of cytotoxic T-lymphocytes in our system. Furthermore, also natural effector mechanisms seem to be effective since we could show that NDV can directly activate peritoneal exudate cells to become tumour cell cytostatic and cytotoxic (data not shown).

Our approach has shown that the concept of viral xenogenization-postoperative-immunotherapy can be successfully applied for a highly metastatic tumour. A lasting immunity could not be achieved in other xenogenization protocols employing herpes simplex virus (Reiss-Gutfreund et al. 1982) or lytic NDV strain Cal (Eaton et al. 1967).

The mechanism of antimetastatic activity in our tumour system requires further elucidation. Natural effector mechanisms could be amplified by stimulation of endogenous interferon synthesis. NDV was shown to activate interferon synthesis in spleen cells and fibroblasts (Ito et al. 1982). The amplification of CTL could also be mediated via activation of T-helper cells, as shown in a Vaccinia virus system (Fujiwara et al. 1984). Thus, in our system both natural and specific effector mechanisms may be contributing to an effective defense against a highly metastatic tumour cell.

Eaton, M. D., Levinthal, J. D. & Scala, A. R., 1967, Journal of the National Cancer Institute, 39 (6), 1089.

Fujiwara, H., Shimuzu, J., Takai, Y., Wakamiya, N. Ueda, S., Kato, S. & Hamaoka, 1984, European Journal of Immunology. 14. 171.

Ito, Y., Nagai, Y. & Maneo, K., 1982, Journal of General Virology, 62, 349.

Kobayashi, H., 1979, Advances in Cancer Research, 30, 279.

Langhorne, J. & Fischer-Lindahl, K. 1981, in: Immunological Methods II, edited by Lefkovits, I. & Pernis, B., (Academic Press), p. 222.

Lefkovits, I., 1979, in: Immunological Methods I, edited by Lefkovits, I. & Pernis, B. (Academic Press), p. 356.

Lotzova, E., Savary, C. A., Freedman, R. S. & Bowen, J. M., 1984, Cancer Immunology and Immunotherapy, 17, 124.

Murray, D.R., Cassel, W.A., Torbin, A. R., Olkowski, Z. L. & Moore, M.E., 1977, Cancer 40, 680.

Reiss-Gutfreund, R. J., Nowotny, N.R., Dostal, V. & Wrba, H., 1982, European Journal of Cancer and Clinical Oncology, 18 (6), 523.

Schirrmacher, V., Fogel, M., Rußmann, E., Bosslet, K., Altevogt, P. & Beck, L., 1982, Cancer Metastasis Reviews, 1, 241.

Schirrmacher, V., Jacobs, W., 1979, Journal of Supramolecular Structures, 11, 105.

Wallack, M. K., Meyer, M., Bourgoin, A.,Dore C., Leftheriotis, E., Carcagne, J. & Koprofski, H., 1983, Journal of Biological Response Modifiers, 2, 586.

A COMPARISON OF THE RESPONSES OF PULMONARY AND SUBCUTANEOUS TUMOURS TO
RADIATION AND CYCLOPHOSPHAMIDE

K.A. SMITH[1], A.C. BEGG[2] AND J. DENEKAMP[1]
[1]Gray Laboratory, Mount Vernon Hospital, Northwood, Middlesex
[2]Netherlands Cancer Institute, Plesmanlaan 121, 1066 CX Amsterdam, The
Netherlands

Keywords : lung metastases, subcutaneous tumours, cyclophosphamide,
          X-irradiation

INTRODUCTION

The response of tumours to treatment aimed at eradicating them can vary
with size or site of growth. The present study was undertaken to compare
the chemosensitivity and radiosensitivity of a tumour growing subcutaneously or as metastatic deposits in the lung. Tumours were treated over a
range of sizes with cyclophosphamide (CY) or X-rays. Graded doses of the
two agents were used to allow dose response curves to be constructed.

MATERIALS & METHODS

The tumour used in these studies was a transplantable anaplastic sarcoma
SaF. It is not immunogenic to the host as determined by an inability to
immunise the host against it. Tumours were implanted subcutaneously by
injecting 10^3 cells in a single cell suspension. At fixed times after
implantation (6,8,10 + 12 days) the mice were either treated with graded
doses of X-rays or CY, or the subcutaneous tumours were excised when they
reached 10 mm to allow lung metastases to develop. The lung tumours were
then treated with X-rays or drug at selected intervals (0,3,6,9 + 12 days)
after surgical excision of the primary.

We have previously shown that excision of the primary at 10 mm leads to
a very high incidence of lung metastases, approaching 100% (Begg & Smith,
1980). Unanaesthetised mice were irradiated locally to the primary tumour,
or locally to the thorax.   240 kV X-rays were used, at a dose rate of 3
Gy min^{-1}. Details of the irradiation arrangements have been published
elsewhere (Sheldon & Hill 1977; Travis et al 1979). After high X-ray
doses (>25 Gy) the animals irradiated to the thorax died at 20-30 days of
oesophageal damage. In order to investigate whether the tumours were well

oxygenated at the time of irradiation the oxygen-mimetic radiosensitizer
misonidazole was used for some of the treatments. This compound sensitizes
only in the absence of oxygen (Adams et al 1976). It was injected i.p.
20-30 minutes before irradiation at a dose of 0.67 or 0.8 mg g^{-1}.

The mice treated with CY were injected i.p. with graded doses, from 40
to 230 mg kg^{-1}.

Tumour response was assessed in terms of growth delay or local control
(in the subcutaneous site), or as cure of the animal (for the multiple lung
metastases). The growth of subcutaneous tumours was assessed by twice
weekly caliper measurements. The time taken to reach 6 mm mean diameter
was used. The presence or absence of lung metastases was determined at
sacrifice, either at 70 days or when mice were sacrificed at the first sign
of respiratory distress.

RESULTS

Figures 1 & 2 show the response of animals treated with X-rays or CY to
the primary tumours. Figure 1 shows the response at 6, 8 or 10 days to

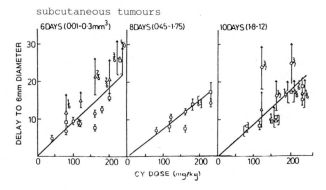

Figure 1. Delay in growth of subcutaneous SaF tumours treated with CY.

graded doses of CY up to the maximum tolerated dose of 230 mg kg^{-1}. The
symbols result from three separate experiments, with 6-8 animals in each
group. In all groups a significant growth delay was seen. Upward arrows
indicate that some tumours were locally controlled - these animals have
been included in this analysis by allotting them an arbitrary time for
regrowth, corresponding to the latest time at which a tumour has been seen
to regrow after any treatment (55 days). There is no detectable difference
in the chemosensitivity of the subcutaneous tumours over the size range
investigated.

Figure 2 shows growth delay data for subcutaneous tumours treated with
X-rays 6 days after implantation (at volumes of 0.3 - 0.4 mm^3). Data are

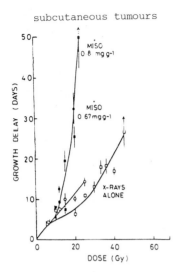

Figure 2. Growth delay induced by irradiation of subcutaneous SaF tumours 6 days after inoculation.

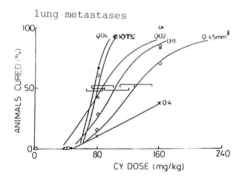

Figure 3. Response of mice bearing multiple pulmonary metastases to CY.

shown from two separate experiments, local control was achieved only at the higher doses. The animals irradiated after receiving misonidazole were much more sensitive than those given X-rays alone, indicating the presence of a large proportion of hypoxic cells in these tumours. A similar displacement of the 2 curves was seen for tumours treated at 12 days (data not shown).

Figures 3 and 4 show the response of the multiple pulmonary metastases to CY or X-rays. The percentage of animals cured of all tumour is plotted against CY or X-ray dose. In Figure 3 data are shown for tumours treated 0-12 days after excision of the primary. The mean tumour volume (determined by sacrificing a sample group at each time is indicated agaist each curve. As expected, the dose of CY needed to cure 50% of animals (TCD50) increased as the mean tumour volume at treatment increased; an increase in the indicated SEM and the shallower slope reflects the greater heterogeneity of response at later times after seeding.

Figure 4 shows the response to X-rays of mice bearing lung metastases treated 6 or 12 days after excising the primary tumour. The two symbols represent two experiments and the closed and open symbols are for mice treated with or without misonidazole. No measurable sensitization by misonidazole was seen in metastases treated at 6 days. This indicates that all the tumour cells at this stage were well oxygenated and radiosensitive. By 12 days the response was much more variable in the two experiments and there was a clear sensitization in both by the addition of miso. The X-ray doses were limited to 20-25 Gy because at higher doses the mice did not survive long enough to determine whether all tumour cells had been eradicated.

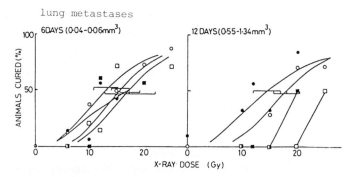

Figure 4. Response of mice with multiple lung metastases to X-rays alone (open symbols) or X-rays + misonidazole (closed symbols).

DISCUSSION

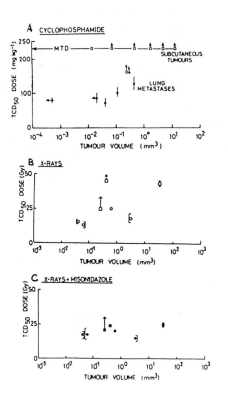

Figure 5. Response of SaF tumours treated as subcutaneous implants or as naturally seeded lung metastases. The dose needed to cure half the animals is plotted as a function of tumour size.

These results show a difference in chemo- and radio- sensitivity with both size and site. The conclusions are summarised in Figure 5. Panel 5A shows the very marked difference in sensitivity to CY at the two sites. For the subcutaneous tumours, it was impossible to achieve any local control or cure with the maximum tolerated dose of the drug over the size range 0.01 - 12 mm^3. By contrast, with non-toxic drug doses, local control was easily achieved in the lung metastases, particularly over the size range 0.001 - 0.1 mm^3. Panel B shows the response to X-rays alone, and again there is an indication of more resistance in the subcutaneous tumours over equivalent size ranges. This difference between the two sites is reduced when misonidazole is added (Panel C), indicating that the difference in sensitivity is mainly a result of the poorer oxygenation of the subcutaneous tumours. The hypoxia, or other associated nutritional deficiences seem to have an even more marked effect on the chemosensitivity than on the radiosensitivity (cf panel A). Other aspects of the vasculature are currently under study at both sites over a variety of tumour sizes in order to investigate the causes of these alterations of radio and chemosensitivity.

REFERENCES

Adams, G.E., Flockhart, I.R., Smithen, C.E., Stratford, I.J., Wardman, P., & Watts, M.E., 1976, Radiation Research 67, 9.

Begg, A.C., 1980, Comparison of natural and artificial lung metastases from a murine tumour of spontaneous origin. In Metastasis: Experimental and Clinical Aspects, edited by K. Hellman, P. Hilgard and S.A. Eccles. (Martinus Nijhoff).

Sheldon, P.W. & Hill, S.A., 1977, British Journal of Cancer 35, 995.

Travis, E.L., Vojnovic, B., Davies, F.E., & Hirst, D.G., 1979, British Journal of Radiology, 52, 67.

COMPARATIVE STUDY OF THE CHEMO-SENSITIVITY OF DIFFERENTLY METASTASIZING LLT LINES

KATALIN PAL, J. TIMAR, L. KOPPER and K. LAPIS
1. Institute of Pathology and Experimental Cancer Research, Semmelweis Medical University, Budapest, Hungary

Keywords: Liver metastasis; HUdR; Immunoresistance; Chemosensitivity

INTRODUCTION

A tumour line (LLT-HH) with increased metastatic capacity was developed from liver metastases (Kopper & Lapis, 1982) which appeared after intrasplenic transplantation of LLT cells (Pal et al. 1983a). Comparative studies of the parent (LLT) and selected (LLT-HH) cells showed no differences in growth rate, or cell kinetic parameters between the two lines. We examined aspects of tumour cell - host cell interactions and found a decrease in the sensitivity of LLT-HH cells to macrophages and NK cells (Pal et al. 1984) and the loss of intracellular junctions between LLT-HH / macrophages and LLT-HH / endothelial cells (Timar et al. 1983). It is probable that these functional changes are dependent on the changes in the cell surface of metastatic cells (Nicolson, 1982, Barnett & Eccles, 1984). In this model we detected the following changes in the cell surface: increased GAG content (Timar et al. 1982), increased sialic acid content (Furesz et al. 1983), increased galactose/galactosamine and mannose/glucosamine expression.

In the experiments described here we examined the comparative chemo-sensitivity of LLT and LLT-HH cells, attempting to find a metastasis-specific agent against the highly metastatic cells.

Materials and Methods

Throughout the study inbred C57/BL mice were used from our institute colony. LLT (Lewis lung tumour) was maintained by intramuscular (hind leg), while LLT-HH / selected line with increased metastatic capacity / by intrasplenic transplantation (Pal et al. 1983). The number of liver metastases was counted under a stereomicroscope.

The drugs used were as follows:

Cyclophosphamide; ASTA; 5-Hexyl-2-desoxyuridine; synthesized in the Institute for Central Chemical Research of the Hungarian Academy of Science, Budapest, Hungary.

Results

Earlier we demonstrated in the muscle-lung 3LL metastasis model (Szabo et al. 1980) and spleen-liver metastasis model (Pal et al. 1983b) that cyclophosphamide was the most effective chemotherapeutic agent against the LLT tumour cells. We examined the cyclophosphamide sensitivity of both LLT and LLT-HH cells in the spleen-liver metastasis model. We did not observe differences in respect to cyclophosphamide sensitivity between the LLT and LLT-HH cells (Table 1).

Table 1. Effect of cyclophosphamide on the growth of LLT and LLT-HH[+].

Tumour line	Number of cells[+]	Group	Evaluation (day)	Number of liver metastases	P
LLT	10^5	CO	11	12.5 ± 14.1	
		CY[++]	11	0.7 ± 1.5	<0.05
LLT	5×10^5	CO	12	48.0 ± 32.31	
		CY	12	2.40 ± 3.36	<0.05
LLT-HH (p.42)	10^3	CO	15	39.3 ± 7.3	
		CY	15	3.0 ± 2.3	<0.05
LLT-HH (p.62)	3×10^3	CO	11	79.4 ± 48.7	
		CY	11	6.6 ± 10.1	<0.05

+ Transplanted intrasplenically
++ Given I.P., 60 mg/kg^{-1}

According to earlier experiments (Lapis et al. 1982) HUdR inhibits galactosyl transferase and this inhibition may be causing changes in the cell surface GAG, glycoproteins, sialic acid which are characteristic of the LLT-HH cell line.

On the basis of these observations we examined the chemo-sensitivity of LLT and LLT-HH cells to hexyldesoxyuridine. This agent only inhibited the metastases of LLT-HH in 4 x 75 mg/kg doses, the metastases of LLT cells were resistant to the treatment (Table 2). Further experiments with 5-hexyl-2-desoxyuridine showed that the treatment was more effective if carried out as soon as possible after tumour cell transplantation and if repeated several times.

Table 2. Effect of hexyldesoxyuridine on the number of liver metastases[+].

Line	Number of cells	Group	Dose mg/kg	Day of treatment	Number of liver metastases	P
LLT[++]	5×10^5	CO			34.7 ± 29.0	
		HUdR	4 x 75	4.5.6.7.	47.7 ± 30.2	n.s.
LLT-HH[++] (p.75)	3×10^3	CO			66.2 ± 53.6	
		HUdR	4 x 75	4.5.6.7.	6.1 ± 10.1	<0.05
LLT[++]	5×10^5	CO			48.0 ± 32.3	
		HUdR	4 x 75	4.5.6.7.	77.0 ± 12.4	<0.05
LLT-HH[+++] (p.92)	10^5	CO			115.0 ± 15.6	
		HUdR	4 x 75	4.5.6.7.	84.4 ± 27.0	<0.05

+   Splenectomy was performed 3 days after transplantation

++   Evaluation was on day 12

+++ Evaluation was on day 8

Examining the properties of HUdR-treated LLT-HH cells it was found that a) the in vivo clonogenicity of LLT-HH cells decreased; b) macrophage resistant LLT-HH cells became macrophage sensitive; c) WGA-binding glucosamine receptors on the cell membrane decreased.

We propose that the specific therapeutic effect of HUdR can be
explained by differences in the cell surfaces of LLT-HH and LLT cells and
by supposing that the treatment changes those cell surfaces parameters
which are responsible for the increased metastatic capacity. This theory
is supported by Rieber & Castillo (1984), who studied the effect of
bromodeoxyuridine on the membrane of B16 metastatic variants.
Nevertheless, further studies are necessary in this regard.

REFERENCES

Barnett, S.C., Eccles, S.A., 1984, Clinical and Experimental Metastasis,
    2; in press.
Furesz, J., Budavary, F., Pal, K., Timar, J., Lapis, K., 1983, Joint
    Congress of ETCS and EURES.
Kopper, L., Lapis, K., 1982, Tumour Progression and Markers. Editors:
    K. Lapis, A. Jeney, M.R. Price, Kugler, Amsterdam. p. 265.
Lapis, K., Jeney, A., Timar, J., Ecsedi, G., Hidvegi, E., Kopper, L., 1982,
    73rd Annual Meeting American Assocation of Cancer Research.
Nicolson, G.L., 1982, Invasion and Metastasis. Editors: L.A. Liotta,
    I.R. Hart, Martinus Nijhoff, The Hague.
Pal, K., Kopper, L., Lapis, K., 1983a, Invasion and Metastasis 3: 174.
Pal, K., Kopper, L., Lapis, K., 1983b, Clinical and Experimental Metastasis
    1: 341.
Pal, K., Kopper, L., Csaszar, A., Timar, J., Rajnai, G., Lapis, K., 1984,
    Invasion and Metastasis (accepted for publication).
Rieber, M., Castillo, M.A., 1984, International Journal of Cancer 33: 765.
Szabo, Zs., Dworak, O., Kopper, L., Lapis, K., 1980, Journal of Cancer
    Research and Clinical Oncology 97: 161.
Timar, J., Kopper, L., Pal, K., Lapis, K., 1983, Pathological Research and
    Practice 177: 47.

MULTIPLE EFFECTS OF NITROSOUREA TREATMENT ARE ASSOCIATED WITH THE AMPLIFICATION OF LUNG METASTASES OF A RAT SARCOMA

C. PAUWELS[1], M.F. POUPON[1], D. NOLIBE[2], E. ANTOINE[1]

[1]IRSC-CNRS, ER 278, BP 8, 94802 Villejuif Cedex, France

[2]CEA, Lab. des Transuraniens, BP 12, Bruyeres Le Chatel, France

Keywords: metastasis, clonogenicity, selection, immunodepression

INTRODUCTION

Nitrosoureas have demonstrated their antimitotic efficiency against a large panel of animal tumors (Goldin, 1981; Imbach, 1981), but repeated observations in our laboratory (Poupon, 1984) showed that chloronitrosourea treatment increased pulmonary metastasis of a rat nickel-induced rhabdomyosarcoma (RMS) while decreasing local tumor growth. We have questioned whether nitrosoureas directly influence tumor cell population growth, selects a more metastatic type of tumor cell, or decreases the natural immune defense of the host, using a water-soluble chloronitrosourea, chlorozotocin.

MATERIALS AND METHODS

Animals: 10-12 weeks old WAG rats from the Institut de Recherches scientifiques sur le Cancer were used and maintained in SPF conditions.

Tumors: induced by s.c. injection of 5×10^4 (9-4/0) cells derived from a primary nickel-induced rhabdomyosarcoma. These cells were maintained in a continuous line in RPMI 1640 supplemented with 10% FCS.

Metastatic dissemination : measured at autopsy when rats were moribund. Tumor nodules at the surface of the lung were counted and their origin confirmed by histology.

Clonogenic assay : 2.5 ml of 0.5% agar (Bacto-Agar, Difco) in RPMI 1640 containing 10% FCS constituted the lower layer. Cells were suspended in a plating layer (1 ml) of 0.3% agar in RPMI 1640 + 10% FCS and applied over the basal layer.

Drugs : Adriamycin :adriblastin of Roger Bellon(France). Chlorozotocin (CZT) : (2-3 (2-chloroethyl)-3 nitrosoureido D-glycopyranose) were used at doses indicated.

Assay for natural cytotoxicity : ^{51}Cr labelled tumor cells were placed in contact with effector cells (lung intracapillary cells) in microtest plates and ^{51}Cr release was assayed after four hours.

Quantitative analysis of in vivo tumor cell arrest and survival :
^{125}IUDR-labelled tumor cells were inoculated i.v. (10^{6} cells per rat),
viable tumor cells in the lungs were determined 24 hours after inoculation
(Fidler, 1970).

RESULTS

Effect of chlorozotocin on tumor growth and metastasis

Chlorozotocin (CZT), given at 10 mg/kg/b.w., weekly for five weeks to
rats bearing a transplanted RMS decreased their survival time, slowed the
local tumor growth rate, decreased the frequency of lymph node invasion,
but enhanced lung metastasis (Table 1).   Other treatments consisting of
one injection of Adriamycin or five lower doses of CZT reduced lung metastasis,
concomitant with a slowing of local tumor growth.

Table 1. Effect of CZT on growth and metastasis of RMS 9-4/0.

	Tumor size* (mm ± SD)	No. of lung nodules± SD	No. rats with lymph node metastases	Survival times (days) ± SD
Physiological saline 5 doses	35 ± 3	16 ± 9	10/10	60 ± 4
CZT 5 doses of 10 mg/kg	23 ± 1	120 ± 25 ($p < 0.01$)	7/10	49 ± 3
CZT 5 doses of 1 mg/kg	31 ± 2	12 ± 4 (NS)	10/10	40 ± 2
Adriamycin 1 dose of 10 mg/kg	22 ± 4	2 ± 1 ($p < 0.01$)	9/10	65 ± 3

p : probability of no difference determined by Wilcoxon's test
NS: not significant. * : tumor size : mean diameters (mm + SD)

Increase of cloning efficiency of tumor cells by CZT in vitro treatment

Salmon's assay (Salmon, 1978) was applied to tumor cells derived from
a series of 7 rat nickel-induced RMS. CZT or adriamycin doses used were in
the range of plasma concentrations obtained after in vivo treatment. The
cloning efficiency of all tumor cells was increased by their incubation with
CZT, while it was decreased by adriamycin. For example, the cloning
efficiency of 46-2 RMS cells was increased from 0.6% to 1.25%, following
1 hour incubation with 0.4 ug/ml CZT. Under the same conditions, ADR
completely prevented the growth of colonies.

Selection by cloning of tumor cell sublines resistant to CZT

Sublines derived from cell colonies grown in agar after incubation with 0.4 mgm/ml CZT, acquired new characteristics. The most surprising was the loss of tumorigenicity of cells grafted into syngeneic rats after 7 CZT selections, while their cloning efficiency was unchanged. This was maintained in further clonings (Table 2).

Table 2. Cloning efficiency : effect of CZT and ADR on cell lines selected by cloning and contact with CZT

No. of clonings in agar with CZT (0.4 ug/ml)	C.E. (%) Control	C.E. (%) with ADR	CZT	Tumorigenicity*
Parental 9-4/0	4.6 ± 0.06	0	5.7 ± 0.1	100%
1	2.7 ± 0.03	–	3.0 ± 0.09	100%
3	2.8 ± 0.05	0	3.8 ± 0.06	–
5	2.6 ± 0.07	0	3.5 ± 0.07	100%
7	2.3 ± 0.04	–	3.5 ± 0.10	0%
8	2.5 ± 0.07	–	3.1 ± 0.08	–
9	2.8 ± 0.12	0	4.0 ± 0.10	0%

C.E. : cloning efficiency. * : 10^6 cells were s.c. injected to 10 rats

Effect of CZT treatment on natural immune defenses of the host

NK lymphocytes are especially numerous in the blood capillary compartment of the lungs (Nolibe, 1981). We observed a decrease in LIC NK cytotoxicity in CZT pretreated rats 24 hours after the last CZT injection, with an incomplete return to normal values after 15 days (Table 3).

Table 3. Effects of CZT on the NK cytotoxicity of lung intracapillary cells (LIC).

CZT treatment	Mean ± SE % cytotoxicity		
	50:1	25:1	12.5:1
Untreated	17.2 ± 1.0	12.3 ± 0.6	7.6 ± 0.8
5 doses of CZT, the last at d-1*	3.1 ± 1.0	2.7 ± 0.7	2.4 ± 0.6
the last at d-15	9.3 ± 1.1	8.0 ± 1.2	6.4 ± 0.3

* Day 0 corresponds to the day of LIC NK activity measurement

In parallel, groups of CZT-treated rats received ^{125}IUDR labelled tumor cells i.v. in order to measure their ability to destroy these cells. With an interval of 24 hours between the last CZT injection and that of the radioactive cells, the lungs of 6/10 rats showed a high count of radioactivity, demonstrating their inability to prevent the implantation of tumor cells.

Table 4. Effect of chlorozotocin treatment of rats on survival of i.v. inoculated [125] IUDR labelled tumor cells in lung.

Group of rats	No. of rats* per group		lung-associated radioactivity 1 day after cell injection	p
Untreated	20		639 ± 38	
Five doses of CZT, the last at d-8*	10		106,612 ± 29,290	0.001
Five doses of CZT, the last at d-1	10	(6)	90,039 ± 19,942	0.001
		(4)	480 ± 33	NS

* Day 0 corresponds to the day of i.v. labelled target cell injection.

DISCUSSION

Increase in pulmonary metastasis after chemotherapeutic treatment is not a new phenomenon; other authors have described such an effect (Milas 1979, van Putten 1975) but no explanation was advanced.

The increase in cloning efficiency seen when RMS cells were incubated with CZT seemed to mimic the in vivo observations, but in vitro selection resulted in a non-tumorigenic line. The amplification of plating efficiency is an original observation which could reflect the selection of more clonogenic cell populations. In vivo selection procedures (not shown) yielded subsets of cells with a more restricted modal number of chromosomes which may have survival advantages.

We also showed that lung intra-capillary NK activity was decreased by CZT, and this may have contributed to the enhanced tumor cell survival in the lungs; however, other events could be implicated in this phenomenon; e.g. damage to lung tissue could directly facilitate implantation of tumor cells.

In conclusion, CZT was shown to influence a variety of tumors and host cell functions, each of which, alone or in combination with others could constitute to the drug-induced enhancement of lung metastases.

REFERENCES

Fidler, I.J., 1970, Journal of the National Cancer Institute, 45, 773.
Goldin, A., 1981, In: Nitrosoureas in Cancer Treatment (Serrou, B., Schein P.S. & Imbach J.L., eds) Amsterdam, Elsevier/North Holland.
Imbach, J.L., Martinez, J., Viry J. et al., 1981, In: Nitrosoureas in Cancer Treatment (Serrou B., Schein, P.S. & Imbach, J.L. (eds) Amsterdam, Elsevier/North Holland.
Milas, L., Malenica, B. & Allegretti, N., 1979, Cancer Immunology & Immunotherapy, 6, 191.
Nolib, B., Berel, A., Masse, R., Lafuma, J., 1981, Biomedicine, 35, 230.
Poupon, M.F., Pauwels, C., Jasmin, C. et al., 1984, Cancer Treat. Reports, 68, 749.
Salmon, S.E., Hamburger, A.W., Soehnlen, B.J. et al, 1978, New England Journal of Medicine, 298, 1321.
Van Putten, L.M., Dram, L.K.J., Van Dierendonck, H.M.C. et al., 1979, Cancer Immunology and Immunotherapy, 6, 191.

RELATIONSHIP BETWEEN IN VITRO EFFECTS AND IN VIVO CONTROL OF METASTASIS
INDUCED BY HYDROCORTISONE IN A RAT RHABDOMYOSARCOMA MODEL

M. BECKER[1], E. MOCZAR[2], S. KORACH[1], V. LASCAUX[1] and M.F. POUPON[1]

[1]IRSC-CNRS ER 278, BP 8, 94802 Villejuif, France
[2]Lab. Tissu Conjectif, Faculté de Médecine, 94010 Créteil, France

Keywords: differentiation, ECM components, control of dissemination

INTRODUCTION

Hydrocortisone (HC) induces differentiation when added to the culture
medium of tumor cells derived from a nickel-induced rhabdomyosarcoma (RMS)
of rat. HC given to rats bearing the same RMS during tumor growth and
after surgical ablation prevented metastatic invasion of lungs and lymph
nodes. The corticoids are well known for their immunosuppressive effects.
but this activity did not fit with the observed effects, i.e. prevention of
metastatic spread. We hypothesize therefore that the benefit of HC
treatment could be due to its direct effect on tumor cells. The induction
of differentiation is associated with cellular changes which we analysed.

MATERIALS AND METHODS

Tumors - A rhabdomyosarcoma (RMS) was induced by i.m. injection of nickel
in a Wistar AG rat. The primary tumor was set up in culture, and a parental
cell line named 9-4/0 was derived and cloned as reported by Sweeney, 1982.
Two sublines were used: 8 and 6 which are of low and high metastatic potential respectively. All lines were cultivated in Dulbecco's modified
medium (DMEM).

Animals - 10-14 week old female inbred Wistar AG rats from the Institut
de Recherches Scientifiques sur le Cancer (Villejuif, France) were used.

Fourteen rats per group received a s.c. injection of 10^5 cells from
RMS subline 6. After 2 weeks a tumor appeared at the injection site.
Hydrocortisone (succinate, Roussel Lab., France) was started on day 21,
added to the drinking water at 25 mg/100 ml in 0.1% alcohol. Daily HC
absorption corresponded on average to 15 mg/kg b.w. Tumors were surgically
excised under barbiturate anaesthesia at 15 mm diameter. HC treatment was
given until the 12th week, then progressively diminished. Autopsies were
done when the rats had respiratory distress. Cured rats were killed and
autopsied at the 16th week.

RESULTS

Effects of HC treatment of rats on metastatic invasion

     HC treatment of rats reduced the number of metastases on the surface of the lungs (table 1). The invasion of axillary or inguinal lymph nodes was delayed and the incidence decreased. At autopsy the para-aortic lymph nodes were less frequently invaded (1/14 versus 7/14 in the control).

Table 1. Effect of HC treatment on pulmonary metastasis from a RMS.

Treatment	Individual counts of lung tumor nodules	Median	P
HC 15 mg/kg	0, 0, 0, 0, 1, 3, 4, 6 10, 15, 21, 31, 31, 42, 62	8	0.001
Control	0, 0, 4, 4, 28, 41, 66 70, 72, 72, 95, 112, 118, 157	68	

Effect of HC on tumor cell proliferation and differentiation in vitro

     Proliferation of lines 9-4/0 and 6 were strongly inhibited by HC, while subline 8 was less affected (Table 2). Differentiation occurred as evidenced by the presence of multinuclear myotubes, resulting from the somatic fusion of several cells (Figure 1b), these structures were rare in untreated cells (Fig. 1a).

Table 2. HC-induced changes in the doubling time of three cell lines.

	Doubling times (hours)	
Lines	Untreated cells	Hydrocortisone-treated cells (0.1 µg/ml)
9-4/0	24	33
subline 8	26	30
subline 6	25	36

5×10^4 cells were seeded in 6 cm Falcon Petri dishes, cultivated in 5 ml 10% FCS supplemented D-MEM, for 5 days in 5% CO_2/air atmosphere.

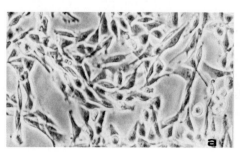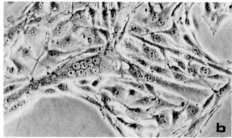

Figure 1. Morphology of tumor cells in culture. a: control; b: with HC

Increased resistance of HC treated cells to natural killer lymphocytes

9-4/0 cells cultivated for 3 days in the presence or absence of HC were labelled with ^{51}Cr (Poupon 1983). HC treated cells were more resistant to NK mediated lysis than untreated tumor cells (table 3).

Table 3. Decreased susceptibility of HC pretreated 9-4/0 tumor cells to the spontaneous lytic activity mediated by splenic lymphocytes

% of lysis	Splenic lymphocytes to tumor cell ratio			
	25	50	100	200
HC treated cells	8 ± 1*	12 ± 1	17 ± 4	28 ± 2
Untreated cells	7 ± 1	20 ± 4	37 ± 1	51 ± 4
p	NS	0.03	0.001	0.002

* mean of triplicates ± standard deviation. ^{51}Cr labelled tumor cells were incubated for 5 hr with lymphocytes. The results are expressed as percent of released radioactivity in wells containing lymphocytes.

Enrichment of glycoprotein and proteoglycan fractions of cell surface components after in vitro HC treatment of cells

9-4/0 cells cultured with or without HC were labelled with ^{3}H-gluco-samine and ^{35}S sulfate. After 5 days the cell surface components were successively extracted by heparin (100 ug/ml) and then by trypsin (2.5 ug/ml). The glycosaminoglycans (GAG) were assayed as described by Wasteson (1973) digested by pronase, and precipitated by cetylpyridinimum chloride (CPC). The glycoproteins and proteoglycans were precipitated by trichloracetic acid (TCA). Subtraction of the radioactive value corresponding to the CPC precipitate (proteoglycan) from the TCA precipitate allowed an evaluation of the glycoprotein content. As shown in table 4, HC treatment of 9-4/0 cells induced an increase of pericellular glycoproteins in the heparin extract, and an increase of proteoglycans, namely heparin and chondroitin sulfates in the trypsin extract. Hyaluronic acid content did not appear to be changed

Table 4. Cell surface glycoproteins and proteoglycans expressed by 9-4/0 cells and its weakly metastatic subline, with or without HC treatment.

Lines		cpm per 10^5 cells	
		HC-treated	untreated
	Glycoproteins	12.000*	5.400
Line 9-4/0	Chondroitin sulfate	5.800	2.300
	Heparan sulfate	5.700	2.000
	Glycoproteins	12.500	13.500
Subline 8	Chondroitin sulfate	8.000	11.000
	Heparan sulfate	5.800	6.000

*the standard deviations did not exceed 10% of the values

DISCUSSION

We show here that hydrocortisone induces tumor cell differentiation (as noted by Furcht, 1979) and decreases metastatic spread. These facts suggest that the degree of differentiation and metastatic capacity are inversely related. The more advanced differentiation of HC treated tumor cells was demonstrated by the presence of typical myotubes, and also by their increased resistance to NK lysis as previously reported (Gidland 1980). The increased cell surface content of heparan and chondroitin sulfates and glycoproteins induced by HC could be due to their increased synthesis or decreased degradation. Highly metastatic cells are capable of degrading extracellular matrix components, (Kramer, 1982) and the loss of this facility under HC treatment could explain the increase in cell surface components, and also their reduced invasive capacity.

In conclusion, it appears that the differentiation of certain tumor cells might be usefully modified and may provide a novel approach to the treatment of metastasis.

REFERENCES

Furcht, L.T., Mosher, D.F., Wendelschafer-Crabb, G. et al., 1979, Cancer Research, 39, 2077.
Gidland, M., Orn, A., Pattengale, P.K. et al., 1980, Nature (London), 292, 848.
Kramer, R.M., Vogel, K.G., Nicolson, G.L., 1982, Journal of Biology Chemistry, 257, 2678.
Poupon, M.F., Judde, J., Pot-Deprun J., et al., 1983, British Journal of Cancer, 48, 75.
Sweeney, F.L., Pot-Deprun, J., Poupon, M.F. et al., 1982, Cancer Research, 42, 3775.
Wasteson, A., Uthne, K. and Westermark, 1973, Biochemical Journal, 136, 1069.

THE EFFECT OF RADIATION DOSE AND EXCISION DELAY ON LMC$_I$ TUMOUR METASTASIS
IN THE RAT

B. DIXON and D. A. BAGNALL
Radiobiology Department, Regional Radiotherapy Centre, Leeds LS16 6QB

Keywords: Metastasis, Radiation, Surgery, Rat

INTRODUCTION

Chemotherapy is often immunosuppressive (Harris et al 1976) and also
may enhance the entrapment of surviving clonogenic cells in host tissues
(Milas & Peters 1984). Neither of these effects should occur with non-
immunogenic tumours when locally irradiated and changes in the incidence of
metastases after delayed surgery should reflect only the further spread of
cells and development of metastases in unaltered host tissues. The TD$_{50}$
for the LMC$_I$ tumour is 12 ± 2 cells (Speakman & Dixon 1981) and is not
increased in "immunised" hosts. Thus the purpose of the experiments
reported in this study of the LMC$_I$ tumour was to determine if further
seeding and the latency of metastases is restored but not enhanced by local
irradiation.

MATERIALS AND METHODS

Isologous female 180-200g Wistar rats with primary tumours growing subcutaneously in the flank, transplanted by the method of Thomlinson (Dixon
& Speakman 1979), were anaesthetized   with 40 MgKg^{-1} sodium amylobarbitone
and their 8-10 mm tumours were locally irradiated with single doses of ^{60}Co
γ-rays (Table 1). Their tumours were then excised 0-30 days later (11-12
per group, Table 1), thereafter scoring animals daily (0-3 months) or
weekly (3-5 months) measuring all superficial metastases that appeared.
All tumour-positive animals were examined for further metastases at post-
mortem. All tumour-negative animals were kept for a 150 days or more after
primary tumour irradiation.

Table 1.   Excision times and radiation doses used.

RT (Gy)	Day and Size (mm) of Irradiated Tumour Excised							
	0	2	5	9	16	20	25	30
0	9±1	13±1	17±1	22±3	-	-	-	-
10	9±1	10±2	11±1	13±1	18±3	-	30±2	-
20	9±1	10±1	11±1	11±1	11±2	-	18±3	23±2
40	9±1	10±1	10±1	10±2	10±2	11±2	12±5	17±3

RESULTS

Primary tumours _in situ_ were progressively delayed in growth with increasing dose of irradiation. After 10 Gy, normal growth was only restored after 6 days, and no significant growth occurred for 14 and 18 days after 20 Gy and 40 Gy respectively (Figure 1).

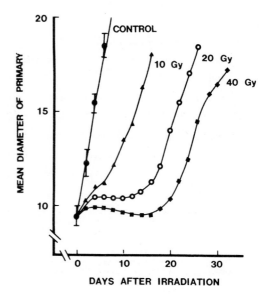

Figure 1.   The Response of the Primary Tumour to Irradiation.

After "early" (i.e. 0-9 day) excisions there was a dose dependant and significant reduction in the overall incidence of metastases (Figure 2) and in the mean number of metastases per affected animal (Table 2). With progressive delay in surgery the percentage of animals with metastases increased (Figure 2) and, in onset, this increase coincided with the restoration in growth of the primary tumour (Figure 1). Also there was no significant reduction in the mean number of metastases per affected animal (Table 2).

The latency (T_{8-10}) of metastases after the early excision of irradiated tumours was increased by 10-14 days and their incidence, except in

the mediastinum was significantly reduced (Table 3). However further delay
in the excision of irradiated tumours did not increase the mean T_{8-10} and
their incidence at each site was the same as after the excision of unirradiated tumours (Table 3). Also the further growth of metastases at all
sites (superficial, abdominal and mediastinal)was characteristic of the
LMC_I tumour (data not shown).

Table 2. Incidence of Metastases After Early or Late Excisions.

	0 - 9 Day Excisions			16 - 30 Day Excisions		
Gy to Primary	Number Excised	% with Mets	Mets/ +ve Rat	Number Excised	% with Mets	Mets/ +ve Rat
0	47	75±6	2.3±0.2	-	-	-
10	47	53±7	2.2±0.2	18	100	2.5±0.3
20	48	40±7	1.6±0.3	25	92±5	2.3±0.3
40	45	55±8	1.3±0.2	52	69±6	2.2±0.2

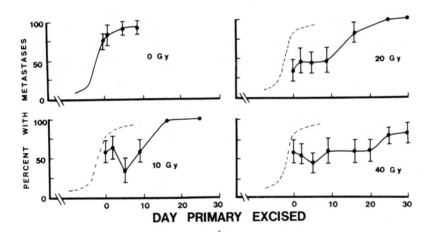

Figure 2. Metastasis and Delay in Surgery after Irradiation.
Control curve ex Dixon and Speakman (1979). All other data
this study.

Table 3. Latency and Incidence of Metastases by Site. (T_{8-10} in Days)

Site of Met	Control Surgery (0-9 Days n = 47)		Radiation plus Surgery			
			(0-9 days, n = 139)		(16-30 days, n = 95)	
	T_{8-10}	%	T_{8-10}	%	T_{8-10}	%
'Muscle'	18±8	26±6	31±5	9±2	36±6	22±4
Inguinal	26±10	28±7	37±12	12±3	44±7	24±4
Aortic	30±12	43±7	40±8	19±6	37±9	41±5
Axilla	38±11	40±7	52±12	22±4	45±8	41±5
Adrenal	50±15	9±4	46±21	4±2	48±14	16±4
Mediast.	52±17	26±6	62±11	19±3	56±10	37±5

DISCUSSION

Whereas cyclophosphamide eliminates all occult metastases (Speakman & Dixon 1981), this was not expected and did not occur after radiotherapy (Figure 2 and Table 2). Nevertheless after early excisions, reductions in the incidence of metastasis positive rats, and in the number of metastases per rat occurred (Table 2), together with an increase in latency (Table 3). These effects may be due to reduced numbers and viability of cells spread by surgery. Tumours removed within 9 days were smaller than in control animals (Table 1) and after 20-40 Gy the fraction of clonogenic cells is reduced by $10^{-3}- 10^{-4}$ (Moore 1976).

Accepting 50% as the real pretreatment level of occult metastases, (Figure 2 and Table 2), then the increase in tumour positive rats and the number of positive sites with delayed surgery may only be attributed to re-seeding occurring after irradiation. However, the distribution of positive sites is the same as after surgery alone, and no further increase in latency was detected (Table 3). Also their growth was the same as the un-irradiated primary tumour and its metastases (Dixon & Speakman 1979). Contrary to the view of Von Essen and Stjernsward (1978) the data thus support the conclusion that primary tumour irradiation only delays further spread of metastases. When regrowth occurs the metastatic process, in all other aspects continues unchanged.

REFERENCES

Dixon, B. & Speakman, H., 1979, Local recurrence and metastasis of excised breast carcinoma in the rat. Journal of the Royal Society of Medicine, 72, 572.

Harris, J., Sengor, D., Stewart, T. & Hyslop, D., 1976, The effect of immunosuppressive chemotherapy on immune function in patients with malignant disease. Cancer N.Y. 37, 1058.

Milas, L., Peters, L. J., 1984, Conditioning of tissues for metastasis formation by radiation and cytotoxic drugs. In Cancer Invasion and Metastasis: Biologic and Therapeutic Aspects, Edited by G. L. Nicolson and L. Milas (Raven Press - New York), p. 321.

Moore, J. V., 1976, The response of a rat mammory tumour to cyclophos-phamide and to subsequent irradiation. Ph.D. Thesis. University of Leeds.

Speakman, H. & Dixon, B., 1981, An experimental approach to chemotherapy for occult metastases: a quantitative model. European Journal of Cancer and Clinical Oncology, 17, 1287.

Von Essen, C. F. & Stjernsward, J., 1978, Radiotherapy and metastases. In Secondary Spread of Cancer, edited by R. W. Baldwin. (Academic Press - London), p. 73.

ORGAN DISTRIBUTION OF METASTASES FOLLOWING INJECTION OF SYNGENEIC RAT
TUMOUR CELLS INTO THE ARTERIAL CIRCULATION VIA THE LEFT VENTRICLE

P. MURPHY, I. TAYLOR and P. ALEXANDER
Depts of Surgery and Medical Oncology, University of Southampton
Southampton General Hospital, Southampton SO9 4XY

Keywords: Adrenal, Brown Fat, Intra-cardiac

INTRODUCTION

The factors that determine which organs develop metastases once
tumour cells have entered the arterial system are not known. To study
this question, the cells from three chemically induced rat tumours, a
sarcoma, an oestrogen dependent breast carcinoma and a hepatoma were injected into the left ventricles of syngeneic hooded Lister rats, and human
melanoma cells into rats immunosuppressed with Cyclosporin A. Unlabelled
cells were given to determine metastatic pattern, radiolabelled cells
to determine distribution and trapping of the tumour cells in the
different organs and radiolabelled Cobalt 57 microspheres to determine
both the percentage distribution of cardiac output and the relative
vascularity of the rat organs.

METHOD

Cell preparation: The tumours were maintained for four to five
passages as subcutaneous transplants after which they were re-established
from frozen stocks. The sarcoma and hepatoma were cultured for 36 hours
and the cells removed from the flasks by incubating with protease for 15
minutes before being washed and injected as a single cell suspension.
These cells were radiolabelled by the addition of 125-Iodeoxyuridine for
the last 24 hours of incubation. The breast carcinoma and human melanoma
were injected without culturing.

Injections: Cells or microspheres were injected through fine
cannulae, passed into the left ventricle via the right carotid artery.

191

RESULTS

Tumour cell distribution: Radiolabelled tumour cells were distributed
amongst the organs in approximately the same ratio as the proportion of
cardiac output received. The exception being lung and liver in which the
proportion of radiolabelled cells was much greater than cardiac output
received. This discrepancy arises because approximately one third of the
cells delivered to muscle, gut etc. are not retained, but traverse these
capillary beds and enter the venous circulation where they are trapped in
lung and liver. (A proportion of the radioactivity found in the liver
stems from cell debris cleared by the reticulo-endothelial system). There
is no evidence for recirculation of tumour cells from measurements of cell
distribution between 0 minutes and 24 hours. (See Table 1).

Table 1. Distribution of Cells Injected into the Left Ventricle.

ORGANS	% DISTRIBUTION OF CARDIAC OUT-PUT.	% DISTRIBUTION OF LABELLED SARCOMA CELLS AT 5 MINUTES	RELATIVE VASCU-LARITY (% CARDIAC OUTPUT/ORGAN/ WEIGHT
Muscle/Bone	37 ± 7	24.7 ± 6.8	0.6 ± 0.1
Kidneys	14.8 ± 4.7	9 ± 2.8	18.2 ± 4.8
Skin	12.5 ± 2.4	6.8 ± 3.5	0.4 ± 0.1
Heart	8.3 ± 3.4	5.8 ± 2	23.5 ± 9.2
Brown Fat	5.1 ± 2.1	5.8 ± 2.8	9.2 ± 4.6
Adrenals	0.4 ± 0.2	0.2 ± 0.1	13 ± 7.3
Lung	1.2 ± 0.3	17.5 ± 5.8	1.4 ± 0.7
Small Bowel	6.4 ± 1.4	4.3 ± 1.1	5.8 ± 1.5
Liver	$0.3 \pm 0.3*$	13.8 ± 2.8	0.1 ± 0.1

*Hepatic artery flow only

Metastatic pattern: The adrenals were the commonest site for tumour
growth following injection of every one of the four tumour cell types.
Bony, (including jaw) and ovarian metastasis was also common. In addition
to the general preference for these three organs, each tumour had individual preferences e.g. sarcoma to brown fat and human melanoma to kidney.
Heart, liver, pancreas, yellow fat, muscle and skin rarely developed
metastasis. Intestines, spleen, brain, thymus, thyroid and testes never
developed metastases. (See Table 2).

Table 2. Metastatic Sites After Left Ventricular Injection of 3×10^5 to 4×10^6 cells.

SITES OF METASTASES	SARCOMA (N=31)	BREAST CARCINOMA (N=27)	HEPATOMA (N=12)	HUMAN MELANOMA (N=5)
Adrenals	100%	100%	100%	100%
Bone	65%	44%	33%	0%
Lung	22%	67%	8%	0%
Brown Fat	87%	7%	0%	0%
Kidneys	0%	0%	0%	60%
Ovaries	3/4	24/27	4/4	0/5

Metastatic efficiency: Not only are the adrenals, bone and ovaries frequent sites for metastasis from large inocula of tumour cells but remain so from the delivery of low numbers of cells. The number of cells received by each organ can be evaluated from the fraction of radioactivity retained following inoculation of labelled cells. From the table it can be seen that as few as 10-30 sarcoma cells trapping in the adrenals produce metastases, but 45,000 trapping in the kidneys fail to do so. (See Table 3)

Table 3. Relative Susceptibility of Kidney and Adrenal.

No. OF CELLS INJECTED INTO LEFT VENTRICLE	No. OR CELLS TRAPPED IN:		INCIDENCE OF METASTASES IN:	
	ADRENAL	KIDNEY	ADRENAL	KIDNEY
10^6	1,000	45,000	12/12	0/12
$10^4 - 3 \times 10^4$	10-30	450-1350	5/9	0/9
10^3	1	45	0/5	0/5

The fraction of cardiac output received clearly does not determine where metastases arise from cancer emboli in the arterial circulation since both adrenals receive only $0.4\overset{+}{-}0.2$% of cardiac output and yet are the most common site of metastases. Similarly the incidence of metastases is not determined by the number of cells trapping in an organ as this parallels cardiac output. The vascularity of an organ (see Table 3) is also not decisive - whilst the organs susceptible to metastases are vascular, some highly vascular organs such as the kidney are generally refractory. From radioautographic studies carried out five minutes after injection of labelled sarcoma cells there is no readily detectable difference in the diameter of the capillary bed in which the cells arrest. The cells are found in the same position as the 15 micron microspheres in the periphery of the adrenal and the glomeruli of the kidney - i.e. at the arterial end of the capillaries.

These studies suggest that organ preference is not determined by mechanical factors. That the biochemistry of the organ may be involved is suggested from experiments (see Table 4) in which dexamethazone allows metastases to arise in organs which are otherwise not involved, such as kidney and liver.   (See Table 4)

Table 4. Effect of Dexamethazone on Sites of Metastasis of 10^5 Sarcoma Cells.

DEXAMETHAZONE PROTOCOL	ADRENAL METASTASES	KIDNEY METASTASES	No. OF METASTASES
None	14/14 animals	0/14 animals	>10
Starting between Day −1 & Day +1	6/6	6/6	3-10
Starting Day +2 to Day +6	5/5	5/5	3-10

(Dexamethazone continued until animal killed. Day 0 = Day of cell injection).

Since kidney metastases developed also when the dexamethazone was started some days after tumour inoculation it seems unlikely that impairment of macrophage function contributes to the dexamethazone effect as any destruction of the injected cells by tissue macrophage would have occurred within one or two days. Rats which had been immunosuppressed by Cyclosporin A (to an extent that allowed xenografts to grow) showed the normal pattern of metastases (i.e. none in the kidney), and this excludes impairment of T-cell function as a factor in the induction by dexamethazone of metastases in kidney and liver. This may be caused by the same mechanism which makes the adrenal a preferred site of metastases, namely high local concentration of corticosteroids.

Adrenal preference is not confined to our model. Tumour cells in the arterial circulation of other species commonly cause adrenal metastases and in patients presenting with non-small cell lung cancer (a tumour which discharges cells directly into the arterial system) the adrenal may be the only sites of metastases. At autopsy of these patients the adrenals are the commonest site of metastases and even at autopsy of those dying with tumours draining to the lung or liver the adrenals are the third or fourth commonest bloodborne metastatic site.

REFERENCES

Budinger, J.M. 1958 Cancer, 11: 106.
Pagani, J. 1984 Cancer, 53: 1058.
Willis, R.A. 1964, Pathology of Tumours. 4th Edition London (Butterworths) p. 175.

METASTASIS OF A MURINE MAMMARY CARCINOMA IN MICE

R. VAN GINCKEL, W. VANHERCK, W. DISTELMANS, M. DE BRABANDER

Janssen Pharmaceutica Research Laboratories, B-2340 Beerse, Belgium

Keywords: mammary carcinoma

INTRODUCTION

A model is described for studying metastasis formation in vivo.

METHODS

CDF$_1$ mice are inoculated with TA$_3$ mammary carcinoma cells (2 x 10^6 cells in a volume of 0.05 ml) into the connective tissue of the tail. Primary tumors appear between day 5-10 after injection of the tumor cells (see figs. 1-5).

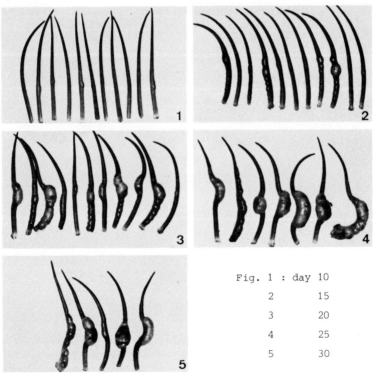

Fig. 1 : day 10
     2   15
     3   20
     4   25
     5   30

RESULTS

All mice examined at day 35 have developed macroscopic metastases at different sites e.g. heart, lungs, paraaortic glands, kidney, liver (see figs. 6-10).

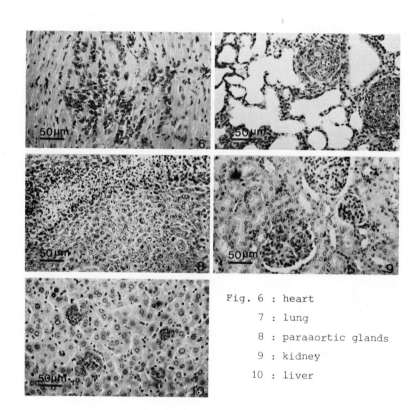

Fig. 6 : heart
     7 : lung
     8 : paraaortic glands
     9 : kidney
    10 : liver

Size and number of metastases are not correlated to the size of the primary tail tumor. The onset of metastasis formation can be defined by amputation of the tail to remove the primary tumor burden at different times after inoculation. Amputation before day 25 inhibits the appearance of macroscopic metastases (mice killed at day 35). Amputation later on does not influence size and number of macroscopic metastases.

CONCLUSION

This model mimics closely the clinical course of metastasis formation, since metastases are not localized in one preferential site but are disseminated all over the body.

REFERENCES
Baserga, R. & Baum, J., 1955 Cancer Research, 15, 52.

A NEW EXPERIMENTAL MODEL OF LYMPH NODE METASTASIS: INJECTION OF TUMOUR CELLS INTO RAT MESENTERIC LYMPH NODES VIA THE AFFERENT LYMPHATICS

R.A. COBB and H.W. STEER

Department of Surgery, Southampton General Hospital, Tremona Road, Southampton SO1 6HU

Keyword: Rat, Lymphatic metastasis, Neoplasms, experimental

INTRODUCTION

Metastasis to lymph nodes is present in 60% of surgical specimens of excised rectal tumours (Dukes 1940), and 60% of patients with colorectal cancer at post mortem (Abrams et. al. 1950) The aim of these experiments was to establish a model of mesenteric lymph node metastasis in the rat in order to study aspects of lymphatic metastasis.

METHODS

Lacteal cannulation

Each rat was anaesthetised using Hypnorm and Diazepam. An upper midline abdominal incision was employed. The terminal ileum was identified and suspended over a water heated perspex chamber, and irrigated with 0.9% saline (at $40^{\circ}C$). Using an operating microscope, a suitable lacteal was selected and exposed by gently dissecting off the overlying visceral peritoneum and mesenteric fat. Presiliconised glass capillaries were drawn out to micropipettes using an electro magnetic micropipette puller, then broken off at a diameter appropriate for the lacteal. These cannulae were filled with the fluid to be inoculated, and placed in an extension arm which was held in a micromanipulator. The lacteal was approached at 20-30 degrees from the horizontal and the cannula was inserted into the lacteal in the direction of the mesenteric lymph node using the micromanipulator. The fluid in the cannula (approximately 50 microlitres) was inoculated into the lacteal over 3-5 minutes.

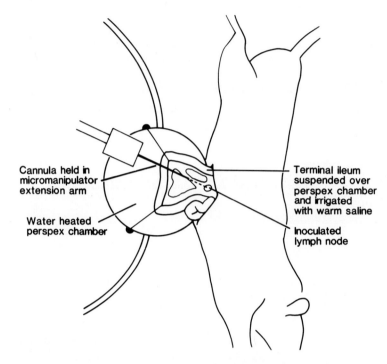

Figure 1. Line drawing of the method of lacteal cannulation.

Thoracic duct cannulation and lymph collection

For experiment 3, the thoracic duct was cannulated according to the method described by Gowans (1959). Thoracic duct lymph was collected in hourly aliquots using an automatic fraction collector into plastic tubes, each containing 0.5 ml of Dulbecco's A+B + 20 units of heparin per ml.

MC 28 sarcoma

This tumour was originally induced with methylchloranthrene at the Chester Beatty Institute in inbred CBH/Ola/Cbi rats, and has been maintained by subcutaneous passage. For these experiments, tumours from the 27th to 32nd passage were disaggregated using protease, and cultured in plastic flasks for 36 hours before harvesting a single cell suspension. ^{125}Iododeoxyuridine was added to the tissue culture flasks when the medium was changed 24 hours before harvesting to obtain labelled cells (experiments 3 & 4).

Autoradiography

Kodak AR 10 strip film was employed, using the technique described by Rogers (1969).

Gamma counts

Gamma   counts were performed on specimens of thoracic duct lymph for one
minute   each   in   an   automatic   well   counter   calibrated   for
^{125}Iododeoxyuridine.

RESULTS

Experiment 1

To   demonstrate   that   MC   28   sarcoma developed in the mesenteric lymph
node following lacteal inoculation of a tumour cell suspension.

Lacteal inoculation with 4 X 10^4 to 3 X 10^5 MC 28 sarcoma cells
Examined 6 to 26 days later

Mesenteric lymph node tumour	15/15 rats
Tumour at any other site	0/15 rats

Experiment 2

To   demonstrate   that   lung tumours develop if viable tumour cells reach
the lungs following lacteal inoculation.

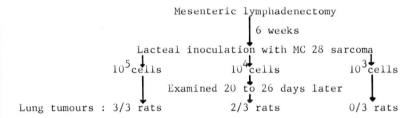

Lung tumours : 3/3 rats

Experiment 3

Autoradiography was performed on serial sections of lymph nodes excised
10   minutes   and   24   hours   following   lacteal   inoculation   with
^{125}Iododeoxyuridine   labelled   MC   28   sarcoma.   This demonstrated that
tumour   cells were present in the marginal and peripheral medullary sinuses
within 10   minutes of injection, and that after 24 hours tumour cells had
not reached further than the peripheral medullary sinuses.

Experiment 4

3   rats   had thoracic duct lymph collected following lacteal inoculation
of ^{125}Iododeoxyuridine labelled MC 28 sarcoma cells.

Radioactivity   appeared   in thoracic duct lymph within 1 hour, peaked at

2-3 hours, and returned to background levels by 6 hours.

The total amount of radioactivity appearing in the thoracic duct lymph represented only 1-2% of the injected dose. Following centrifugation of the lymph samples, 100% of the radioactivity was found in the supernatants and none in the cell pellets.

DISCUSSION

There has been one report of attempted injection of tumour cells into rat mesenteric afferent lymphatics (Madden & Gyure 1968). The results in this paper indicated that translymphnodal passage of tumour cells occurred in 80% of animals. However, examination of the method described suggests that the lymphatics cannulated were efferent from, and not afferent to the mesenteric lymph nodes.

The finding of small amounts of radioactivity in the supernatant fraction of thoracic duct lymph following lacteal inoculation of ^{125}Iododeoxyuridine labelled MC 28 sarcoma represents either free ^{125}Iododeoxyuridine in the inoculum, or cell lysis in the lymph node.

Our experiments have shown that:

1. MC 28 sarcoma developed in the mesenteric lymph node but at no other site following lacteal inoculation of a tumour cell suspension.

2. Lacteal inoculation of tumour cells to animals which had undergone previous excision of mesenteric lymph nodes developed lung tumours.

3. MC 28 sarcoma cells did not reach the thoracic duct up to 24 hours following afferent lymphatic injection.

CONCLUSION

Early translymphnodal passage of MC 28 sarcoma does not occur.

We are using this experimental model to study the cellular immune response of mesenteric lymph nodes to inoculated tumour cells.

REFERENCES

Abrams, H.L., Spiro, R. & Goldstein, N., 1950, Cancer,3 ,74.
Dukes, C.E., 1940, Journal of Pathology, 50, 527.
Gowans, J.L., 1959, Journal of Physiology, 146, 54.
Madden, R.E. & Gyure L., 1968, Oncology, 22, 281.
Rogers, A.W., 1969, Techniques of Autoradiography, 2nd ed.
   (Elsevier Publishing).

LYMPH NODE METASTASIS FOLLOWING SUBCUTANEOUS IMPLANTATION OF THE RC TUMOR

M. VANDENDRIS[1] , P. DUMONT[2] , P. SEMAL[2] , R. HEIMANN[3] ,
R. VANHOOF[4] , and G. ATASSI[2]

[1]Department of Urology, Brugmann University Hospital, Brussels
[2]Department of Experimental Chemotherapy, Bordet Institute, Brussels
[3]Department of Pathology, Bordet Institute, Brussels
[4]Pasteur Institute, Brussels

Keywords: lymph node metastases - tumor model - chemotherapy

INTRODUCTION

Human cancers spread commonly to the local lymph nodes. On the other hand, animal tumor models metastasize less frequently and rarely show lymphatic metastases. For that reason, most works on metastasis have been done with models of hematogenous metastasis. Few experimental murine models of lymph node metastasis have been described and most of these have flaws such as erratic metastasis (Sato 1961, Franchi et al. 1968), metastases of too small size (Tsukagochi & Sakurai 1970) or marked immunogenicity (Finlay-Jones et al. 1980, Hagmar & Ryd 1978). This report describes a suitable murine model of lymph node metastasis which may be used for experimental investigations.

TUMOR AND PATTERN OF METASTASIS

The RC renal adenocarcinoma used in the experiments is a poorly immunogenic undifferentiated tumor. It was maintained in CDF1 mice by serial subcutaneous (sc) and intraperitoneal transfers (Vandendris et al. 1983). The tumor showed a constant and reproductible behavior and was able to develop metastases. In previous experiments, the RC tumor had responded to different classes of chemotherapeutic agents and to clinically active drugs which had been reported inactive against P388 and/or L1210 leukemias.

The sc inoculation of 10^7 RC tumor cells in the dorsal part of
the foot produced a primary tumor which metastasized early to the
popliteal and para-aortic lymph nodes (Vandendris et al. 1984). The high
number of cells inoculated made the metastatic process constant and
reproducible. Metastases rapidly appeared and all mice in which tumor excision was performed on day 6 died with evidence of dissemination (figure 2).
All tumor-bearing mice developed bulky para-aortic lymph node metastases
and showed simultaneously a marked enlargement of the spleen. The growth
curves of the nodes and the spleen were roughly parallel (figure 1).

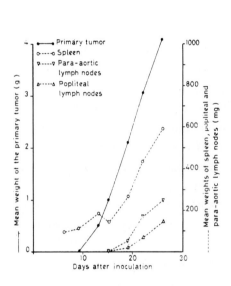

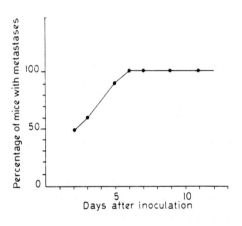

Figure 1. Growth curve of the
primary tumor, spleen, and lymph
node metastases. Standard
deviations have been omitted
for clarity.

Figure 2. Percentage of mice
with metastases as a function
of the time between inoculation
and tumor excision. Mice were
inoculated sc in the foot with
10^7 tumor cells.

Microscopically, tumor cells appeared at first in the peripheral
sinus of the lymph node and spread down in the radial sinuses, invading
progressively the node. At a later stage of tumor dissemination, a
massive microscopic involvement was observed in the liver, the spleen
and the lungs.

CHEMOTHERAPEUTIC EXPERIMENTS

The experimental protocol for chemotherapy of metastases was performed as follows: 10^7 tumor cells were inoculated sc in the foot and groups of mice were treated on days 1 and 8 postimplant with adriamycin (4mg/kg) or vincristine (1 mg/kg). In 2 treated groups, the tumored leg was amputated on day 11. Treated and control tumor-bearing mice were killed and examined after 18 days. To evaluate the efficacy of the treatment, the parameters used were the mean weights of primary tumor, para-aortic lymph nodes and spleen. In a second experiment, mice in which the tumored leg was amputated on day 13, were treated peri-operatively with vincristine (1mg/kg) and the assay was based on the same criteria.

TABLE 1. EFFECT OF VINCRISTINE OR ADRIAMYCIN, WITH OR WITHOUT ADJUVANT SURGERY, AGAINST PARA-AORTIC LYMPH NODE METASTASES - EARLY TREATMENT.

	Average primary tumor weight (g)	Mean weight of the lymph nodes (mg)	Mean weight of the spleen (mg)
Control mice	3.701	94.3	275
Vincristine	2.441	11.2	198
Adriamycin	2.495	21.8	203
Vincr.+ surgery	–	3.9	127
Adriam. + surgery	–	1.6	129

In the first experiment (early treatment), the drugs produced only a slight regression of the primary growth but entailed a significant decrease of lymph node metastases at autopsy (Table 1). Combined with surgery, vincristine and adriamycin produced an apparent cure in most of the cases. In the second experiment, vincristine was administered only at the time of amputation: no cure was observed and only a moderate reduction in the mean weights of the lymph node metastases and the spleen could be seen.

CONCLUSION

The RC tumor implanted in the foot produces bulky lymph node
metastases in a regular way and following a constant and reproducible
pattern, entailing the invasion of the popliteal and para-aortic lymph
nodes. A massive microscopic invasion of the spleen , the liver and the
lungs occurs simultaneously. The tumor shows a low immunogenicity. These
characteristics are in accordance with criteria defined for a suitable
model of lymph node metastasis (Carr 1983). The constancy of lymph
node invasion makes the model useful for investigating the mechanism of
lymphatic metastasis. Furthermore, the high sensitivity of the RC tumor
to chemotherapeutic agents should allow the selection of drugs targetted
to lymph node metastases.

REFERENCES

Carr. I., 1983, Cancer Metastasis Reviews, 2, 307.
Finlay-Jones, J.J., Bartholomaeus, W.N., Fimmel, P.J., Keast, D., &
        Stanley, N.F., 1980, Journal of the National Cancer Institute, 64, 1363.
Franchi, G., Reyers Degli Innocenti, I., Rosso, R. & Garattini, S., 1969
        International Journal of Cancer, 3, 765
Hagmar, B., & Ryd, W., 1978, Acta Pathologica et Microbiologica
        Scandinavica (A), 86, 231.
Sato, H., 1961, Cancer Chemotherapy Reports, 13, 33
Tsukagochi, S., & Sakurai, Y. 1970. Cancer Chemotherapy Reports, 54, 311
Vandendris, M., Dumont, P., Heimann, R., & Atassi, G., 1983, Cancer
        Chemotherapy and Pharmacology, 11, 182.
Vandendris, M., Dupont, P. Semal, P. Heimann, R. & Atassi, G. 1984
        Clinical & Experimental Metastasis, (in press   )

PROBLEMS AND PROSPECTS IN THE CONTROL OF METASTASIS

U. KIM
Department of Pathology, Roswell Park Memorial Institute,
Buffalo, NY 14263, USA

Keyword: Invasion, Angiogenesis, Anticoagulation, Immunotherapy

The study of the biological, biochemical and immunological characteristics of metastasizing and nonmetastasizing rat mammary carcinomas, together with a better understanding of the mechanism of tumor-host interaction in the development of metastasis, may provide us with means to experimentally manipulate the behavior of tumor cells to alter their metastatic potential. Let us examine some of the problems and prospects involved.

Surgical excision

Unlike most murine tumors that metastasize via the venous return to the lung following surgical amputation of the tumor-bearing limb, early excision of the hematogenously metastasizing rat mammary adenocarcinoma TMT-50 prevents the development of lung metastasis. In contrast, it is extremely difficult to prevent the lymphogenous ones from metastasizing or recurring by the same procedure. However, the earlier they are excised, the longer it takes for the metastasis to develop. These findings suggest the possibility that some of the Stage I human breast cancers with a long-term "cure" have hematogenously spreading potential.

Anti-invasion

It has been postulated that invasive tumor cells have enhanced motility associated with increased levels of contractile proteins in the form of microtubules and microfilaments (Gabbiani & Csank-Brassert 1976). Mareel and associates (1980) reported that the mitotic spindle poisons, vinca alkaloid compounds, not only have anti-mitotic activity, but also prevent migration of murine fibrosarcoma cells in vitro and in vivo. However, since these drugs also inhibit cell division, the "restrained" movement of sarcoma cells may be caused indirectly by the overall growth retardation of tumors. Our attempts to demonstrate any significant concentration of myosin in the metastasizing rat mammary carcinoma cells have not been successful (Dunington et al. 1984).

Tanaka and colleagues (1981) noted the complete prevention of lung metastasis in mice implanted with Lewis lung carcinoma with an anti-fibrinolytic agent, tranexamic acid, seemingly by blocking the tumor cells in the primary from entering the neighboring blood vessels. It is unlikely that any such cells were present in the systemic circulation at the time of treatment, otherwise the drug would have helped them to aggregate and settle in the lung, thus producing an effect opposite to the one the investigators achieved. Time, therefore, would seem to be the critical factor in administering such drug, which is obviously a difficult task in cancer patients. Furthermore, the notion that certain proteolytic enzymes must break down the basement membrane collagen in order to initiate the invasive process may be applicable only to a limited number of tumors, for most human and animal mammary cancers that metastasize naturally already have either defective or no basement membrane barriers (Gusterson et al. 1982; Dunington et al. 1984), suggesting that enzymatic degradation of basement membranes may not be the essential ingredient for tumor invasion.

Anti-angiogenesis

Heparin released from mast cells has been recognized as the principal angiogenesis factor associated with solid tumors. Taylor & Folkman (1982) successfully inhibited the growth and metastasis of various murine tumors by blocking their angiogenesis with protamin, a potent anti-heparin compound. However, further studies are necessary to elucidate its mechanism of action, for heparin has been tried in the control of experimental tumor metastasis by many investigators. Jirtle (1981) found the rate of blood flow in the metastasizing rat mammary tumors to be 2-5 times lower than in the nonmetastasizing control ones, as measured by the rate of retention of radio-labelled latex microspheres by tumor vasculature. Such lower blood flow rate may interfere with optimal drug delivery as well as with the oxygen tension needed to make them more radiosensitive. Kaelin and associates (1984) were successful in increasing the blood flow in these malignant tumors with calcium entry blocking agents, overcoming that inherent therapeutic difficulty. On the other hand, a lower blood flow rate and a decreased protein/phospholipid ratio in their plasma membranes seem to render the tumors more sensitive to hyperthermia (Yatvin et al. 1982). In addition, the capacity to withstand the higher atmospheric oxygen tension

in the lung capillary may be essential for tumor cells to traverse the lung
into the arterial circulation and colonize distant organs. Indeed, most
lymphogenously metastasizing cells seem to have such capacity.

Anticoagulation

Many investigators have shown a significant reduction in the number of
tumor deposits in the lung of laboratory animals implanted i.v. with dispersed tumor cells by the administration of a variety of anticoagulants,
including heparin and coumarin derivatives (Maat & Hilgard 1981), and more
recently by prostacyclin (Honn et al. 1983). Gasic and associates (1978)
provided the rationale for this type of therapy by demonstrating the
platelet-aggregating capacity of plasma membrane vesicles isolated in vitro
from human and animal tumors. However, it is questionable whether this
kind of intrapulmonary tumor colonization is a true representation of hematogenous lung metastases that arise spontaneously in animals bearing an
extrapulmonary solid tumor (Stackpole 1981). On the contrary, in certain
tumors anticoagulation may even promote cell dissemination beyond the lung.
The lymphogenously metastasizing rat mammary tumors tend to slip through
the capillary network of the lung without being trapped, colonizing the
bone and other parenchymatous organs.

Activation of resident macrophage

Stimulation of the reticuloendothelial system, notably that of resident
macrophages, has been found to inhibit the hematogenous lung metastases by
various immunoadjuvants such as BCG, C. parvum and bacterial cell-wall
skeleton. This led to the development of N-acetyl-muramyl-dipeptide (MDP),
one of the most immunopharmacologically active moieties of bacterial
peptidoglycan (Wachsmuth & Dukor 1981). The effectiveness of MDP, incorporated in liposomes and injected i.v. into tumor-bearing animals to activate
the alveolar macrophage in situ for the prevention of lung metastasis, was
reported by Fidler et al. (1981). Since all blood-borne tumor cells pass
through the lung, the arming of the resident macrophage to intercept them
as they enter the pulmonary artery may be the best method of eradication.
However, it is not certain whether the activated macrophage can destroy the
lymphogenously metastasizing cells that have already resisted the cytotoxic
cells in the regional lymph node before entering the lung.

T-cell deficient environment of athymic nude mice

Nude mice are notoriously resistant to xenografts of malignant human
tumors and naturally metastasizing rat mammary carcinomas, but not to those

of conventional laboratory animal tumors. Such selective graft resistance, as well as the ability of these mice to frequently prevent the development of metastasis, has been attributed primarily to NK. Suppression of T-cells with cyclosporin A in intact rats bearing a metastasizing mammary tumor causes significant retardation of tumor growth and metastasis, but has no effect on the nonmetastasizing ones (Kim et al. 1984). This suggests that certain levels of T-cell suppression, or a T-cell deficient state, may be a favorable host condition in the control of cancer spread. However, the optimum T-cell deficient state, equivalent to that of athymic nude mice, may be difficult to achieve. In addition, the antigenic modulating capacity of tumor cells, together with the easy adaptability to their environment, places a major constraint on the development of effective anti-tumor and anti-metastatic measures.

REFERENCES

Dunington, D. J., Kim, U., Hughes, C. M., Monaghan, P., Ormerod, E. J. & Rudland, P. S., 1984, Journal of the National Cancer Institute, 72, 1984.

Fidler, I. J., Sone, S., Fogler, W. E. & Barnes, Z. L., 1981, Proceedings of the National Academy of Science, USA, 78, 1684.

Gabbiani, G. & Csank-Brassert, J., 1976, American Journal of Pathology, 83,457.

Gasic, G. J., Boettiger, D., Califano, J. L., Gasic, T. B., & Stewart, C.J., 1978, Cancer Research, 38, 2950.

Gusterson, B. A., Warburton, M. J., Mitchell, D., Ellison, M., Neville, A. M. & Rudland, P. S., 1982, Cancer Research, 42, 4763.

Honn, K. V., Busse, W. D. & Sloane, B. F., 1983, Biochemical Pharmacology, 32, 1.

Jirtle, R. L., 1981, European Journal of Cancer, 17, 53.

Kaelin, W. G. Jr., Shrivastav, S. & Jirtle, R. L., 1984, Cancer Research, 44, 896.

Kim, U., Shin, S-I. & Cohen, S. A., 1984, Selective suppression of T cell function in normal rats simulating the T-independent antitumor and anti-metastatic reaction of nude mice against metastasizing rat mammary carcinomas. In Immune-deficient Animals, edited by B. Sordat (Karger, A. G., Basel), p.235.

Maat, B. & Hilgard,P., 1981, Cancer Research & Clinical Oncology, 101, 275.

Mareel, M., Storm, G., Debruyne, G., & Van Cauwenberg, R., 1980, Anti-invasive effect of microtubule inhibitors. In Microtubules and Micro-tubule Inhibitors, edited by M. De Brander (Elsevier, North Holland Biomedical Press, Amsterdam), p.535.

Tanaka, N., Ogawa, H., Tanaka, K., Kinjo, M. & Kohga, S., 1981, Invasion & Metastasis, 1, 149.

Taylor, S. & Folkman, J., 1982, Nature, 297, 307.

Wachsmuth, E. D. & Dukor, P., 1981, Immunopathology of muramyl-peptides. In Proceedings of the International Symposium on Immunomodulation by Microbial Products & Related Synthetic Compounds, edited by Y. Yamamura & S. Kotani (Excerpta Medica, Amsterdam), p.60.

Yatvin, M. V., Vorpahl, J. & Kim, U., 1982, Differential response to heat by metastatic and non-metastatic rat mammary tumors. In Hyperthermia, edited by H.K. Bicher & D.F. Bruley (Plenum Press Corp., New York), p.177.

METASTASIS FROM METASTASES: AN ANIMAL MODEL

J.D. CRISSMAN[1], K.V. HONN[2,3] and B.F. SLOANE[2,4]
[1]Departments of Pathology[1], Radiation Oncology[2], Biological Sciences[3]
and Pharmacology[4],
Harper-Grace Hospitals and Wayne State University, Detroit, MI 48201 USA

Keywords: spontaneous metastasis, experimental metastasis

INTRODUCTION

     Metastasis from metastases unquestionably contributes to the pro-
gression of malignant neoplasms. Ketcham et al. (1969) and Hoover and
Ketcham (1975) demonstrated that metastases release viable tumor cells
into the circulation. In the 1975 study this was demonstrated by joining
a parabiotic recipient to a syngeneic animal with established metastases
from a primary tumor which had been removed. This resulted in the
establishment of metastases in the recipient animal. Evidence that
metastases from metastases contribute to the lethal organ burden in the
lung has also been presented by Raz (1984). Most clinicians agree that
metastases contribute to the metastatic cascade, but do not feel that
this is of primary importance in the progression of human cancer. To
evaluate the contribution of metastases to metastasis, we developed two
animal model systems.

METHODS

     An amelanotic variant (Bl6a) of the Bl6 melanoma was obtained from
the Division of Cancer Treatment (NCI) tumor bank and propagated in
syngeneic mice as previously described (Honn et al., 1984). Viable
tumor cells were isolated from subcutaneous tumors by sequential collagenase dispersion and centrifugal elutriation as previously described
(Sloane et al., 1981).

     Lung metastases were produced in 10 wk old male C57BL/6J mice by
two methods. In the first model lung metastases were established by
intravenous injection (tail vein) of 10^3 Bl6a melanoma cells (TVM). The

second model was established by foot pad injection of 10^6 B16a melanoma cell (FPM). The leg was subsequently amputated on d. 15 post tumor cell injection.

Fetal lung, kidney and gonad tissue was removed from near term C57BL/6J mice and implanted in the posterior thigh muscle of the recipient animals as described by Kinsey (1960). Implantation was performed 5 d. post tail vein injection of tumor cells or 5 d. post surgical removal of the primary tumor. At 5 d. no circulating tumor cells were present as determined by the survival time of ^{125}IUdr labeled B16a cells. The animals were sacrificed by cervical dislocation 3-5 wk after fetal tissue implantation. The leg containing the fetal tissue was fixed in 10% buffered formalin and the thoracic lungs were fixed in Bouins solution. Surface thoracic lung tumors were quantitated macroscopically and tissue sections of thoracic lung and fetal implants were prepared after paraffin embedding. The areas of thoracic lung, fetal tissue and B16a melanoma metastases were quantitated using the BioQuant Image Analysis System (R&M Biometrics, Nashville, TN).

Tail vein injections of tumor cells were performed at 1-4 wk post fetal lung implantation. The animals were sacrificed 2 wk post tumor cell injection. The fetal lung was histologically evaluated to determine when revascularization of the implants occurred. For the TVM, 10^3-10^5 tumor cells were injected to determine the number of cells required for establishment of secondary metastases in the implanted fetal lung. In the FPM, 5×10^5 and 1×10^6 tumor cells were injected and amputation performed at intervals from 8-21 d. In both models, the thoracic lungs were removed and surface and cross-sectional metastases quantitated.

RESULTS

Vascularization of the fetal lung occurred from 2-3 wk post implantation. Thirty percent of animals developed tumor colonies in the fetal lung when B16a cells were injected tail vein at 2 wk post lung implantation and 100% at 3 wk post lung implantation. Preliminary studies determined that the optimum number of B16a cells to produce thoracic lung colones as well as permit sufficient survival time to develop secondary metastases was 10^3 in the TVM. Likewise, in the FPM with amputation at 15 d. injection of 10^6 B16a cells resulted in a 100% incidence of thoracic lung metastases and sufficient survival time for metastases to develop in the implanted fetal lung.

Secondary metastases (Figure 1) were identified in the fetal lungs in

76% of the animals in the TVM and 78% in the FPM (Table 1). In the TVM
the average number of metastases in the cross section of the implanted
lung was 3.88 and the ratio of metastasis area/fetal lung area was 3.17.
The interval between implantation and termination was 5 wk which appeared
to be a sufficient period for extensive growth of the secondary metastases. In the FPM the average number of metastases was 4.89 and the
ratio of metastasis area/fetal lung area was 0.11 after a 5-6 wk interval.
In the FPM the secondary metastases were slightly more frequent but
smaller. In general, the animals with the largest areas of metastases
in the thoracic lung also demonstrated large areas of metastases in
the fetal lung suggesting that a selection for rapidly growing tumors
occurred in most of the animals.

The secondary metastases were always found in the parenchyma of the
implanted fetal lung. Implantation of fetal kidney, bowel, and gonad
tissues resulted in small secondary metastases in two animals with
implanted testes. No secondary metastases were found in the remaining
tissues.

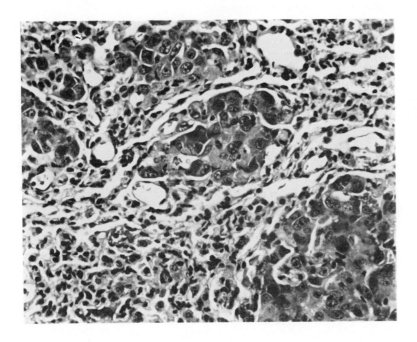

Figure 1. Photomicrograph of the implanted fetal lung with several foci
of secondary metastases originating from the thoracic lung metastases.
The tumor cells are larger, with hyperchromatic anaplastic nuclei as
compared to the surrounding fetal lung tissue. Air spaces are not
readily identifiable in the implanted lung as it has never been expanded.

Table 1. Metastases from metastases.

	Tail Vein Model	Foot Pad Model
No. of animals	17	9
No. with metastases	76%	78%
No. of metastases	3.88	4.89
Metastatic area (mm^2)	17.94	3.63
Metastatic area/lung area	3.17	0.11
Interval after implants	5 wk	5-6 wk

DISCUSSION

Sugarbaker et al. (1971) were unable to demonstrate metastasis from metastases at 28 d. post implantation of newborn tissues (lung). In contrast, our study demonstrated metastasis from metastases in the FPM at 40 d. and in the TVM at 35 d. post implantation of fetal lung.

The primary cause of cancer deaths today is metastasis. Therefore, new therapies will have to be directed at the destruction of existing metastases and the interruption of the metastatic cascade. The models described in this study may be useful in screening drugs capable of inhibiting metastasis from metastases.

REFERENCES

Honn, K.V., Onoda, J.M., Diglio, C.A., Carufel, M.M., Taylor, J.D. & Sloane, B.F., 1984, Clinical and Experimental Metastasis, 2, 61.
Hoover, H.C. & Ketcham, A.S., 1969, Annals of Surgery, 169, 297.
Kinsey, D.L., 1960, Cancer 11, 674.
Raz, A., 1984, Clinical and Experimental Metastasis, 2, 5.
Sloane, B.F., Dunn, J.R. & Honn, K.V., 1981, Science 212, 1151.
Sugarbaker, E.V., Cohen, A.M. & Ketcham, A.S., 1971, Annals of Surgery, 174, 161.

THE EFFICIENCY OF TRAPPING OF BLOOD BORNE CANCER CELLS BY THE ORGAN OF FIRST ENCOUNTER IN EXPERIMENTAL RAT TUMOURS

P. MURPHY, J. FLEMING, I. TAYLOR and P. ALEXANDER

Depts. of Surgery, Medical Oncology & Nuclear Medicine, University of Southampton, Southampton General Hospital, Southampton SO9 4XY

Keywords: Transpulmonary Passage, Intraportal, Intracardiac

Bloodborne tumour cells are shed, depending on the site of the primary tumour either into the portal vein and thence to the liver or into the vena caval system and on to the lung. Exceptionally, tumour cells may be carried via vertebral venous plexuses directly to bone (Batson, 1940). Dissemination beyond the organ of first encounter can occur either from cells that have succeeded in traversing the capillary beds of these organs to gain access to the systemic arterial circulation or from cells released by metastases growing in these organs of first encounter and not from the primary. If metastasis is a step wise process with initial localisation to the organ of first encounter, then local adjuvant therapy directed to this organ at the time of removal of the primary may result in cure. This investigation sets out to determine the probability of tumour cells derived from different syngeneic rat tumours traversing the lung or liver capillary beds to cause generalised metastasis by studying the sites of metastases and the trapping of radiolabelled tumour cells after intravenous, intra-portal and left ventricular injection of tumour cells.

METHODS

All experiments used 180-290 gram syngeneic hooded Lister rats which were bred at Southampton from Chester Beatty Research Institute breeding stock in which the tumours were originally induced. The sarcoma had been produced by a subcutaneous implant of methylcholanthrene, the hepatoma by feeding dimethylazobenzene and the breast carcinoma with a subcutaneous implant of oestrogen. The tumour cells were removed from the culture vessel either mechanically or with trypsin. Injections of cells were carried out in conscious animals. Intravenous cannulae were inserted via the right jugular vein and left ventricular cannulae via the right carotid artery on the day prior to injection. Intraportal vein injections were performed by direct venepuncture under ether anaesthesia.

RESULTS

Sites of Growth

The table shows that after i.v. inoculation of tumour cells the lungs were the only site of tumour growth, even after injection of more than a million cells which is 50 times the dose needed to induce lung tumours in 50% of the animals (TD_{50}). When tumour cells were given intraportally (again at 50 to 100 times the TD_{50} dose, growth of tumour was almost entirely restricted to the liver (Table 1). In the two cases in which lung growths occurred in addition to liver growth, there was gross peritoneal spread suggesting leakage at the time of inoculation.

Table 1.

Sites of tumour growth following injection into rats of syngeneic tumour cells ($3x10^5$ to $4x10^6$) intravenously (i.v.) into the portal vein (i.po.) or into the left ventricle (i.c.).

	Sarcoma			Hepatoma			Mammary Carcinoma		
	i.v.	i.po.	i.c.	i.v.	i.po.	i.c.	i.v.	i.po.	i.c.
Lung	20/20	0/6	7/31	4/4	1/5	1/12	10/10	1/5	18/27
Liver	0/20	6/6	1/31	0/4	5/5	0/12	0/10	5/5	0/27
Adrenal	0	0	31/31	0	0	12/12	0	0	27/27
Bone	0	0	20/31	0	0	4/12	0	0	12/27
Brown fat	0	0	27/31	0	0	0	0	0	2/27
Ovaries	0	0	3/4	0	0	4/4	0	0	24/27
Skin	0	0	4/31	0	0	0	0	0	0
Skeletal muscle	0	0	0	0	0	0	0	0	0
Gut	0	0	0	0	0	0	0	0	0
Kidney	0	0	0	0	0	0	0	0	0

    Following left ventricular injection of tumour cells, the adrenal was the commonest site for tumour growth, occurring in almost every rat that developed metastases. Bony growths were common but skeletal muscle and kidney metastases were not seen. Brown fat growths were almost entirely confined to the rats injected with sarcoma cells. Lesions were multiple in adrenal, brown fat and bone, but usually single when occurring in less favourable sites.   The organ selectivity did not vary detectably in the range of 10^4 to 2×10^6 cells. With a dose of 10^3 cells three of four rats developed tumours and these were restricted to bone and brown fat without the development of adrenal lesions.

Injection of radiolabelled tumour cells: Following i.v. or i.po. injection of IuDr labelled cells, which had been freed from cell debris by Ficoll gradient purification, more than 97% of the injected radioactivity was trapped in lung or liver respectively. 89% of the radioactivity found in the lung immediately after injection of radiolabelled sarcoma tumour cells is lost from this organ within 16 hours. This disappearance is not associated with recirculation of viable tumour cells to other organs, but is a consequence of cell damage. The activity builds up initially in the liver and then as a result of autolysis appears as free iodide. If the cells had been slowly released over 24 hours into the systemic circulation they would be distributed as observed after left ventricular inoculation, (see below) but this was not the case.

Following left ventricular injection the distribution of radioactivity in different organs immediately after injection of labelled sarcoma cells parallels the cardiac output received by these organs as measured by the microsphere method except that a greater fraction of the cell associated radioactivity appears in lung and liver than corresponds to the cardiac output. The differences between cardiac output and distribution of radio- labelled tumour cells suggests that approximately 30% of the cancer cells traverse the capillary beds of muscle, kidney, skin and gut etc., to be trapped via the venous circulation in lung or liver. Arrest in lung or liver from the venous circulation is complete.

DISCUSSION

For the experimental tumours studied growth was restricted almost completely to lung and liver following intravenous and intraportal injec- tion. This localisation we considered to be due to effective trapping in these organs because the same tumour cells when given via the left ventri- cle were capable of effectively colonising other organs. By comparing the largest number of cells which when given intravenously produced no tumours outside the lung with the smallest number of cells which when delivered arterially produced tumours in bone or adrenal, it is possible to set an upper limit for the fraction of cells that have passed through the lung with their reproductive capacity intact. For such an estimate to be valid all animals need to be examined for tumours at approximately the same time. We have done this with the sarcoma cells between days 18-21 following

2×10^6 cells intravenously and 3×10^4 cells intracardiacally. The former only had lung tumours while three of four of the latter all had large adrenal and other growths. From this data we conclude that less than

$$\frac{3 \times 10^4}{2 \times 10^6} \times 100\% = 1.5\% \text{ can have traversed the lung intact.}$$

That the actual value is probably much lower is indicated by the experiments with radioactively labelled cells when trapping in the lung exceeded 98% and there was no evidence that intact labelled cells passed through the lung into the arterial circulation.

These observations accord with those of others (e.g. Tarin & Price, 1979: Wallace *et al.*, 1978: Fidler, 1970) who found following i.v. injection tumours were either only seen in the lung or when occurring in other organs did so at a time when they could have occurred as a metastasis which stemmed from a lung lesion. The data in experimental animals seem to mirror those seen in man where, on the basis of detailed post-mortem studies, Willis, 1964 and Bross *et al.*, 1975, have questioned whether carcinoma and sarcoma cells traverse the lung and emphasise the importance of metastases from metastases for spread beyond the lung. The presence of bone metastases without lung lesions seen particularly with prostate and breast cancer do not necessitate transpulmonary passage as they could develop via direct vertebral plexuses.

REFERENCES

Batson, O. V., 1940, Annals of Surgery, 112: 138-149 .

Bross, I.D., Viadana, E., Pickren, J., 1975. Journal of Chronic Disease, 28, 149 .

Fidler, I.J., 1970. Journal of the National Cancer Institute, 45, 773.

Tarin, D., Price, J.E., 1979. British Journal of Cancer, 39, 740.

Wallace, A.C., Chew, E., Jones, D.G., 1978. Pulmonary Metastases. Ed. Weiss, L., Gilbert, H.A. Boston: Hall & Co.

Willis, R.A., 1964. Pathology of Tumours. 4th Edition, London, Butterworths, 179.

THE EFFECT OF A PRIMARY TUMOUR AND ITS METASTASES ON THE
LODGEMENT OF CIRCULATING TUMOUR CELLS

G. SKOLNIK[1], U. BAGGE[2] and P. HILGARD[3]
Departments of [1]Surgery I and [2]Anatomy, University of Göteborg, Sweden and
[3]Department of Cancer Research, Asta-Werke, Bielefeld, West Germany

Keywords: primary tumour effects; lodgement of circulating cells; Razoxin

INTRODUCTION

The arrest and lodgement in the microvasculature of tumour cells released
from a primary neoplasm are crucial events in metastasis formation. To investigate the mechanisms involved in the microvascular arrest and lodgement
of circulating tumour cells and to perform quantitative analyses of these
processes, it is necessary to use an experimental model in which a defined
number of tumour cells can be delivered to an organ via the blood stream.
Obviously, this can be achieved only by intravascular tumour cell injection.
This experimental model might be considered to mimic the dissemination of
tumour cells that occurs following surgery on solid tumours. It may be ar-
gued, however, that when tumour cells are injected into normal, tumour-free
animals, the direct or indirect influence of the primary tumour on tumour
cell dissemination is not evaluated. The aim of the present study was therefore to analyse the effect of a primary tumour and its metastases on the
lodgement of tumour cells injected into the circulation.

MATERIAL AND METHODS

Male hooded rats of the Lister strain, weighing about 200 g, were used.
In tumour-bearing animals a syngeneic, transplantable, methylcholantrene-
induced fibrosarcoma (known to metastasize to lymphatic nodes) was implanted
in the right hind leg with trochar technique. Razoxin treatment in the tumour
bearing rats was started in conjunction with the tumour implantation. Both
these and the tumour-free rats were treated with Razoxin 30 mg/kg body wt
and day for 3 weeks, after which the lodgement experiments were performed.
Tumour cell suspensions were prepared from the same tumours and labelled
with ^{125}I-5-iodo-2-deoxyuridine as described in a previous paper (Skolnik et
al. 1980). Tumour cells were injected i.v. or intraportally under anesthesia.

The animals were killed 3 hours after the tumour cell injection and the number of lodged tumour cells in the lungs and the liver was determined as described previously (Skolnik et al. 1980).

RESULTS

   In tumour-free rats treatment with Razoxin 30 mg/kg body wt./day for 3
weeks prior to tumour cell injection had no effect on body weights and it
did not influence significantly tumour cell lodgement (Table I). In rats
treated with Razoxin from the time of tumour implantation, no metastases
were observed in the lymphatic nodes. The weight of the primary tumours was
reduced by about 30% and the tumours had a marked surface pallor as compared
to tumours in the group without treatment. Table I shows that when tumour-
bearing rats were injected with tumour cells, lodgement was increased with
35% in the liver and 55% in the lungs as compared with rats in the control
group. Razoxin treatment of tumour-bearing rats caused an increased lodgement with 79% in the liver and 161% in the lungs as compared to controls.
All these differences are statistically significant.

Table I. Number of lodged ^{125}I-labelled tumour cells in the liver and lungs
3 hours after intraportal resp. i.v. injection of 5×10^5 cells.

	LIVER Mean+SEM	LUNGS Mean+SEM
CONTROL	17446+ 455	12727+ 386
RAZOXIN (no tumour)	17956+ 362	12987+ 588
TUMOUR-BEARING	23550+1063	19771+1034
TUMOUR + RAZOXIN	31161+ 892	33240+1314

DISCUSSION

   The observation that the surgical removal of a local primary tumour can
be followed by an accelerated growth and increased incidence of distant metastases has led to the conclusion that the primary tumour by its tumour
load exerts an inhibitory effect on the growth of its spontaneous metastases.
As this effect is observed even in immune-suppressed animals, the suppression of metastases by the primary tumour might be mediated via a non-immune
mechanism (Gorelik et al. 1982).

   The arrest and lodgement of circulating tumour cells in the microvasculature are key events in metastasis formation. While the vast majority of
arrested cells are rapidly destroyed as reported by Fidler (1970),some cells
survive providing a critical reservoir from which metastases may develop.

There is evidence that the host factors responsible for the destruction of malignant cells play their principal role during the first hours after tumour cell arrest (Glaves 1980). Thus it was regarded to be of importance to investigate further the effect of a primary tumour and its metastases on the lodgement phase.

The results from previous investigations on the influence of a primary tumour on the early lodgement of i.v. injected tumour cells have been contradictory. Weiss et al.(1974)reported decreased localization of fibrosarcoma cells, whereas there was an increased localization of lymphosarcoma cells in the lungs of tumour-bearing mice as compared to tumour-free mice 1 hour after i.v. tumour cell injection. It was therefore concluded that the presence of growing primary tumour modifies the pattern of initial arrest of circulating tumour cells. Fidler et al.(1977) reported an increased retention of i.v. injected tumour cells, while, in contrast, Sadler & Alexander (1976) showed a decreased lung retention of tumour cells in tumour-bearing animals. These contradictory results are obviously difficult to explain.The hypothesis by Glaves (1980) is that the presence of a growing tumour can variously inhibit (Normann et al.1979) or enhance (Saba & Antikatzides 1975) components of the reticuloendothelial system, thereby modifying the retention patterns of i.v. injected tumour cells.

In the present study a metastasizing fibrosarcoma caused a significant increase of the lodgement in both the lungs and liver after i.v. or intraportal injection of syngeneic tumour cells. In order to investigate if distant metastases from the primary tumour had any specific effect on the lodgement process, the chemotherapeutic agent Razoxin was used as a tool to inhibit spontaneous metastasis formation. Razoxin has been reported to cause an almost complete suppression of metastasis formation (Hellmann & Burrage 1969), probably through direct effects on the primary tumour by preventing the escape of malignant cells into the blood stream (Salsbury et al.1974).

Razoxin is a cytostatic drug, and pretreatment with other cytostatic drugs, in particular cyclophosphamide, has in previous investigations been found to cause a significant increase in the number of tumour nodules in the lungs after i.v. tumour cell injection (van Putten et al.1975). The nature of the mechanisms behind this drug effect is not known, but most authors agree,that it is primarily non-immunologic and that it most likely results from local damage of the lung leading to an increased retention of tumour cells.

In the present study Razoxin did not cause any enhancement of tumour cell lodgement in tumour-free rats, which seems to exclude a specific pharmacological effect of Razoxin similar to that of cyclophosphamide. When given to tumour-bearing rats, Razoxin caused, however, an increase in tumour cell

lodgement that was even more pronounced than in rats with metastasizing tumour. Since Razoxin is a potent depressor of humoral immunity and has a moderate suppressive effect even on cell-mediated immunity (Hellmann 1972),
the most probable explanation for its increasing effect on lodgement in tumour-bearing animals would be through suppression of the immune response in
animals sensitized to tumour antigens by the presence of a growing solid
primary tumour. Accordingly, in the abscence of a primary tumour, Razoxin
should not have any effect on tumour cell lodgement, which is in agreement
with the findings of the present study.

Another hypothesis to be considered to explain the effect of Razoxin on
the lodgement in tumour-bearing rats would be its prevention of metastasis
formation. When distant metastases are present, an increased tumour load
might have an inhibitory effect on lodgement of circulating tumour cells.
By preventing the establishment of distant metastases, and possibly also by
its reducing effect on the primary tumour size, Razoxin would decrease the
tumour load and thus indirectly promoting tumour cell lodgement.

REFERENCES
Fidler, I.J.,1970, Metastasis: Quantitative analysis of distribution and
    fate of tumour emboli labelled with ^{125}I-5-iodo-2-deoxyuridine. Journal
    of National Cancer Institute 45, 773.
Fidler,I.J., Gersten,D.M. & Riggs,C.W.,1977, Relationship of host immune
    status to tumour cell arrest, distribution and survival in experimental
    metastasis. Cancer 40, 46.
Glaves, D., 1980,Metastasis:Reticuloendothelial system and organ retention
    of disseminated malignant cells. International Journal of Cancer 26, 115.
Gorelik,E., Segal,S., Shapiro,J., Katzav,S., Ron,Y. & Feldman, M.1982, Inter-
    actions between the local tumour and its metastases. Cancer Metastasis
    Reviews 1, 83.
Hellmann, K. & Burrage K., 1969, Control of malignant metastases by ICRF 159.
    Nature 224, 273.
Hellmann, K., 1972, Proceedings of the Royal Society of Medicine 65, 264.
Normann,S.J., Schardt,M. & Sorkin, E., 1979, Cancer progression and monocyte
    inflammatory dysfunction: relationship to tumour excision and metastasis.
    International Journal of Cancer 23, 110.
Saba, T. & Antikatzides,T.G., 1975, Humoral mediated macrophage response
    during tumour growth. British Journal of Cancer 32, 471.
Salsbury, A.J., Burrage, K. & Hellmann, K., 1974, Histological analysis of
    the antimetastatic effect of (+)-1,2-Bis (3,5-dioxopiperazine-1-yl) pro-
    pane. Cancer Research 34, 843.
Skolnik,G., Alpsten, M. & Ivarsson,L., 1980, The influence of trauma, dext-
    ran 1000 and dextran 40 on the lodgement of circulating tumour cells.
    Journal of Cancer Research and Clinical Oncology 97, 241.
Sadler, T.E. & Alexander P., 1976, Trapping and destruction of blood-borne
    syngeneic leukemia cells in lung, liver and spleen of normal and leukemic
    rats. British Journal of Cancer 33, 512.
van Putten,L.M., Kram L.K.J., Van Dierendonck, H.H.C., Smink,T. & Füzy M,
    1975, International Journal of Cancer 15, 588.
Weiss, L., Glaves, D. & Waite, D.A., 1974, International Journal of Cancer
    13, 850.

THE EFFECT OF BREATHING 8% OXYGEN ON THE FATE OF INTRAVENOUSLY INJECTED
RODENT SARCOMA CELLS

R. CLARKE, P. V. SENIOR and P. ALEXANDER

Dept. of Medical Oncology, University of Southampton, Southampton General
Hospital, Southampton SO9 4XY

Keywords: Hypobaric Oxygen, Autolysis in Lung

INTRODUCTION

Many experiments have demonstrated that, following intravenous injection, the majority of sarcoma, carcinoma and melanoma cells arrested in
the lungs die there and do not develop into lung metastases. One of the
processes responsible for the death of cancer emboli in the lung may be
the toxicity of oxygen at concentrations encountered in oxygenated blood.
(Alexander & Eccles, 1984). Tumour cells normally grow extravascularly
where the oxygen pressure is in the region of 20 mm. Hg., which corresponds to a concentration in the atmosphere of 12%. We have examined the
sensitivity to oxygen at arterial concentrations of rodent tumour cells
obtained directly from the animal (and not maintained for long periods in
culture) *in vitro*, using both a short term, five day proliferation assay
and a longer term soft agar clonogenic assay. The sensitivity of such
cancer cells to oxygen *in vivo* was studied by comparing the fate of sarcoma cells trapped in the lung following intravenous injection in animals
breathing 8% and normal oxygen concentrations. Two end-points were used;
The autolysis in the lungs of trapped radiolabelled tumour cells was
measured and the number of tumour colonies developing in the lungs of
animals injected with unlabelled tumour cells.

METHODS

Tumours: Three mouse tumours and two rat tumours were used, being
induced in syngeneic animals bred in our colony (FS6 in C57/B1, B16 in
C57/B1, FS19 in CBA mice, and MC26 and MC28 in Hooded Lister rats), whose
biological properties have been described (Eccles, Heckford & Alexander,
1980). Single cell suspensions were produced by mechanical disaggregation

by a solution of protease and ribonuclease for 1½ hours at room temperature.

Proliferation assay: Cells were resuspended in DMEM supplemented with foetal calf serum, glutamine, antibiotics and fugizone at cell concentrations from 4×10^4 to 5×10^5/ml. Six 0.1 ml. replicates of each cell concentration were added to 96 well micro-titre plates and incubated at $37\,^{\circ}$C in either 20% or 5% oxygen concentration in 5% CO_2 and nitrogen. Plates were fixed with buffered formol saline at one, three and five days. Cell density was estimated optically following methylene blue staining. (Martin, F., Martin, M., Jeanine J., Lecneau, A., 1978).

Soft agar clonogenic assay: Cells were resuspended in CMRL 1066 supplemented with horse serum glutamine, vitamin C, asparagine, 0.3% agar and antibiotics at cell concentrations from 10^3 to 10^5/ml. The cells were plated out in 30 mm. vented petri dishes at 1 ml./dish. Three replicates per cell concentration were incubated at $37\,^{\circ}$C in 5% or 20% CO_2 and nitrogen. Clones were counted 2-3 weeks later and a minimum of 50 cells per cluster being accepted as a clone.

Autolysis in the lung of trapped tumour cells: Cells were radiolabelled *in vitro* with iodo-deoxyuridine. One day prior to the injection of the cells a cannula was implanted into the right jugular vein of male hooded Lister rats. 0.1 mls. (10^4 cells) of the cell suspension was injected via the cannula and half the rats immediately placed in a chamber continually gassed with 8% O_2 in N_2 and the others left to breathe air. Three rats were killed after two minutes and cohorts of three were killed from both groups at four hours, eight hours and twenty-four hours. (Animals were transferred from 8% O_2 to air after eight hours). The lungs, liver and kidney were removed and the radioactivity in each organ counted and the percentage of the initial radioactivity injected determined.

Lung colony formation: Cells from mouse and rat sarcomas were resuspended in Hanks Salts and injected i.v. via the cannula at concentrations of 10^4, 10^3 and 10^2 in a total volume of 0.1 ml. Three animals per cell concentration were placed in 8% O_2 and N_2 as above, for six hours, then left in air. One month later, or when one of the highest dose animals became ill, the high dose group was killed and if lung colonies were found the next lower concentrations were killed. The number of colonies visible in the lungs was counted.

RESULTS

In vitro: In the proliferation assay, at cell concentrations up to

3×10^5/ml., cells from all sarcomas tested grew better in 5% O_2 than in 20% O_2. Typical results for FS19 and MC26 are shown in Figure 1.

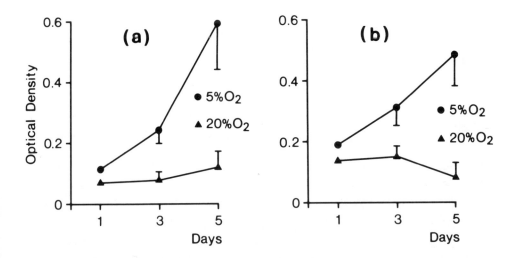

Fig. 1a. MC26 rat sarcoma (1×10^5 cells/ml.): Fig. 1b. FS19 mouse sarcoma (1×10^5 cells/ml.). Bars indicate 95% confidence limits of six replicates.

In the soft agar clonogenic assay, clonal growth of the tumour cells tested (FS6, B16 MC28) was greater in dishes incubated in 5% O_2 than those in 20% O_2. See Table 1.

Table 1. Clonogenic Assay in 5% and 20% Oxygen.

TUMOUR	No. OF CELLS PER DISH	AVERAGE No. OF CLONES PER DISH 5% O_2	20% O_2
FS6	10^4	236 (2.4)	35 (0.4)
	5×10^3	156 (3.1)	10 (0.2)
	10^3	12 (1.2)	1 (0.1)
MC28	5×10^4	104 (0.2)	69 (0.14)
B16/CB1	5×10^3	500 (10)	11 (0.22)
	10^3	108 (11)	2 (0.2)
	5×10^2	42 (8.4	3 (0.6)

(Average Cloning Efficiency in Brackets)

In vivo: Figure 2 shows a typical result for MC28 rat sarcoma for the rate of autolysis of cells trapped in the lung, which occurs more rapidly in animals breathing air than 8% oxygen.

Figure 2. Rate of disappearance of radioactivity in the lung following i.v. injection of I^{125} labelled MC28 rat sarcoma cells in rats breathing air or 8% O_2.

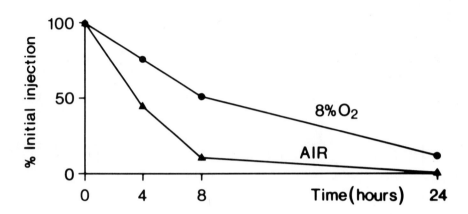

Table 2 shows that the number of colonies found in animals breathing 8% O_2 for six hours is greater than that found in animals breathing air.

Table 2. Effect of Oxygen Concentration Breathed in the Six Hours After i.v. Injection on the Number of Lung Colonies.

TUMOUR	No. OF CELLS INJECTED	No. OF LUNG COLONIES PER	
		8% O_2	AIR
FS19 *in vivo*	10^4	18/14/16	0/0
passage 11	10^3	1/1/1	0/0/0
FS19 *in vivo*	10^4	65/16/13	6/5/2
passage 19	10^3	3/0/0	0/0/1
MC28 *in vivo*	10^5	34/50	5/2/5
passage 29			

DISCUSSION

Tumour cells derived directly from rodent sarcomas and a mouse melanoma grow less well in cultures equilibrated with air than with an atmosphere containing 5% oxygen. *In vivo,* the sarcoma cells are cleared less rapidly from the lungs and form more lung colonies in animals breathing 8% oxygen than air and this supports the view that oxygen toxicity contributes to the death within the lungs of cancer emboli.

REFERENCES

Alexander, P. & Eccles, S. A., 1984. Cancer Invasion & Metastases. Edited Nicolson, G. & Milas, L. (Raven Press), p.293
Eccles, S. A., Heckford, S. & Alexander, P., 1980. British Journal of Cancer, 42: 252.
Martin, F., Martin, M., Jeanine, J. & Lecneau, A., 1978. European Journal of Immunology, 8: 607-611.

ARTIFICIAL AND SPONTANEOUS METASTASIS FORMATION: CORRELATIONS WITH TUMOR CELL PROPERTIES

J.P.VOLPE[1], N.HUNTER[1], I.BASIC[1], L.C.STEPHENS[2], & L. MILAS[1]

[1]Department of Experimental Radiotherapy and [2]Division of Veterinary Medicine and Surgery, M. D. Anderson Hospital and Tumor Institute, Houston, TX

Keywords: tumor cell properties; lung colony forming efficiency; spontaneous metastasis

INTRODUCTION

Malignant properties of tumors, including propensity for metastatic spread, are commonly assessed on the basis of histologic grading. However, the ability of tumors to give metastasis depends on many factors including certain properties of tumor cells that cannot be identified with histological analysis (Fidler et al. 1978; Milas et al. 1983). Such properties, including cell volume, DNA content, and cell clumping, have been found to influence the metastatic ability of tumor cells (Liotta et al. 1976; Fidler et al. 1978; Suzuki et al. 1980), but the extent of their contribution to the metastatic process is unknown and may vary among different tumors. It is, therefore, important to identify properties of tumor cells that correlate best with metastasis. We have investigated the extent of correlation between several properties of 12 syngeneic tumors and the ability of these tumors to give spontaneous lung metastases or to colonize the lung upon i.v. injection. In addition, the ability of the lung colony forming efficiency (LCFE) to correlate with spontaneous metastasis was investigated. This report is a preliminary communication of our ongoing studies.

MATERIALS AND METHODS

The six sarcomas (SA) and six carcinomas (CA) syngeneic to C3Hf/Kam mice used in this investigation include: NFSA, FSA, FSA-II, SA IIa, SA-NHI, SA-4020, MCA-4, MCA-K, MCA-35, HCA-I, and ASCA-SG. All of these tumors arose spontaneously, except for FSA, which was chemically induced. LCFE was determined by injecting 2×10^5 viable tumor cells (determined by trypan blue exclusion) i.v. into the tail vein of 10-12-week-old female mice. Spontaneous lung metastasis was assayed by injecting i.m. 5–10×10^5 viable tumor cells in a volume of 10–$20 \, \mu l$ into the legs of 9-12-week-old female mice, amputating the primary tumor at 12 mm, and scoring the lungs for the presence of metastases at the appropriate time after amputation.

The time it took a tumor to grow from 6 to 12 mm was used as the tumor doubling time. Histologic grading was analyzed using tissue sections stained in hematoxilin and eosin. The relative malignancy of the tumors, evaluated separately for sarcomas and carcinomas, was determined by ranking them as 1, 2, or 3 for the cytologic features of plemorphism, mitoses, and differentiation along with the growth characteristics of growth pattern, invasion, and necrosis. Cell volume was determined on samples of 1–5×10^4 cells/ml by a multichannel analyzer (Channelyzer II) and a Coulter counter. DNA content was assayed by flow microfluorometry (ICP II, Phywe Co.). Immunogenicity was assessed by the ability of specifically sensitized mice to resist the engraftment of viable tumor cells and was expressed as the ratio of TD_{50} values in immunized over control mice.

Spearman's rank correlation coefficients (r) were obtained and adjusted to account for the degrees of freedom by the statistical program Minitab (Pennsylvania State release). Significance and p values were determined from the nonadjusted coefficients (Zar 1974).

RESULTS

Figure I shows the correlation between spontaneous metastasis and LCFE, which is the only correlation significantly different from zero at the 5% error level. However, if the error level is increased to $p < .1$, then 7 other correlation coefficients differ from zero. Table I is a summary of the correlation coefficients showing the relationship between the properties studied and spontaneous metastasis or LCFE. The histologic subcategories are not listed in the table, but include these characters that correlate with metastasis: the mitotic ranking of the sarcoma ($r = -.66$, $.05 < p < .1$), the differentiation ranking of the sarcomas ($r = .66$, $.05 < p < .1$), the plemorphic ranking of the adenocarcinomas ($r = .61$, $p > .1$), and the growth pattern of sarcomas ($r = .39$). The following histologic subcategories correlated with LCFE: the ranking of plemorphism of the sarcomas ($r = .57$, $.05 < p < .1$), the ranking of the histologic grade of the sarcomas ($r = .46$, $p = .1$), and the differentiation of the sarcomas ($r = .31$). All other correlations were at or near zero.

Figure I.   The correlation between the ranks of spontaneous lung metastasis and
             lung colony forming efficiency (LCFE).

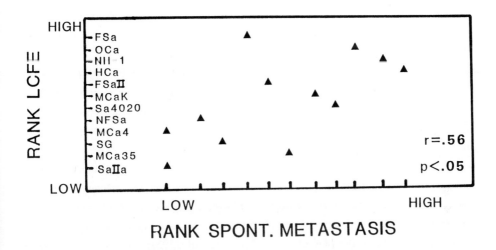

Table I.   The correlation coefficients of the properties studied and spontaneous
            (SP) lung metastasis and lung colony forming efficiency (LCFE).

	CORRELATION[a]						
SP,	LUNG METASTASIS				LCFE		
	Sa	Ca	Total		Sa	Ca	Total
Doubling time	0	0	0		0	0	0
Histologic grading[d]	.23	0			.46[c]	0	
Cell volume	.75[b]	0	.35[c]		0	0	0
DNA content	NA	NA	0		NA	NA	0
Immunogenicity	0	0	0		0	0	0
% Nonsingle cells	.45[c]	0	0		0	0	0
% Nonviable cells					0	0	-36[b]

[a]r is adjusted for degrees of freedom

[b]$.05 < p < .1$

[c]$p = .1$

[d]Subcategory correlations are described in the text

DISCUSSION

The results of this preliminary study show that only a few of the properties studied correlated with either spontaneous metastasis formation or LCFE. Only histological grading, cell volume, and percent of nonsingle cells had some degree of correlation with spontaneous metastases of sarcomas, and only histologic grading and percent of nonviable cells correlated with LCFE. Interestingly, none of the properties studied correlated with either spontaneous metastasis formation or LCFE of carcinomas, with the exception of cellular pleomorphism, which correlated with spontaneous metastasis ($r = .61$, $p > .1$). Therefore, these data imply that although a single property of a tumor may greatly influence the outcome of metastasis, there will be considerable variation between tumors. It is likely that more valid correlations would be obtained if more tumors were analyzed. Also, our studies examined the correlation between LCFE and spontaneous metastasis, which we consider important because of the widespread use of LCFE as a model of metastasis. Reports in literature are controversial, but the studies were mainly limited to one or a few tumor systems (Kripke et al. 1978; Stackpole 1981; Sweeney et al. 1982; Unemori et al. 1984). Here we found that although the LCFE of an individual tumor may or may not predict the ability for metastasis, the overall correlation using 12 different tumors was significant. However, it should be noted that even this correlation explained only 31% of the variability of spontaneous metastasis ($r = .56$, $r^2 = .31$).

REFERENCES

Fidler, I.J., Fersten, D.M., and Hart, I.R., 1978, Advances in Cancer Research, 28, 149.

Kripke, M.L., Gruys, E., and Fidler, I.J., 1978, Cancer Research, 38, 1962.

Liotta, L.A., Kleinerman, J., and Saidel, G.M., 1976, Cancer Research, 36, 889.

Milas, L., Peters, L.J., and Ito, H., 1983, Clinical and Experimental Metastasis, 1, 309.

Stackpole, C.W., 1981, Nature, 289, 798.

Suzuki, N., Williams, M., Hunter, N.M., and Withers, H.R., 1980, British Journal of Cancer, 42, 765.

Sweeney, F.L., Pot-Deprun, J., Poupon, M.F., and Chouroulinkov, I., 1982, Cancer Research, 42, 3776.

Unemori, E.N., Ways, N., and Pitelka, D.R., 1984, British Journal of Cancer, 49, 603.

Zar, J.H., 1974, Biostatistical Analysis (Prentice-Hall, Inc.).

INITIAL STEPS OF COLONIZATION OF THE LUNG BY TWO TUMOUR CELL VARIANTS WITH DIFFERENT METASTATIC CAPACITIES

N. PAWELTZ, P. AULENBACHER, H.O. WERLING and E. SPIESS
Institute of Cell and Toumor Biology, German Cancer Research Center,
D-6900 Heidelberg, FRG

Keyword: Lung colonisation: embolisation

INTRODUCTION

Recent publications concerning cell behavior and characteristics demonstrate a wide diversity of tumour cell properties. One of the most important tumour cell characteristics is their metastatic capacity, which involves primary invasion, dissemination, secondary invasion and growth of daughter tumours. Several systems with different metastatic abilities have been described (Mareel, 1983). In 1983 Matzku and his colleagues selected two rat tumour cell variants which originated from a sarcoma of BDX rats. They display very different metastatic behaviors (Matzku et al., 1983) since the ASML variant is highly metastatic to the lung via the lymphatic vessels, while the AS variant shows only a weak ability to metastasize. However, tumours can be found within the lung after intravenous inoculation of the two variants. We have characterized these variants morphologically and cytogenetically. There is a pronounced difference in their surface structure, the karyograms, their adhesion, spreading and aggregating behavior. When these variants are confronted with excised endothelium of the aorta, the low metastasizing variant is strongly adherent, spreads, penetrates the endothelium through gaps and induces endothelial cells to retract. The highly metastasizing cells, however, are only loosely adherent and remain spherical and inactive (Aulenbacher et al., 1984). These unequal behaviors in vitro suggest that there might also be differences in the colonization of the lung.

MATERIALS AND METHODS

Approximately 5×10^6 AS and ASML cells were suspended in their culture medium and then inoculated into BDX rats via the tail vein. The lungs were removed from the animals after an initial perfusion with fixative at 12, 30 and 60 min after inoculation and then prepared for electron microscopy. For scintigraphic studies, the tumour cells were labelled with In^{111} and injected into the rats. The distribution pattern of labelled cells was then determined by means of a gamma-camera at various time intervals.

RESULTS

The first accumulation of the In^{111}-labelled tumour cells can be found mainly within the lung and to a lesser extent in the liver. The radio-activity gradually disappears from the lung and concomitantly increases within the liver and spleen. There is no significant difference in the distribution pattern between the two tumour cell variants except that the AS cells leave the lung more slowly than ASML. Thus, we conclude that after an initial arrest only a small number of tumour cells remain within the lung.

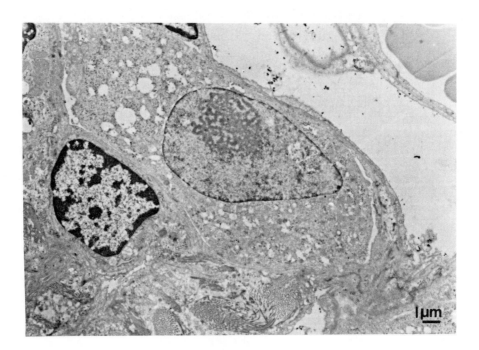

Figure 1. An AS cell within a capillary.

Ultrastructural analysis shows that the majority of tumour cells are destroyed within the lung. Although we could find some cell debris in

contact with leukocytes, we cannot explain the mechanism of destruction.
Possibly the radioactivity in the liver and in the spleen originates from
cell debris rather than from living cells.

However, some tumour cells remain intact and begin to settle in the lung.
Initially the AS cells can be found as single cells within the capillary
lumen (Figure 1). They are mostly attached to the endothelial cells and
fill the lumen completely. In later stages the capillaries become inflated.
No indications of an extravasation process of the tumour cells can be found
at the onset of colonization. The formation of protrusions on one end of
the cell resembles an uropod of stimulated lymphocytes. This indicates an
active mobility of the AS cells within the vessel.

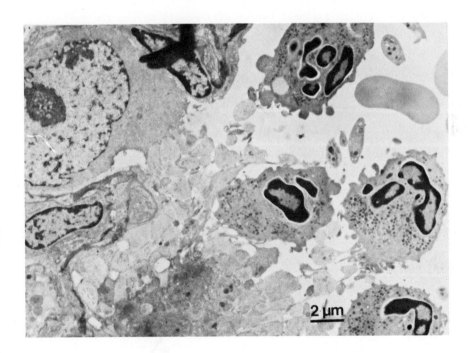

Figure 2. An AS cell is surrounded by platelets and leukocytes forming
          an embolus.

During the beginning of the colonization by ASML cells, some platelets
are attached to or near tumour cells. At slightly later stages, a fibrin

clot is formed which includes tumour cells, platelets and a few leukocytes (Figure 2). This clot is then surrounded by a circle of leukocytes resembling an inflammation reaction. The emboli induced by ASML cells increase in size and obstruct the capillaries; they then break through capillary walls giving rise to larger accumulations. Signs of extravasation are not observed in these preparation.

DISCUSSION

Previously we have demonstrated that the two tumour cell variants ASML and AS differ in their surface ultrastructure, settling and spreading behavior, aggregation capacities and karyograms (Paweletz et al., 1984; Werling et al., 1984). While the ASML variant is rather inactive compared to AS cells, the cytogenetic properties suggest a stronger malignancy in ASML cells than in the AS variant. When the AS cells are grown in an *in vitro* confrontation system they exhibit an invasive activity which is not observed in the highly metastasizing ASML cells (Aulenbacher et al., 1984). We have shown that both variants behave differently during the initial steps of colonization in the lung. It is well known that malignant cells can induce coagulation leading to the formation of emboli which obstruct the lung capillaries (Gasic, 1984). These foci then give rise to a secondary tumour. AS cells behave differently during colonization and show no signs of embolus formation. Therefore, both tumour cell lines behave differently *in vivo* and *in vitro*. These experiments show that it is difficult to make predictions for *in vivo* behavior based on *in vitro* observations. Active invasion ability under *in vitro* conditions is not a prerequisite for successful metastasis *in vivo*.

REFERENCES

Aulenbacher, P., Werling, H.O., Paweletz, N. & Spiess, E., 1984, *Anti-cancer Research* 4, 75.
Gasic, G., 1984, *Cancer Metastasis Review*, 3, 99.
Matzku, S., Komitowski, D., Mildenberger, M. & Zoller, M., 1983, *Invasion and Metastasis*, 3, 109.
Mareel, M., 1983, *Cancer Metastasis Review*, 2, 201.
Paweletz, N., Werling, H.O., Aulenbacher, P., & Spiess, E., 1984, *Scanning Electron Microscopy* II, 783.
Werling, H.O., Ghosh, S., & Spiess, E., 1984, *Journal of Cancer Research and Clinical Oncology* 107, 172.

INTERACTIONS BETWEEN NORMAL HUMAN FIBROBLASTS AND CARCINOMA CELLS IN MONOLAYER CULTURE

E.C. CHEW, T.K., LAM and H.J. CHAN-HOU

Department of anatomy, The Chinese University of Hong Kong, Shatin, N.T., Hong Kong

Keyword: Human Fibroblast - carcinoma cell confrontation

A distinctive feature of malignant cells is their capacity to infiltrate and form secondary tumours (metastases) at local and distant host sites. Many investigations into the interactions of normal mesenchymal and malignant cells in monolayer culture have demonstrated the penetration of malignant cells into the territory occupied by mesenchymal cells (Knyrim & Paweletz, 1977; Kramer & Nicolson, 1979; Benke & Paweletz, 1984). However, the mechanisms by which tumour cells invade normal host tissues are poorly understood. In this communication, we present the sequence of interactions between normal human fibroblasts and carcinoma cells in monolayer culture and the possible mechanisms involved.

MATERIALS AND METHODS

The tumour cell line (NPC/HK1) was established from a differentiated squamous carcinoma of the nasopharynx (Huang et al., 1980). Human embryonic fibroblasts and the NPC/HK1 cells were maintained in RPMI-1640 medium supplemented with 10% fetal calf serum to which 100 IU/ml penicillin, and 100 ug/ml streptomycin, were added. They were incubated at $37^{\circ}C$ in an atmosphere of 5% CO_2 in air. The confluent sheets of tumour cells and fibroblasts were confronted with fibroblasts and malignant cells respectively, in suspension. The cells were allowed to interact for 3, 6, 12, 48, and 72 hours after confrontation. The specimens were fixed in 2.5% glutaraldehyde in cacodylate buffer, dehydrated, critical point dried, coated with gold-palladium and examined with a Joel JSM-35CF scanning electron microscope at 15 kV.

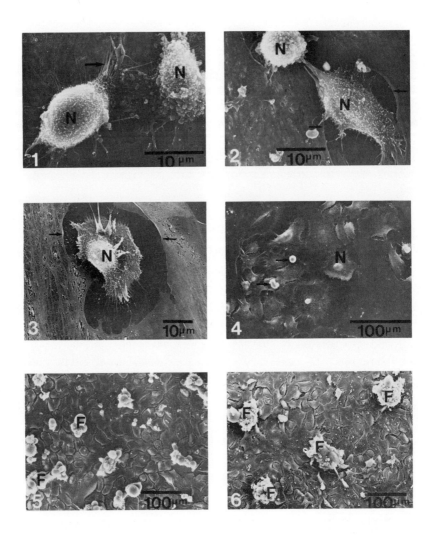

Figures 1 - 4. NPC/HK1 cells (N) resting on a confluent layer of normal embryonic fibroblasts. NPC/HK1 cells invade the monolayer. 1. After 3 hours of confrontation. NPC/HK1 cell has fine filopodia (arrow). 2. After 6 hours of confrontation. By inducing slight retraction of fibroblasts (arrows). 3. After 12 hours of confrontation. By inducing further retraction of fibroblasts (arrows). 4. After 3 days of confrontation. An aggregate of NPC/HK1 cells in a crater. Spherical cells may indicate dividing tumor cells (arrows).

Figures 5 - 6. Normal embryonic fibroblasts (F) resting on a confluent layer of NPC/HK1 cells. Normal fibroblasts do not invade the monolayer. 5. After 6 hours of confrontation. Normal fibroblasts (F) attach to the underlying tumor cells. 6. After 3 days of confrontation. Normal fibroblasts (F) remain rounded on the flattened tumor cells.

Results

   The morphological events occurring after confrontation of normal
fibroblasts and tumor cells in two different *in vitro* conditions over a
period of 72 hours have been evaluated by scanning electron microscope.
At 3 hours after seeding of tumor cells on the confluent layer of
fibroblasts, the tumor cells became attached to fibroblasts by fine
filopodia. Most of the tumor cells remained rounded but some began to
spread on top of the fibroblasts. A slight retraction of fibroblasts was
also noted (Fig. 1). At 6 hours after inoculation, further retraction of
fibroblasts was observed. The tumor cells penetrated the fibroblast
monolayer and spread on the underlying extracellular matrix (Fig. 2).
From 9 - 12 hours after confrontation, the craters produced by retraction
of fibroblasts enlarged and the tumor cells became more flattened (Fig 3).
At day 3, larger craters with even more flattened tumor cells were found
and some spherical tumor cells, probably undergoing division, began to
appear (Fig 4). In contrast, when normal fibroblasts were seeded on the
confluent layer of tumor cells, they behaved differently. At 3 - 6 hours
after inoculation, the fibroblasts became attached to the underlying
tumor cells by thin filapodia and tended to form small aggregates
(Fig. 5). Nevertheless, even after 2 to 3 days of incubation, the
fibroblasts remained rounded and aggregated. No penetration of the
fibroblasts and retraction of turor cells were seen (Fig. 6).

Discussion

   We have clearly demonstrated that after addition to a monolayer of
normal embryonic fibroblasts, NPC/HK1 can induce retraction of
fibroblasts and directly penetrate them. The retraction of fibroblasts
results in the formation of craters and the tumor cells penetrate and
spread on the extracellular matrix in these craters. The penetration of
fibroblasts by tumor cells can occur singly or in aggregates. But when
normal fibroblasts were seeded on a confluent layer of tumor cells, the
fibroblasts, either singly or in aggregates, may also attach to the
underlying tumor cells. However, the fibroblasts do not penetrate the
flattened tumor cells and no retraction of tumor cells was observed. It
was found that when small glass particles were seeded on the top of Wi38
fibroblasts in culture, no retraction of underlying fibroblasts was seen
(Benke and Paweletz, 1984). When HeLa cells were seeded on a monolayer
of pre-exisiting monolayer of Wi38 fibroblasts and when B16 melanoma
cells were added on a confluent bovine aortic endothelial cells,

retraction of underlying cells has been noted (Benke et al., 1984; Kramer
and Nicolson, 1979). In previous studies which include our own, it has
been established that following inoculation of tumour cells into the
peritoneal cavity of rodents, a retraction and rounding up of mesothelial
cells preceded tumour invasion (Birbeck and Wheatley, 1965; Kaneshima et al.
1976; Chew et al., 1982). Aulenbacher et al. (1984) found that the tumour
cell variant (As-cells) exhibited a dramatic invasive behavior, while there
was no sign of invasion in the ASML-variant which was highly metastatic via
the lymph vessels. In view of the phenomena observed both in vitro and in
vivo, it is suggested that tumour cells produce a 'retractive factor' which
causes the underlying normal cells to retract in order to facilitate invasion of tumour cells. This factor may also inhibit the spread and invasion
of normal fibroblasts on top of the flattened tumour cells. Although the
nature of this factor is not clear, it seems likely that it may act on the
cytoskeleton of normal fibroblasts to cause the contraction of these cellular elements.

REFERENCES

Aulenbacher, P., Wenling, H.O., Paweletz, N. and Spiess, E. (1984),
   Invasive activities of metastasizing and nonmetastasizing tumour cell
   variants in vitro. Anticancer Research 4: 75
Benke, R., and Paweletz, N. (1984), Scanning electron microscopic observations on cells grown in vitro. VII, HeLa cells can penetrate Wi38
   fibroblasts. European Journal of Cell Biology 33: 52
Birbeck, M.S.C. and Wheatley, D.N. (1965), An electron microscopic study
   of the invasion of ascites tumour cells into the abdominal wall. Cancer
   Research 25: 490
Chew, E.C., Ooi, E.C.V., Lam, O.W. and Kwan, S.M. (1982), A scanning
   electron microscopic study on the inital invasion of Ehrlich ascites (EA)
   tumour cells in peritoneal layer. Proceedings of the 40th meeting of the
   Electron Microscopy Society of America. Bailey, G.W. (Ed.) 228
Huang, D.P., Ho, J.H.C., Poon, Y.F., Chew, W.C., Saw, D., Lui, M., Li, C.L.,
   Mak, L.S., Lai, S.H. and Lau, W.H. (1980), Establishment of a cell line
   (NPC/HK1) from a differentiated squamous carcinoma of the nasopharynx.
   International Journal of Cancer 26: 127
Kaneshima, S., Kudo, H., Kosaka, H., Iitsuka, Y., Kimachi, H. and Takenchi,
   T. (1976), A scanning electron microscopic study on implantation of
   Ehrlich ascites tumour cells in the peritoneal layer. Yonago Acta Medica
   20: 101
Knyrim, K. and Paweletz, N. (1977), Cell interactions in a 'bilayer' of
   tumour cells. A scanning electron microscopic study. Virchows Archives
   B. Cellular Pathology 25: 309
Kramer, R.H. and Nicolson, G.L. (1979), Interactions of tumour cells with
   vascular endothelial cell monolayers: A model for metastatic invasion
   Proceedings of National Academy of Science U.S.A. 76: 5704

MULTIPLE PHENOTYPE DIVERGENCE OF MAMMARY ADENOCARCINOMA CELL CLONES

D. WELCH[1] D. EVANS[2], S. TOMASOVIC[2], D. KRIZMAN[2], L. MILAS[2], and G. NICOLSON[2]
[1] Cancer Research Unit, The Upjohn Company, Kalamazoo, Michigan, USA
[2] The University of Texas-M.D. Anderson Hospital, Houston, Texas, USA

Keywords : Tumor Progression, Metastasis, Phenotypic drift, Heterogeneity

INTRODUCTION

Cell clones isolated from the 13762NF mammary adenocarcinoma are unstable when subcultured _in vitro_. As these cells are grown, their metastatic potential, sites of metastases, cell surface properties and sensitivities to ionizing radiation, hyperthermia and chemotherapy agents shift as a function of _in vitro_ passage number. The magnitude and direction of these shifts are reproducible using different cryoprotected cell stocks and phenotypic drift is independent between phenotypes (Neri & Nicolson 1981, Welch et al. 1983, Welch, Neri & Nicolson 1983, Welch & Nicolson 1983).

Using the B16 melanoma, others (Poste, Doll & Fidler 1981) have demonstrated that cloned cell lines diverge as they are passaged _in vitro_ or _in vivo_ causing tumor heterogeneity. However, this apparently random generation of cell subpopulations is seemingly in conflict with the notion of preprogrammed tumor progression observed in the 13762NF system.

In order to determine whether the reproducible phenotypic shift of 13762NF cell clones is the result of a _en bloc_ shift of all cells within the population, or clonal divergence, we subcloned local tumor-derived clone MTF7 at low and high _in vitro_ passage numbers. The subclones were analyzed for : metastatic potential, _in vitro_ morphology, karyotype, ploidy, growth rate, and sensitivity to ionizing radiation, hyperthermia and 5-fluoro-2'-deoxyuridine (FUdR).

MATERIALS AND METHODS

Cells were grown in alpha-modified minimum essential medium (AMEM, Gibco 410-2000) supplemented with 10% FBS in Corning tissue culture plates. MTF7 cells were detached with a 0.25% trypsin solution; resuspended in complete AMEM; and subcloned by plating cells onto 96 well flat

bottom plates. Randomly selected subclones from low and high passage
cultures of MTF7 were expanded for freezing and experimentation.

   Experimental metastasis assays were performed by injection of 50,000
cells/0.2 ml into the lateral tail vein of age-matched, syngenic Fischer
344 female rats. Lung colonies were quantitated 23 days post-inoculation
as previously described (Welch, Neri & Nicolson 1983).

   Sensitivity to radiation (137_{Cs}), hyperthermia ($45^{o}C$) and FUdR were
determined by a standard colony formation assay to assess cell killing.
Data were analyzed by previously published methods (Welch et al. 1983,
Welch & Nicolson 1983).

RESULTS

In vitro properties

   MTF7 cells at low passage (T11) and high passage (T35) yielded subclones of different morphologies. Doubling times (DT) ranged between
16.8-17.4 hr except for one subclone, MTF7 (T35).2 (DT = 26 hr). Saturation
densities ranged between 1.2 - 2.2 x 10^5 cells/cm^2 for all MTF7 subclones.
Each of the subclones shared marker chromosomes in addition to markers
unique to a particular subclone.

Experimental metastatic potential

   MTF7 (T11)-derived subclones were heterogeneous (0-> 100 metastases per
lung) in their abilities to colonize lung following intravenous injection
(Figure 1). Likewise, subclones of MTF7 (T35) were heterogenous for the
number, (3 to > 600 metastases per lung) total volume and size distribution
of metastases.

Sensitivities to ionizing radiation, hyperthermia and FUdR

   Sensitivity was assayed at two levels: (1) ability to accumulate and/or
repair sublethal damage (D_q) and; (2) inherent sensitivity, (D_o) (Figures
2 and 3). MTF7 (T11) was homogeneous (no significant subsets, p<0.05) in
their sensitivities to ionizing radiation (D_o = 1.6 to 2.0 Gy; D_q = 0 to
2.3 Gy). When these same subclones were analyzed for their sensitivity to
hyperthermic treatment, the dose-response parameters were significantly
different (D_o = 5.2 to 10.0 min; D_q = 0.8 to 12.3 min). Sensitivity to
FUdR treatment was also significantly different (slope = -0.70 to -1.59 of
linear portion of a log-log dose-response curve; y-intercept = 1.31 x 10^2
to 47.80 x 10^2). At high passage, MTF7 (T35), was heterogeneous for all
survival curve parameters for ionizing radiation (D_o = 1.2 to 2.1 Gy, D_q =
1.8 to 4.9Gy), hyperthermia (D_o = 3.6 to 6.3 min; D_q = 3.7 to 9.3 Gy) and

FUdR (slope = -0.77 to -0.93; y-intercept = 4.64×10^2 to 8.83×10^2).

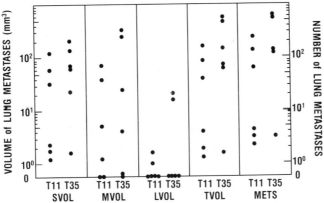

Figure 1. Experimental metastatic potential for MTF7 (T11) and MTF7 (T35) subclones. TVol, total metastasis volume (mm^3); SVol, volume of lung metastasis produced by lesions < 1mm in diameter; MVol, volume of lung metastases produced by lesions between 1 and 3 mm in diameter; LVol, volume of metastases > 3mm in diameter; METS, total number of surface lung colonies. Data points are mean value for each subclone.

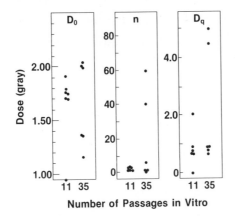

Figure 2. Ionizing radiation survival curve parameters for MTF7 subclones. Data are computer analyzed using a non-linear regression model (Welch et al. 1983). Data points are mean value for each subclone.

DISCUSSION

Our results clearly domonstrate the rapid generation of 13762NF cell subpopulations with diverse phenotypes from a cloned cell population. furthermore, the phenotypic composition of the clone MTF7 population changed during passage in vitro. It is this change that probably results in the previously described drift. Our data suggest that a preprogrammed divergence or common selective pressure yields a reproducible cell mixture. Whether cellular divergence is indeed preprogrammed remains to be determined.

These results also suggest certain implications in the design of therapy. Since tumour cells are capable of self-regeneration of heterogeneity, particularly with respect to sensitivity to various therapy and metastatic potential, it may be necessary to compensate for tumour instability in order to successfully treat malignant neoplasms. Therapy should be designed to reduce the potential for instability, limiting the evolution of highly malignant and therapy-resistant subpopulations.

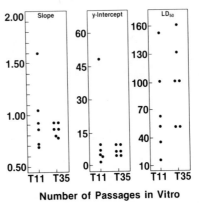

Figure 3. FUdR survival curve parameters for MTF7 subclones. Data are computer analyzed along the linear portion of log-log dose-response curve (Welch & Nicolson 1983). Data points are mean value for each subclone.

REFERENCES

Neri, A. & Nicolson, G.L., 1981, Phenotypic drift of metastatic and cell surface properties of mammary adenocarcinoma cell clones during growth in vitro, Internation Journal of Cancer, 28:731.
Poste, G., Doll, J., and Fidler, I.J., 1981, Interactions among clonal subpopulations affect stability of the metastatic phenotype in polyclonal populations of B16 melanoma cells. Proceedings of the National Academy of Sciences (USA), 78:6226.
Welch, D.R., Milas, L., Tomasovic, S.P. and Nicolson, G.L., 1983, Heterogeneous response and clonal drift of sensitivities of metastatic 13762NF mammary adenocarcinoma clones to gamma radiation in vitro. Cancer Research, 43:6.
Welch, D.R., Neri, A., Nicolson, G.L., 1983, Comparison of 'spontaneous' and 'experimental' metastasis using rat 13762 mammary adenocarcinoma metastatic cell clones. Invasion & Metastasis, 3:65.
Welch, D.R. and Nicolson, G.L., 1983, Phenotypic drift and heterogeneity in response of metastatic mammary adenocarcinoma cell clones to Adriamycin, 5 fluoro-2'-deoxyuridine and methotrexate treatment in vitro. Clinical and Experimental Metastasis, 1:317.

AN IN VITRO STUDY OF TUMOUR INVASION TO COMPARE METASTATIC AND NON-METASTATIC CELLS

C.T. BASSON[1] and E. SIDEBOTTOM[2]
[1]Yale School of Medicine, New Haven, CT.06510
[2]Sir William Dunn School of Pathology, Oxford OX1 3RE

Keyword: Invasion   Metastasis

INTRODUCTION

Invasion is a necessary, although not sufficient, prerequisite for metastasis. It is important at several stages of the metastatic cascade, notably the initial extension of the primary tumour, the penetration of blood vessels and lymphatics and the ultimate colonization of the secondary site. A reliable, reproducible in vitro system for the investigation of tumour cell invasion would clearly be of great value in helping to unravel the mechanisms involved, and might lead to rational therapy to delay or prevent the onset of metastatic disease.

Several possible systems have been described (Liotta & Hart, 1982) but none has yet proved to be entirely satisfactory. Interesting, though inconsistent, results have been obtained with pieces of human amnion cultured in vivo as the target tissue (e.g. Felix et al., 1982; Thorgeissen et al., 1982). This membrane has many desirable qualities for this type of work: it is easily obtained in large quantities; it consists of a single layer of epithelial cells anchored on a basement membrane, which in turn rests on a connective tissue stroma. It is robust, survives well on storage or culture and is easy to handle and process. The epithelium can be removed to provide an acellular sheet composed of a basement membrane and stroma.

We have previously reported that our matched pairs of metastatic and non-metastatic hybrid melanoma cell lines differ in their tendency to invade at the site of a primary tumour (Sidebottom & Clark, 1983). In collaboration with Mareel we have shown that both cell lines invade in the cultured embryonic heart fragment assay but that no distinction can be made between their invasive patterns. It was therefore of interest to see if the in vivo behaviour could be reproduced in the in vitro amnion invasion system.

METHODS AND RESULTS

Pieces of human amnion were prepared and mounted in chambers essentially as described in Russo et al. (1981). Either an intact epithelial surface, a denuded basement membrane or a stromal surface was exposed to a suspension of the appropriate tumour cells for 2 to 5 days. We used not only the F87 hybrid melanoma lines 6T2 and 4T1 but also B16 BL6 murine melanoma, HT1080 human fibrosarcoma, and A2058 human melanoma in the experiments. Each line was assayed in duplicate, a) without serum, b) with 10% foetal calf serum, c) with acid treated foetal calf serum (to inactivate serum proteases), and d) with 1% fetuin/I.T.S. (insulin, transferrin, selenium) serum replacement supplement. The fetuin/I.T.S. supplemented tests were also run with the chemo-attractant F.M.L.P. at 10^{-7}M to 10^{-9}M. All the cell lines tested adhered to the three different target surfaces although often only a small minority of the applied cells did so. No cell line gave unequivocal evidence of complete penetration of either intact or denuded membrane. However, some qualitative differences in the proliferative and invasive patterns of 4T1 (non-metastatic) and 6T2 (metastatic) cells were noted. These are summarized in the table, together with results obtained with the other cell lines.

Passive invasion implies that some tumour cells have proliferated on the epithelium, caused degeneration of the underlying cells and thus come to lie on the basement membrane. This effect was seen with all cell lines other than 6T2. Active invasion was recorded when tumour cells were present between the epithelium and the basement membrane. Examples were seen of tumour cells apparently pushing between adjacent epithelial cells although only a small proportion of adherent cells were able to penetrate the epithelium and none went on to penetrate the basement membrane.

On denuded basement membrane some tumour cells produced defects which we refer to as local degradation. Some 'locally invasive' cells migrated into the plane of the basement membrane via these defects and extended processes into the stroma but again no cells passed completely through the basement membrane and the stroma.

Interactions of tumour cells with stromal surfaces of the amnion were sometimes difficult to interpret. All cell lines adhered and all except 4T1 showed some convincing examples of local degradation and local invasion. However, separation of stroma from basement membrane, and folding of membranes during processing sometimes deposited cells in positions that they had clearly not reached by active invasion. These problems are discussed elsewhere (Basson, 1984, Basson & Sidebottom, 1984).

Table 1. Tumour cell interactions with amnion surfaces.

		Tumour Cell Lines				
		4T1	6T2	BL6	A2058	HT1080
	Adhesion	+	+	+	+	+
Epithelium	Passive Invasion	+	−	+	+	+
	Active Invasion	−	+	+	+	−
	Adhesion	+	+	+	+	+
Basement	Local degradation	−	+	+	+	+
Membrane	Local invasion	−	+	+	+	+
	Complete invasion	−	−	−	−	−
	Adhesion	+	+	+	+	+
Stroma	Local degradation	−	+	+	+	+
	Local invasion	−	+	+	+	+
	Complete invasion	−	?	?	−	?

DISCUSSION

The amnion assay, in our hands, did not produce the complete penetration of the amnion reported by Liotta's group. Nevertheless we can distinguish between the histopathology of invasion into the amnion by non-metastatic 4T1 and metastatic 6T2 cells. However the discrepancies between data from different laboratories coupled with interpretative problems arising from histological artefact indicate that this assay is not yet the quick, simple, quantitative, in vitro test originally hoped for.

REFERENCES

Basson, C.T., 1984, In vitro models of tumour cell invasion. M.Sc. thesis, Oxford University.

Basson, C.T. & Sidebottom, E. 1984. Manuscript in preparation.

Felix, H. et al., 1982, Scanning Electron Microscopy,2,741.

Liotta, L.A. & Hart, I.R., 1982, editors. Tumour Invasion and Metastasis. (Martinus Nijhoff).

Russo, R.G. et al., 1982, p.172 in Tumour Invasion and Metastasis. editors Liotta, L.A. & Hart, I.R.

Sidebottom, E. & Clark, S.R. 1983, British Journal of Cancer,47,399.

THE INFLUENCE OF SUCCINYL CONCANAVALIN A ON THE MIGRATION AND INVASION
IN VITRO OF NBT II

W. SCHROYENS* and R. TCHAO
Department of Pathology, The Medical College of Pennsylvania, 3300 Henry
Avenue, Philadelphia, Pa. 19129 USA
*Current Address: Medizinische Klinik, Justus Liebiq Universität,
Klinikstrasse 36, 6300 Giessen, FRG

Keyword: migration, invasion, in vitro, succinyl concanavalin A

INTRODUCTION

   Studies on the migratory behaviour of tumor cells in culture have received much attention because tumor invasion is thought to be in part due
to their altered control of locomotion (Mareel 1980). This behaviour has
been mostly studied in monolayer cultures. Concanavalin A, which binds to
the cell membrane, has been shown to inhibit migration of macrophages
(Kumagai & Arai 1973), ascites lymphoma cells and carcinoma cells (Friberg
et al. 1972), neural crest cells (Moran 1974), and wounded Vero cell monolayers (Simpson & Mason 1977) in vitro, and in vivo to inhibit the migration of epidermal cells during wound closure in newts (Donaldson &
Mason 1977). For our experiments succinylated concanavalin A (s-Con A), a
less toxic derivative of concanavalin A (Gunther et al. 1973), was used as
a tool to study the role of cellular migration in invasion. We report here
on the reversible inhibition of the migration of an epithelial cell line
NBT II by s-Con A in a two-dimensional culture system while in a three-
dimensional culture model no inhibition of invasion was observed.

METHODS

   The NBT cell line is derived from a chemical-induced urinary bladder
carcinoma in the Wistar rat. Its characteristics as a squamous cell
carcinoma in vivo and in vitro have been described (Toyoshima et al. 1971).
In preliminary experiments, 10^5 NBT II cells were seeded in T25 culture
flasks (Falcon, Oxnard, Ca.) in minimal Eagle's medium supplemented with
15% fetal calf serum, 0.05% glutamine and antibiotics. They were treated
for five days with different doses (50,100,250,500,1000µg/ml) of s-Con A
(United States Biochemical Co., Cleveland, Ohio) dissolved in the medium to

determine optimal dosage. All concentrations inhibited cell migration.
At 1000μg/ml cells lost their adhesiveness. For further experiments we
chose 200μg/ml. Next, NBT II cell aggregates were obtained by putting a
4 ml cell suspension (10^6 cells/ml) in a 25 ml Erlenmeyer flask. It was
gassed with 5% CO_2 in air, sealed with a rubber stopper, and rotated on a
gyratory shaker, 120 rpm at 37°C. Aggregates were collected 24 hours later.
For the two-dimensional system, they were seeded and left to attach to the
surface of stationary Falcon flasks. Treatment with s-Con A was for various periods up to six days. To study invasion we used the chick embryo
heart model (Mareel et al. 1979). Precultured 9 to 11 day old chick embryo
heart fragments, 4 mm in diameter, were confronted with the tumor aggregates on semi-solid medium. They were incubated for two hours, transferred
to a 6 ml Erlenmeyer flask with 2 ml of s-Con A-treated and untreated
culture medium, placed on a gyratory shaker at 120 rpm, 37°C, and gassed
with 5% CO_2 in air for up to seven days.

RESULTS

    In the two-dimensional system, the control cultures showed cells had
migrated from the aggregate six hours after seeding. The edge of the NBT
II island was irregular and broken as individual cells separated and moved
away from the mass. The cells continued to spread and after three days
occupied the substrate as a spreading sheet with some single peripheral
cells. After six days, the area covered had increased about twenty times.
The average diameter of the outgrowing colony of cells was calculated from
measurements on pictures made with time-lapse photography at 24 hour intervals. In the presence of s-Con A, migration of NBT II was suppressed
immediately. When medium containing s-Con A was replaced by s-Con A-free
medium to which 10 mM ⍺-methyl mannose was added, the inhibition of migration was reversed. The cells started to spread again after two hours.
    Due to our interest in invasion, we proceeded to study the effect of
s-Con A on the invasiveness of NBT II, knowing that it inhibited reversibly
the migration of NBT II in the two-dimensional system. The invasiveness
of NBT II in the chick embryo heart model has been described (Schroyens et
al. 1984). When the histology of the heart fragment plus NBT II maintained
with and without s-Con A was compared, no difference in the extent of invasion was observed. In all cultures fixed after 4 and 7 days, groups of
NBT II and some single cells were found in the heart fragment. NBT II
cells could be easily recognized in the heart muscle by their large nuclei
and nucleoli. Although slight variations in the relative amounts of NBT II

inside the heart were observed in individual cultures, the pattern of NBT II occupation was consistent. Invasion under the peripheral capsule of the heart fragment was a common feature.

To show that s-Con A was still present on the invading cells, immuno-peroxidase staining for con A was done. Multiple controls of various types were added to ensure specificity of the reaction. Tissue sections from s-Con A-free cultures were negative. Cultures treated with s-Con A showed that peripheral NBT II cells, as well as those inside the fragment, stained positively. The positive reaction of the cytoplasm of NBT II cells can be explained by pinocytosis of the membrane-bound lectin, analagous to the cell entry mechanism described for another lectin in fibroblasts (Nicolson et al. 1975).

DISCUSSION

The central question of this study was to examine the role of active tumor cell motility in the process of invasion. Tumor cell motility has been studied in vitro by a variety of assays which fall into 2 basic groups. Techniques such as the aggregate culture assay, agarose drop assay and wound-culture assay measure migration in 2 dimensions. For measurements of migration in 3 dimensions, there are the Boyden chamber assay, three-dimensional matrix culture, and organ culture. In an attempt to delineate the role of tumor cell motility in invasion, we studied one from each group. Previously, it was shown that s-Con A inhibited the migration in two dimensions of dense cultures of 3T3 and SV40-3T3 cells (Mannino et al. 1981). To our knowledge there have been no studies on the effect of s-Con A on epithelial cells.

The delay of the reversibility of the effect of s-Con A on the in-hibition of locomotion by adding ∝-methyl mannose, a sugar that spec-ifically inhibits the binding of s-Con A, indicates that this effect of s-Con A on the migration of NBT II correlates to its binding to the cell membrane. The data suggests that s-Con A inhibits migration possibly by increasing the lateral adhesion between NBT II cells. The parameters that determine the adhesiveness of one cell to another in culture are not well understood, and the recognition and adhesion is a multi-step process (Edel-man 1983). The mechanism by which concanavalin A and s-Con A increase lateral adhesion between cells is also unknown. S-Con A may cross link cells physically, but an alternative explanation could be that it induces changes in the plasma membrane leading to an increase in intercellular ad-hesion. It has been suggested that s-Con A does not work by binding to,

and removing from the medium the necessary factors for cell motility (Ballmer et al. 1980). Peroxidase-anti-peroxidase staining of culture flasks
which contained s-Con A did not stain positively, excluding the possibility
that s-Con A binds the cells to the plastic.

Embryological experiments have shown that the position of cells and
their contact with other tissue largely determine their locomotive behaviour (Vakaet et al. 1980). We have previously observed that the mode
of NBT II cell motility can be influenced by the substrate, such that on
glass, single cells do not translocate, while on collagen they migrate
individually (Tchao 1982). It is therefore conceivable that bringing the
invasive cells in contact with connective tissue could alter cell behaviour
and overcome the inhibitory effects of s-Con A. We must conclude that the
motility of tumor cells in vitro is different for different in vitro culture systems. This is not surprising since several factors contribute to
cell locomotion. Our results question the correlation between tumor cell
motility in a two-dimensional system and the invasive behaviour of these
cells in three dimensions, and implies that the ability or inability of
cells to migrate on plastic does not necessarily reflect their invasiveness
in vitro.

REFERENCES
Ballmer, K., Mannino, R.J. & Burger, M.M., 1980, Experimental Cell
    Research, 126, 311.
Edelman, G.M., 1983, Science, 219, 450.
Donaldson, Donald J. & Mason, James M., 1977, Experimental Zoology, 200,
    55.
Friberg, S., Golub, S., Lilliehöök, B. & Cochran, A., 1972, Experimental
    Cell Research, 73, 101.
Gunther, Gary R., Wang, J., Yahara, I., Cunningham, B. & Edelman, G.,
    1973, Proceedings of the National Academy of Sciences USA, 70, 1012.
Kumagai, K. & Arai, S., 1973, Journal of the Reticuloendothelial Society,
    13, 507.
Mannino, Raphael J., Ballmer, K., Zeltner, D. & Burger, M.M., 1981, The
    Journal of Cell Biology, 91, 855.
Mareel, M., Kint, J. & Meyvisch, C., 1979, Virchow Archiv B Cell
    Pathology, 30, 95.
Mareel, M., 1980, International Review of Experimental Pathology, 22, 65.
Moran, D., 1974, Experimental Cell Research, 86, 365.
Nicolson, G.L., Lacorbiere, M. & Hunter, T.R., 1975, Cancer Research, 35,
    144.
Schroyens, W., Bruyneel, E., Tchao, R., Leighton, J. & Mareel, M., 1984,
    Invasion and Metastasis, Vol. 3, Nos. 2 & 3, 160.
Simpson, W.A. & Mason, James M., 1977, Growth, 41, 147.
Tchao, R., 1982, Cell Motility, 4,333.
Toyoshima, K., Ito, N., Hiasa, Y., Kamamoto, Y. & Makiura, S., 1971,
    Journal of the Cancer Institute, 47, 979.
Vakaet, L., Vanroelen, C. & Andries, L., 1980, in Cell Movement and
    Neoplasia, edited by M. DeBrabander et al., (Pergammon), p. 65.

INHIBITORS OF GLYCOPROTEIN SYNTHESIS AND PROCESSING : A NEW CLASS OF ANTIINVASIVE AGENTS ?[*]

M. MAREEL[1], C. DRAGONETTI[1] and R. HOOGHE[2]

[1]Laboratory of Experimental Cancerology, Department of Radiotherapy and Nuclear Medicine, University Hospital, De Pintelaan 185, B-9000 Ghent, Belgium

[2]Department of Radiobiology, SCK-CEN, B-2400 Mol, Belgium

[*]Supported by Grants from the Kankerfonds van de Algemene Spaar- en Lijfrentekas and from the Nationale Loterij (39.000/983), Belgium

Keywords : Glycoproteins, invasion, organ culture

INTRODUCTION

Inhibitors of tumour invasion are useful tools for the analysis of the mechanisms of invasion and might have a therapeutic value. Using an organ culture assay we have described 3 classes of anti-invasive agents : Microtubule inhibitors inhibit invasion through interference with the cytoplasmic microtubule complex (Mareel and De Mets 1984), flavonoids through alteration of the extracellular matrix of the host tissue (Bracke et al. 1984), and alkyl-lysophospholipids through alteration of cytomembrane fluidity (Storme et al. 1985). Several authors have suggested that cell surface carbohydrates are related to the malignant phenotype (Van Beek et al. 1973; Irimura & Nicolson 1981). We have, therefore, examined the effect of agents that are expected to interfere with glycoprotein synthesis and/or processing on the invasion of MO_4 mouse fibrosarcoma cells in vitro.

MATERIALS AND METHODS

MO_4 cells

MO_4 cells are virally transformed C_3H mouse cells (Billiau et al. 1973) that are invasive in vitro (Mareel et al. 1979) and metastatic in vivo (Meyvisch & Mareel 1982). These cells are maintained on tissue culture plastic substrata in Minimum Essential Medium Eagle (modified) with Earle's salts and non-essential amino acids (EMEM, Flow Laboratories Ltd, Irvine, Scotland) supplemented with 10% fetal calf serum, 0.05% (w/v) L-glutamine, and 250 I.U. penicillin/ml (hereafter called culture medium).

Assay for invasiveness

MO_4 cell aggregates (diameter = 0.2 mm) were confronted with precultured 9-

day-old embryonic chick heart fragments (diameter = 0.4 mm) and incubated on a Gyratory shaker at 120 rpm (Mareel et al. 1979). After 4 and 8 days confronting pairs were fixed and processed for histology and immunohistochemistry as described earlier (Mareel et al. 1981). For a semiquantitative analysis of the interaction between the MO_4 cells and the heart tissue we used the grading published by Bracke et al. (1984) : Grades III and IV meet the criteria of invasion.

Viability of heart tissue was assessed by preculture of fragments with incubation alone, as described for confronting pairs. After 4 days they were washed and explanted in Nunclon Delta SI 24-well multidishes (Nunclon, Roskilde, Denmark). These cultures (6 in each experiment) were followed under an inverted microscope for 1 to 3 weeks.

Drugs

Tunicamycin (NSC 177382, provided by the Natural Products Branch, Division of Cancer Treatment, NCI, Bethesda, Md) was dissolved in NaOH 0.01M (0.5 mg/ml) and further diluted in culture medium to final concentrations between 0.1 and 1.0 µg/ml. 2-deoxy-D-glucose (Merck, Darmstadt, F.R.G.) and β-OH-norvaline (Sigma, St. Louis, Mo) were dissolved in culture medium at concentrations of 1 to 100 mM and 0.01 mM to 1.0 mM respectively. Monensin (Calbiochem-Behring, La Jolla, Ca) was dissolved in ethanol (1 mg/ml) and further diluted in culture medium to concentrations between 0.01 and 1.0 µg/ml. 1-deoxynojirimycin (provided by D. Schmidt and E. Truscheit, Bayer-A.G., Wuppertal, F.R.G.) and swainsonine (provided by P. Dorling, School of Veterinary Studies, Murdoch University, Murdoch, Western Australia) were dissolved in culture medium to concentrations of 1 to 10 mM and 0.1 to 0.4 µg/ml respectively. Marcellomycin (obtained from M. Rozencweig, Bristol Laboratories, Syracuse, N.Y.) was dissolved in Ringer's solution (10 µg/ml) and further diluted in culture medium (0.003 to 0.1 µg/ml). Drugs were added at the onset of the culture period. After 4 days, cultures were washed and further incubated for 4 days without drug either on Gyratory shaker (assay for invasiveness) or in multidishes (assay for viability). All cultures were done in triplicate. Controls with the solvent alone were included for each drug.

RESULTS

The effect of various agents on the invasion of MO_4 cells into chick heart in organ culture is summarized in Table 1.

An example is shown in Figure 1. Tunicamycin (1.0 µg/ml); 2-deoxy-D-glucose (100 mM), β-OH-norvaline (1 mM), and Monensin (0.1 µg/ml) inhibited invasion. 1-deoxy-nojirimycin (10 mM), swainsonine (0.4 µg/ml) and Marcellomycin (0.1 µg/ml) had no effect on invasion. All antiinvasive agents and Marcellomycin inhibited the growth of

Table 1.   Semiquantitative evaluation of the interaction between MO_4 cells and precultured chick heart fragments in organ culture.

Drug (concentration)	Grading after	
	4 days	4 + 4 days[a]
None	III,IV	IV
tunicamycin (1.0 µg/ml)	II	III,IV
2-deoxy-D-glucose (100 mM)	II	III,IV
β-OI I-norvoline (1.0 mM)	II	IV
Monensin (0.1 µg/ml)	II	IV
1-deoxynojirimycin (10.0 mM)	III,IV	IV
swainsonine (0.4 µg/ml)	IV	IV
Marcellomycin (0.1 µg/ml)	IV	IV

[a]4 days in presence of drug followed by washing out and further incubation for 4 days without drug.

confronting pairs. Both inhibition of invasion and of growth were reversible. Treated precultured heart fragments did not differ from untreated controls as they produced growing cultures after explantation in multidishes, except for tunicamycin and Marcellomycin.

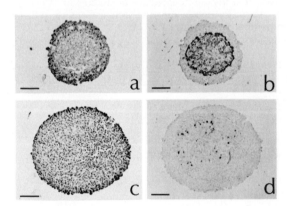

Figure 1.   Lightmicrographs from confrontations of MO_4 cells with a heart fragment, incubated for 4 days with 0.1 µg Monensin/ml (a and b), and for 4 days with 0.1 µg Monensin/ml followed by washing and further incubation for 4 days without drug. Staining with H & E (a and c) and with an antiserum against chick heart (b and d). Scale bars = 100 µm.

DISCUSSION

The present experiments in vitro pointed to a new class of antiinvasive agents. Comparison of the antiinvasive agents described here with other inhibitors of cell proliferation (Mareel et al. 1982) and with Marcellomycin (Morin & Sartorelli 1984) makes it unlikely that inhibition of growth was responsible for inhibition of invasion. Reversibility of the antiinvasive effect and outgrowth of cells from pretreated heart fragments indicated that antiinvasiveness could not be ascribed to a specific cytotoxicity. Interference with glycoprotein synthesis and/or processing is a common aspect of tunicamycin (Guarnaccia et al. 1983), 2-deoxy-D-glucose (Melchers 1973), β-OH–norvaline (Polonoff et al. 1983), and Monensin (Machamer & Cresswell 1984). It is, therefore, tempting to speculate that this aspect of drug action is responsible for inhibition of invasion. Interestingly, swainsonine (Elbein et al. 1982) and 1-deoxynojirimycin (Saunier 1982) which are expected to interfere with trimming of sugar residues required for the formation of complex carbohydrates did not affect invasion.

REFERENCES

Billiau, A., Sobis, H., Eyssen, H. & Van Den Berghe, H., 1973, Archiv für die gesamte Virusforschung, 43, 345.
Bracke, M.E., Van Cauwenberge, R.M.-L. & Mareel, M.M., 1984, Clinical and Experimental Metastasis, 2, 161.
Elbein, A.D., Dorling, P.R., Vosbeck & Horisberger, M., 1982, Journal of Biological Chemistry, 257, 1573.
Guarnaccia, S.P., Shaper, J.H. & Schnaar, R.L., 1983, Proceedings of the National Academy of Sciences USA, 80, 1551.
Irimura, T. & Nicolson, G.L., 1981, Journal of Supramolecular Structure and Cellular Biochemisjtry, 17, 325.
Machamer, C.E. & Cresswell, P., 1984, Proceedings of the National Academy of Sciences USA 81, 1287.
Mareel, M.M., Bruyneel, E.A., De Bruyne, G.K., Dragonetti, C.H. & Van Cauwenberge, R.M.-L., 1982, Growth and invasion: separate activities of malignant MO4 cell populations in vitro. In Membranes in Tumour Growth, edited by T. Galeotti et al. (Elsevier Biomedical Press), p.223.
Mareel, M.M., De Bruyne, G.K., Vandesande, F. & Dragonetti, C., 1981, Invasion and Metastasis, 1, 195.
Mareel, M.M. & De Mets, M., 1984, International Review of Cytology, 90, 125.
Mareel, M., Kint, J. & Meyvisch, C., 1979, Virchows Archiv Cell Pathology, 30, 95.
Melchers, F., 1973, Biochemistry, 12, 1471.
Meyvisch, C. & Mareel, M., 1982, Invasion and Metastasis, 2, 51.
Morin, M.J. & Sartorelli, A.C., 1984, Cancer Research, 44, 2807.
Polonoff, E., Machida, C.A. & Kabat, D., 1982, Journal of Biological Chemistry, 257, 14023.
Saunier, B., Kilker, R.D., Tkacz, J.S., Quaroni, A. & Hersovics, A., 1982, Journal of Biological Chemistry, 257, 14155.
Storme, G.A., Berdel, W.E., van Blitterswijk, W.J., Bruyneel, E.A., De Bruyne, G.K. & Mareel, M.M., 1984, Cancer Research (In Press).
Van Beek, W.P., Smets, L.A. & Emmelot, P., 1973, Cancer Research, 33, 2913.

IN VITRO RESPONSE OF MURINE METASTATIC VARIANTS TO HUMAN PLATELET DERIVED
GROWTH FACTOR (PDGF)

A. POGGI, E. VICENZI, G. FERRARI and M.B. DONATI
Istituto di Ricerche Farmacologiche Mario Negri, Via Eritrea, 62, 20157
Milano, Italy

Keywords: platelet derived growth factor

INTRODUCTION

Blood platelets seem to influence the sequence of events leading to
tumor cell dissemination and metastasis formation (Donati & Poggi 1980).
Stimulated platelets would release the content of their α-granules
(Niewiarowski & Paul 1981). Among released proteins, a small polypeptide
named Platelet Derived Growth Factor (PDGF) is worth mentioning. This
peptide is a potent mitogenic factor for normal cells of mesenchymal
origin, acting at concentrations of 10^{-10}-10^{-9}M. PDGF is the major
constitutive growth factor present in serum (Stiles 1983).

It is not clear whether PDGF is able to stimulate also the growth of
cancer cells. Virally transformed fibroblasts show a reduced dependence
on serum for in vitro proliferation (Scher et al 1978). In contrast,
several tumor cells of non viral origin have been found sensitive to the
mitogenic effects of platelet lysates or to platelet factors different
from PDGF (Hara et al 1980; Kepner & Lipton 1981).

The purpose of our study was to investigate the effects of human
platelet extract and purified PDGF on in vitro growth of two metastatic
variants of a murine fibrosarcoma.

MATERIAL AND METHODS

Human platelet extract was prepared from fresh platelet concentrates
(Poggi et al 1984). Highly purified human PDGF was a generous gift of
Dr. Åke Wasteson, Linköping, Sweden. PDGF stock solution was diluted in
medium containing 0.1% bovine serum albumin (BSA).

Two metastatic variants (M4 and M9) of a benzopyrene induced murine fibrosarcoma (mFS6) were studied. The two sublines are characterized by a markedly different metastatic ability in vivo, M_4 being the more invasive (95% metastatic incidence to the lungs) and M_9 the less (no metastasis) (Giavazzi et al 1980). Tumor cells, obtained by collagenase digestion of the tumor, were plated in RPMI 1640 medium plus 10% fetal bovine serum (FBS).

DNA synthesis was measured as methyl-^{3}H-thymidine (^{3}H-TdR) incorporation by the cells. Tumor cells (5×10^4 cells/well) were plated in 24 well Costar plates in RPMI medium plus 10% FBS. After 48 hours, fresh medium with the test samples was added and the cells incubated for further 24 hours. Then ^{3}H-TdR was pulsed for 6 hours and TCA precipitable radioactivity was counted (Poggi et al 1984).

To test cell proliferation, tumor cells (2×10^4 cells/well) were plated in RPMI medium plus 10% FBS. After 48 hours, serum free medium with test samples was added. Cells were detached by trypsin and counted by a Coulter Counter at 3 day intervals.

RESULTS AND DISCUSSION

The effect of human platelet extract and purified PDGF on the ^{3}H-TdR incorporation by tumor cells was studied. Increasing concentrations of human platelet extract (27.5, 275 and 550 µg/ml) induced a dose dependent increase of ^{3}H-TdR in M_9 cells (2.0 ± 0; $6,1 \pm 0.1^{**}$; $8.1 \pm 0.2^{**} \times 10^4$ CPM/well respectively, compared to serum free medium, $1,6 \pm 0.1 \times 10^4$ CPM/well; $^{**}p < 0.01$ at Dunnett t test). This effect was less marked and not dose related in M_4 cells ($38.0 \pm 3.3^*$; 36.4 ± 3.5; $49.0 \pm 1.8^{**} \times 10^4$ CPM/well respectively, compared to serum free medium, $29.1 \pm 1.0 \times 10^4$ CPM/well; $^*p < 0.05$, $^{**}p < 0.01$ at Dunnett t test). M_4 cells showed a higher percentage of cells in S phase (54%) compared to M_9 (37%), as determined by cytofluorometric analysis, in basal conditions. This difference in cell cycle might explain the lower sensitivity of M_4 cells to platelet extract.

Highly purified PDGF was then tested in the same assay (Figure 1). A 2.5 fold increase in M_9 cells and 1.5 fold increase in M_4 cells was obtained by addition of purified PDGF (5 ng/ml). These data confirmed an enhanced PDGF dependence of the low metastatic line compared to the other line.

When the effect on cell proliferation was tested (Table 1), M_4 cells showed a statistically significant increase in cell number in the presence of FBS, platelet extract and PDGF, but also in the presence of the PDGF carrier, BSA. M_9 cells were not stimulated by addition of platelet

Table 1. Effect of human platelet extract and purified PDGF on M_4 and M_9 cell proliferation.[a]

	M_4	M_9
O	4.4 ± 0.6	0.6 ± 0.1
BSA (0.1%)	6.6 ± 1.0 ±[b]	1.0 ± 0.2 **
FBS (5%)	7.4 ± 0.4 **	2.6 ± 0.3
PLAT. EXTR. (115 µg/ml)	8.4 ± 0.5 **	0.8 ± 0.2 **
PDGF (5 ng/ml)	9.3 ± 0.4	2.8 ± 0.1

[a] Data expressed as cell number x 10^5/well (mean ± S.E. of 3 data). Cell number at day O was 3.7 ± 0.2 x 10^5/well for M_4 and 1.3 ± 0.1 x 10^5/well for M_9 cells.

[b] * $p < 0.05$

** $p < 0.01$ at Dunnett t test

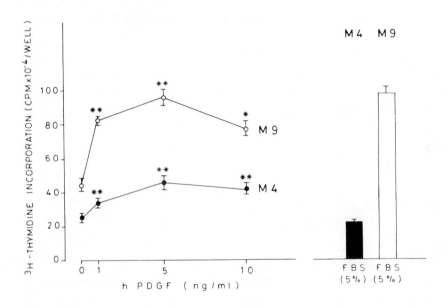

Figure 1. Effect of purified human PDGF (h PDGF) at different protein concentrations (1-10 ng/ml) on ^{3}H-TdR incorporation in M_4 and M_9 cells. Data are expressed as CPM x 10^3/well (mean ± S.E. of 3 data). Statistical analysis was performed separately on each cell line, considering serum free medium as control (O). Aside is shown the effect of 5% FBS in the same assay.

* $p < 0.05$

** $p < 0.01$ at Dunnett t test

extract or BSA. In contrast, purified PDGF (5 ng/ml) induced a statistically significant rise in cell number, like FBS (5%). In addition, 1-10% FBS caused a concentration-dependent increase in cell proliferation in M_9 but not in M_4 cells, in a manner similar to PDGF (data not shown).

In conclusion, we found that two metastatic variants of a murine fibrosarcoma were both sensitive to the mitogenic effects of crude human platelet extract and purified PDGF. PDGF was remarkably more active on the tumor cell line with lower metastatic ability (M_9) than on the line with higher activity (M_4). These results are in agreement with the observations of Currie (1981) who found an inverse correlation between the immunogenicity of metastatic tumors and their PDGF dependence for in vitro growth. We cannot exclude that other serum factors (like fibronectin) may have a differential effect on the growth of the two cell lines, since FBS mimicked the effect of PDGF. Moreover, differences in the cell cycle were found among the two lines. It is also possible that M_4 cells would release in their medium a self stimulating growth factor, that might account for the reduced serum and PDGF dependence of this cell line.

Taken all together, our study underlines the concept that cells with different metastatic potential may have different growth requirements in vitro. This may offer the opportunity for further characterization of relevant properties of metastatic cells in vivo.

ACKNOWLEDGEMENTS
    This paper was partially supported by Italian National Research Council (Progetto Finalizzato "Oncologia"), by an International Project Italia-USA (CNR n. 83.01460.04) and by Associazione Italiana per la Ricerca sul Cancro. The authors wish to thank Dr. S. Niewiarowski (Temple University, Philadelphia, USA) for stimulating discussion. Ivana Garimoldi and Vincenzo De Ceglie helped prepare this manuscript.

REFERENCES
Currie, G.A., 1981, British Journal of Cancer, 43, 335.
Donati, M.B. & Poggi, A., 1980, British Journal of Haematology(Annotation)
    44, 173.
Giavazzi, R., Alessandri, G., Spreafico, F., Garattini, S., Mantovani, A.,
    1980, British Journal of Cancer, 42, 462.
Hara, Y., Steiner, M. and Baldini, M.G., 1980, Cancer Research, 40, 1212.
Kepner, N. & Lipton, A., 1981, Cancer Research, 41, 430.
Niewiarowski, S. & Paul, D., 1981, Platelets in Biology and Pathology 2,
    edited by Gordon (Elsevier/North Holland Biomedical Press) p. 91.
Poggi, A., Rucinski, B., James, P., Holt, J.C., Niewiarowski, S., 1984,
    Experimental Cell Research 150, 436.
Scher, C.D., Pledger,W.J., Martin, P., Antoniades, H., Stiles, C.D., 1978,
    Journal of Cellular Physiology, 97, 371.
Stiles, C.D., 1983, Cell, 33, 653.

ANTIMETASTATIC THERAPY WITH CALCIUM ACTIVE COMPOUNDS

K.V. HONN[1], J.M. ONODA[1], J.D. TAYLOR[2] and B.F. SLOANE[3]

[1]Departments of Radiation Oncology, [2]Biological Sciences and [3]Pharmacology, Wayne State University, Detroit, Michigan 48202 USA

Keywords: calcium channel blockers; calmodulin antagonists; platelet aggregation

INTRODUCTION

Interaction between tumor cells and platelets are thought to facilitate metastasis either by enhancing tumor cell arrest in the microvasculature and tumor cell adhesion to the blood vessel wall (Honn et al. 1984a) or by platelets shielding tumor cells from cytotoxic immune destruction (Gorelik et al. 1984). Although the mechanisms by which platelets might enhance metastasis are not yet fully delineated, several laboratories have demonstrated that both human and animal tumor cells can induce platelet aggregation in vitro and that i.v. injection of tumor cells results in thrombocytopenia in vivo. Gasic et al. (1968,1973) reported that in the presence of thrombocytopenia (induced by neuraminidase or antiplatelet antiserum) the number of lung colonies produced upon tail vein injection of TA3 ascites tumor cells was reduced.

Both intracellular and extracellular Ca^{2+} seem to be required for irreversible platelet aggregation (Owen et al. 1980, Owen & LeBreton 1981). Calcium channel blockers (CCB) prevent the influx of extracellular Ca^{2+} in several cell types, and have recently been shown to inhibit ADP-, epinephrine- and collagen-induced platelet aggregation in vitro (Onoda et al. 1984a). Calmodulin antagonists (CMA) also inhibit platelet aggregation in vitro (Levy 1983). The antiplatelet abilities of CCB and CMA suggest that they might be effective inhibitors of tumor cell-platelet-endothelial cell interactions in vitro and in turn of metastasis in vivo.

METHODS

B16 amelanotic melanoma (B16a) and Walker 256 carcinosarcoma (W256) tumors were passaged, dispersed and the cells elutriated as previously described (Honn et al. 1984b). Final monodispersed tumor cell suspensions were > 90% viable with < 3% host cell contamination. Human platelet rich plasma, washed rat platelets and rat cerebral endothelial cells were prepared as previously described (Honn et al. 1984b). Platelet aggregometry studies, platelet enhanced tumor cell adhesion to endothelial cell studies and "experimental" (lung colony formation) and spontaneous metastasis studies were performed as previously described (Honn et al. 1984b).

RESULTS AND DISCUSSION

Five CCB of the dihydropyridine class (felodipine, FL; nimodipine, NM and nifedipine, NF) the phenylalkylamine class (verapamil, VP) and the benzothiazepine class (diltiazem, DZ) in addition to two CMA (calmidazolium, CZ and trifluoroperazine, TP) inhibited in a dose dependent manner the induction of platelet aggregation (TCIPA) by B16a and/or W256 tumor cells. The IC_{50}'s for inhibition of B16a TCIPA were: NM, 85 μM; NF, 400 μM; DZ, 350 μM and VP, 340 μM. The IC_{50}'s for inhibition of W256 TCIPA were: NM, 900 μM; NF, 1450 μM; FL, 880 μM; CZ, 66 μM and TP, 136 μM. The degree of inhibition was dependent on the strength of the stimulus. For example, W256 cells are considerably more thrombogenic than B16a cells and NM inhibition of TCIPA by equivalent numbers of tumor cells (IC_{50} B16a = 85 μM vs IC_{50} W256 = 900 μM) reflects this fact.

CCB and CMA inhibit in vitro TCIPA at suprapharmacological doses which probably cannot be achieved in vivo, however, they affect platelet function in vivo (see Onoda et al. 1984b) and inhibit metastasis (see below). One possible explanation is that in vivo CCB and possibly CMA may act on platelets in concert with endogenous antiaggregatory agents such as PGI_2. Onoda et al. (1984a,b) have demonstrated that the combination of suboptimal concentrations (i.e., unable to singularly inhibit platelet aggregation) of PGI_2 (0.25 - 1.0 pg/ml) and NM (10 μM) act synergistically to inhibit ADP, thrombin and tumor cell induced platelet aggregation.

We have reported that rat platelets enhance the adhesion of rat W256 cells to monolayers of normal rat endothelial cells under non-aggregatory and aggregatory conditions (Honn et al. 1984c). Two CCB of the dihydropyridine class were tested for their abilities to inhibit the platelet-enhanced W256 cell adhesion to endothelium. NM and FL at a dose of 100 μM inhibited platelet-enhanced W256 cell adhesion under both non-aggregatory and aggregatory conditions. In contrast NF at a dose of 100 μM did not significantly inhibit platelet-enhanced W256 cell adhesion under non-aggregatory conditions but did inhibit adhesion by 38% under aggregatory conditions (Onoda et al. 1984b; Honn et al. 1984b,c). We have recently demonstrated that representatives of the phenylalkylamine and benzothiazepine classes of CCB also inhibit platelet-enhanced tumor cell adhesion to endothelium.

Since we have previously demonstrated that compounds which inhibit interactions among tumor cells, platelets and endothelial cells in vitro have antimetastatic properties when administered in vivo (Honn et al. 1983), we tested CCB and CMA for antimetastatic activity in vivo using spontaneous and "experimental" metastasis models.

A single administration of NM (10 mg/kg body wt, p.o.) 1 hr prior to and 1 hr post intravenous injection of elutriated B16a tumor cells resulted in a 57% decrease in lung colony formation whereas NF at the same dose decreased lung colony formation by 33% (Honn et al. 1984b). NM and FL were compared at a dose of 0.1 mg/kg and were found to inhibit lung colony formation by 34% and 43% respectively. DZ was ineffective at 1 mg/kg but inhibited lung colony formation 40% at 40 mg/kg. VP was ineffective at 1 and 10 mg/kg.

Daily administration of dihydropyridine class CCB (10 mg/kg body wt, p.o.) to mice bearing subcutaneous B16a tumors resulted in a 72% (NM), 70% (FL) and 40% (NF) reduction in spontaneous pulmonary metastasis. The benzothiazepine CCB (DZ) was ineffective at 1 and 10 mg/kg. However, DZ at a dose of 40 mg/kg reduced spontaneous metastasis by 75%. VP was ineffective at 1 and 10 mg/kg. The CMA, TP inhibited spontaneous metastasis by 74% at 10 mg/kg p.o. None of the compounds tested had a significant effect on the weight or volume of the primary tumors. The above results suggest that the calcium active compounds (i.e., CCB and CMA) may represent a generic class from which successful antimetastatic agents can be developed.

REFERENCES

Gasic, G.J, Gasic, T.B. & Stewart, C.C., 1968, Proceedings of the
National Academy of Sciences USA, 61, 46.

Gasic, G.J., Gasic, T.B., Galanti, N., Johnson, T. & Murphy, J., 1973,
International Journal of Cancer, 11, 704.

Gorelik, E., Bere, W.W. & Herberman, R.B., 1984, International Journal
of Cancer, 33, 87.

Honn, K.V., Busse, W.D. & Sloane, B.F., 1983, Biochemical
Pharmacology, 32, 1.

Honn, K.V., Menter, D.G., Onoda, J.M., Taylor, J.D. & Sloane, B.F.,
1984a, Role of prostacyclin as a natural deterrent to tumor
cell metastasis. In Cancer Invasion and Metastasis:
Biologic and Therapeutic Aspects, edited by G.L. Nicolson and
L. Milas (Raven Press), p. 361.

Honn, K.V., Onoda, J.M., Pampalona, K., Battaglia, M., Neagos, G.,
Taylor, J.D., Diglio, C.A. & Sloane, B.F., 1984b, Biochemical
Pharmacology (in press).

Honn, K.V., Onoda, J.M., Diglio, C.A., Carufel, M.M., Taylor, J.D. &
Sloane, B.F., 1984c, Clinical and Experimental Metastasis, 2, 61.

Levy, J.V., 1983, Federation of European Biochemical Societies,
154, 212.

Onoda, J.M., Sloane, B.F. & Honn, K.V., 1984a, Thrombosis Research,
34, 367.

Onoda, J.M., Sloane, B.F., Taylor, J.D. & Honn, K.V., 1984b, Calcium
channel blockers: Inhibitors of tumor cell-platelet-endothelial
cell interactions. In Hemostatic Mechanisms and Metastasis, edited
by K.V. Honn and B.F. Sloane (Martinus Nijhoff), p. 244.

Owen, N.E., Feinberg, H. & LeBreton, G.C., 1980, American Journal of
Physiology, 239, H483.

Owen, N.E. & LeBreton, G.L., 1981, American Journal of Physiology,
241, H619.

ANTIMETASTATIC THERAPY WITH THROMBOXANE SYNTHASE INHIBITORS

J.M. ONODA[1], B.F. SLOANE[2], and K.V. HONN[1]

[1]Department of Radiation Oncology, 210 Science Hall, Wayne State Univ., Detroit, Michigan 48202 USA

[2]Department of Pharmacology, Wayne State University, Detroit, Michigan USA

Keywords: metastasis, thromboxane synthase inhibitor

INTRODUCTION

Platelets may play a crucial role in the metastatic process by enhancing tumor cell arrest and adhesion to the endothelial lining of the micro-vasculature, and possibly by protecting adherent tumor cells from the host immune system (macrophages, natural killer cells) by forming a protective "cocoon" of platelets and fibrin around adherent tumor cells. Gasic et al (1968) demonstrated that platelet reduction (thrombocytopenia) would decrease tumor colony formation induced by the intravenous injection of tumor cells, whereas Gorelik et al (1984) reported that activated (by Poly IC) host immune cells (natural killer cells) decreased pulmonary tumor colony formation induced by the intravenous injection of tumor cells. Therefore, the ability of aggregated platelets to protect tumor cells from host immune defenses may be as crucial for successful metastasis as the ability of aggregated platelets to aid in tumor cell arrest and adhesion. Agents which are capable of inhibiting platelet aggregation have been demonstrated to inhibit metastasis. These include such calcium active compounds as prostacycline (Honn et al, 1981), calcium channel blockers (Honn et al, 1983, 1984) and phosphodiesterase inhibitors (Maniglia et al, 1982). Thromboxane synthase inhibitors, TXSI, have been demonstrated to inhibit platelet biosynthesis of thromboxane A2 (TXA2) but have not been consistent in their ability to inhibit platelet aggregation in vitro (Bertele et al, 1981; Schumacher & Lucchesi, 1983). It has been suggested that in the enclosed system of an aggregometry cuvette, the inhibitory actions of TXSI would cause an increase in the levels of PGH2, the precursor of TXA2; and at elevated levels, PGH2 may mimic the aggregatory

actions of TXA2 (Rybiki & Le Breton, 1983).   Nevertheless, TXSI are
effective in their ability to inhibit platelet biosynthesis of TXA2 in vivo
(McGuire & Wallis, 1983) and have proven antithrombotic actions in vivo
(Gorman et al, 1983; Lefer et al, 1983).   The present study was designed
to determine the effects of the thromboxane synthase inhibitor CGS 14854
on tumor cell-platelet interactions in vitro and metastasis in vivo.

METHODS

Tumor Lines

   Walker 256 carcinosarcoma (W256) and B16 amelanotic melanoma (B16a) were
obtained from the National Cancer Institute (USA) tumor bank.   Tumors were
passaged by s.c. injection of cellular brei into allogeneic female hosts
(Sprague-Dawley rats) for W256 and into syngeneic male hosts (C57BL/6J mice)
for B16a.   Purified W256 and B16a cellular suspensions were prepared from
s.c. tumors by sequential collagenase digestion followed by centrifugal
elutriation as previously described (Sloane et al, 1982).

Platelet Preparation

   Human platelet rich plasma (PRP) was prepared as previously described
(Onoda et al, 1984) and tumor cell induced platelet aggregation (TCIPA)
studies were performed as described by Menter et al, 1984.

Metastasis Studies

   Spontaneous and 'experimental' metastasis studies were performed as
described by Honn et al, 1984.   Dispersed and elutriated B16a tumor cells
were injected into the tail vein of syngeneic mice ('experimental'
metastasis) and the mice were administered CGS 14854 (orally) one hour
prior to and one hour post tumor cell injection; or B16a tumor cells were
implanted s.c. to form a primary tumor with the resultant development of
secondary pulmonary metastases (spontaneous metastasis) with drug treatment
starting one day after tumor cell implantation and continuing once/day for
the length (28d.) of the experiment.

RESULTS AND DISCUSSION

   CGS 14854 inhibits platelet biosynthesis of TXA2 in a dose-dependent
manner although it (CGS 14854) failed to significantly inhibit TCIPA.   The
IC_{50} values for inhibition of TXA2 biosynthesis are approximately 1 uM and
5 uM, respectively, for platelets stimulated by B16a and W256 tumor cells.
In vivo, oral administration of a single 50 mg/kg dose of CGS 14854 will
prolong the bleeding time of treated mice to approximately 250% of control
mice (n=6).   We tested CGS 14854 for in vivo antimetastatic effects in both
the 'experimental' and spontaneous metastasis model systems.   In both

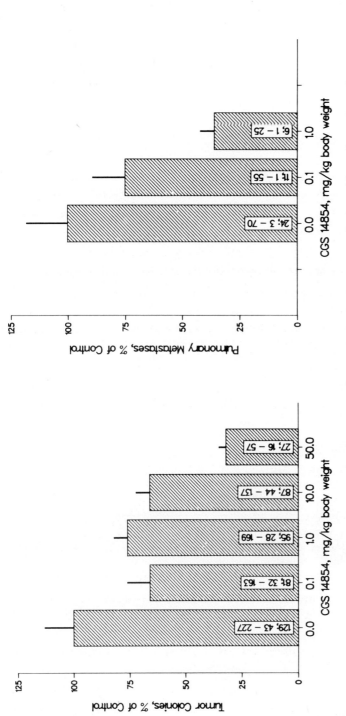

Figure 1. (left) Inhibition by CGS 14854 of 'experimental' pulmonary metastasis of the B16 amelanotic melanoma. Values (n=12) are expressed as a % of control x̄ ± SEM from a representative experiment. Values are significantly different from control (p<.01) as determined by the Kruskal-Wallis test for the 50 mg/kg dose. Values for median; ranges are included within the bars. Control x̄ = 112 pulmonary tumor colonies.

Figure 2. (right) Inhibition by CGS 14854 of spontaneous pulmonary metastasis from a s.c. B16 amelanotic melanoma. Values (n=12) expressed as a % of control x̄ ± SEM from a representative experiment. Values are significantly different from control (p<.01) as determined by the Kruskal-Wallis test for the 1.0 mg.kg dcse. Values for median; ranges are included within the bars. Control x̄ = 26 pulmonary metastases.

model systems, CGS 14854, in a dose-dependent manner, inhibited pulmonary metastases (Figures 1 & 2). At a dose of 1 mg/kg, a greater inhibition of metastasis was observed in the spontaneous metastasis model system than was observed in the 'experimental' model system. Low doses of CGS 14854 may be insufficient to profoundly inhibit tumor colony formation induced by a large bolus injection of tumor cells whereas in the spontaneous model system, the daily administration of CGS 14854 was sufficient to inhibit the continuous, but possibly lower levels of B16a cells entering the host circulatory system.

We have previously reported that inhibitors of tumor cell-platelet interactions in vitro have potent antimetastatic effects in vivo (Honn et al, 1981, 1983, 1984). In this study we report that the thromboxane synthase inhibitor CGS 14854 inhibits tumor cell induced platelet bio-synthesis of TXA2 in vitro, prolongs tail bleeding time in vivo, and has significant antimetastatic effects in two different model systems in vivo.

REFERENCES

Bertele, V., Cerletti, C., Schieppati, A., Di Minno, G. & De Gaetano, G., 1981, The Lancet, 1057.
Diglio, C.A., Grammas, P., Giacomelli, F., & Wiener, J., 1982, Laboratory Investigations, 46, 544.
Gasic, G.J., Gasic, T.B., & Stewart, C.C., 1968, Proceedings of the National Academy of Science, U.S.A., 61, 46.
Gorelik, E., Bere, W.W., & Herberman, G.H., 1984, International Journal of Cancer, 33, 87.
Gorman, R.R., Johnson, R.A., Spilman, G.H., & Aikens, J.W., 1983, Prostaglandins, 26, 325.
Honn, K.V., Cicone, B., & Skoff, A., 1981, Science, 212, 1270.
Honn, K.V., Onoda, J.M., Diglio, C.A., & Sloane, B.F., 1983, Proceedings of the Society for Experimental Biology and Medicine, 174, 16.
Honn, K.V., Onoda, J.M., Diglio, C.A., Carufel, M.M., Taylor, J.D. & Sloane, B.F., 1984, Clinical and Experimental Metastasis, 2, 61.
Lefer, A.M., Burke, S.E. & Smith, J.B., 1983, Thrombosis Research, 32, 311.
Maguire, E.D. & Wallis, R.B., 1983, Thrombosis Research, 32, 15.
Maniglia, C.A., Tudor, G., Gomez, J. & Sartorelli, A.C., 1982, Cancer Letters, 16, 253.
Menter, D.G., Onoda, J.M., Taylor, J.D. & Honn, K.V., 1984, Cancer Research, 44, 450.
Onoda, J.M., Sloane, B.F. & Honn, K.V., 1984, Thrombosis Research, 34, 367.
Rybiki, J.P. & Le Breton, G.C., 1983, Thrombosis Research, 30, 407.
Schumacher, W.A. & Lucchesi, B.R., 1983, The Journal of Pharmacology and Experimental Therapeutics, 277, 790.
Sloane, B.F., Honn, K.V., Dadler, J.G., Turner, W.A., Kimpson, J.J. & Taylor, J.D., 1982, Cancer Research, 42, 980.

THE PROSTACYCLIN-THROMBOXANE BALANCE AND EXPERIMENTAL METASTASES: QUESTIONS
FROM PHARMACOLOGICAL STUDIES

E. VICENZI, V.M. VALORI, A.P. BOLOGNESE DALESSANDRO, A. NIEWIAROWSKA,
D. ROTILIO and M.B. DONATI
Istituto di Ricerche Farmacologiche Mario Negri, Milano, Italy

Keywords: prostacyclin, thromboxane

The interactions between tumour cells and the components of the haemostatic system, such as platelets, clotting factors and the vessel wall have been suggested to play a role in metastasis dissemination (Donati et al, 1982). However, it still remains difficult to establish a clear relationship between cancer cell activities and their invasive potential, expecially in spontaneous metastasis models.

We have recently characterized some sublines with different metastatic potential, derived from a benzo(a)pyrene induced-fibrosarcoma (Mantovani, 1978; Delaini et al, 1981). We have measured on these two cell sublines several activities possibly involved in their interaction with platelets and/or fibrin, including tissue factor activity and plasminogen activator (Colucci et al, 1981; Coen et al, 1983). Moreover, the highly metastatic cells produced significantly higher TxB2 levels ($p < 0.01$) and lower PGI2 activity ($p < 0.01$) than the non metastatic line (Table 1).

TABLE 1.
Generation of thromboxane B2, 6-keto-PGF1 and prostacyclin activity by mFS6 metastatic variants (means $\pm$ SEM of 5-7 values per group).

CELL TYPE	METAST. INC. %	TxB2 nmoles/l/ 2×10^7 cells	6-KETO-PGF1 nmoles/l/ 2×10^7 cells	PGI2 ACTIVITY nmoles/l/ 2×10^7 cells
mFS6	55	0.61 ± 0.08	0.81 ± 0.06	ND
M4	95	1.21 ± 0.20	0.51 ± 0.08	< 0.20
M9	0	0.17 ± 0.06	3.57 ± 0.48	2.11

These data support the suggestion that changes in Arachidonic Acid (AA) metabolites may be associated with changes in the metastatic potential of the cells.

To get further support to this concept, we attempted to re-orient pharmacologically the AA metabolism of mFS6 sublines in order to change their metastatic potential. For this purpose, we studied dazmegrel, a specific TxA2 synthase inhibitor. This had been previously found to depress TxB2 production in platelets from rats, rabbits, guinea pigs and humans. Treatment of platelets with this drug or other TxA2 synthase inhibitors produced a re-orientation of AA metabolism towards other prostaglandins (Bertelé et al. 1984; Defreyn et al. 1982). When cells freshly collected from the highly metastatic tumour M4 were incubated with dazmegrel "in vitro", a concomitant though not spectacular depression of TxB2 and increase of 6-keto-PGFl, was observed (Fig. 1).

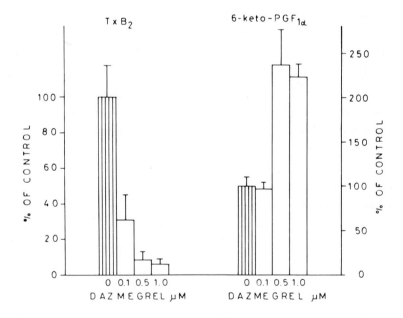

Figure 1. Generation of TxB2 and 6-keto-PGFl, by cells freshly harvested from M4 tumour in the presence of increasing concentrations of dazme rel. Means ± SEM of three experiments.

Several feasibility studies were performed in C57 Bl/6J mice to find out a suitable treatment schedule to maintain a consistently measurable biochemical effect. As a consequence of these studies, dazmegrel was administered by gavage (150 mg/kg b.w. twice a day) from the day of tumour cell implantation (day zero) until the sacrifice of the animals. As shown in Table 2, this treatment schedule decreased serum TxB2 level to less than 10% of the controls. Table 2 indicates that treatment with dazmegrel during the whole period of tumour development failed to affect any of the parameters of tumour and metastasis growth considered.

TABLE 2.

Tumour and metastasis growth and serum TxB2 in mice bearing M4 fibrosarcoma: effect of treatment with dazmegrel (150 mg/kg b.w. twice a day) from day 0 to sacrifice of the animals (means ± SEM).

EXPERIMENTAL GROUP	N	SERUM TxB2 (pmoles/ml)	TUMOUR WEIGHT (mg)	METAST. WEIGHT (mg)	METAST. NUMBER
CONTROL	26	33.4±8.4	7132±284	22.6±4.6	15.2±2.7
TREATED	24	3.0±0.8	6841±266	24.1±5.9	15.2±3.8

p < 0.01 (Student's t test)

Taken all together, these data suggest that a selective inhibition of Thromboxane generation does not affect the metastatic potential of cells with a high TxB2 level. Indeed, metastases can develop in animals with very low platelet TxB2 production as well as in controls. Moreover, the reorientation of AA metabolism induced by dazmegrel in "in vitro" experiments could not be clearly shown "ex vivo". Further experiments should clarify whether this was due to some methodological problem in cancer cell preparation or to difficult access of dazmegrel to tumour tissue "in vivo".

Acknowledgements

This work was partially supported by Italian National Research Council (Project "Oncologia"),the Gustavus and Louise Pfeiffer Research Foundation, Los Angeles, Calif.,USA and the "Associazione Italiana per la Ricerca sul Cancro". We thank Dr. Giovanni de Gaetano for stimulating discussions. Vincenzo and Felice de Ceglie and Ivana Garimoldi helped prepare this manuscript.

REFERENCES

Bertelé, V., Falanga, A., Tomasiak, M., Chiabrando, C., Cerletti, C. and
    de Gaetano, G., 1984, Blood, 63, 1460.
Coen, D., Bottazzi, B., Bini, A., Conforti, M.G., Mantovani, A., Mussoni,
    L. and Donati, M.B., 1983, International Journal of Cancer, 32, 67.
Colucci, M., Giavazzi, R., Alessandri, G., Semeraro, N., Mantovani, A. and
    Donati, M.B., 1981, Blood, 57, 389.
Defreyn, G., Deckmyn, H. and Vermylen, J., 1982, Thrombosis Research, 26,
    389.
Donati, M.B., Rotilio, D., Delaini, F., Giavazzi, R., Mantovani, A. and
    Poggi, A., 1982, Animal models for the study of platelet-tumour cell
    interactions. In: Interactions between Platelets and Cancer Cells,
    edited by G.A. Jamieson (Alan R. Liss, Inc. New York) p. 159.
Mantovani, A., 1978, International Journal of Cancer, 22, 741.

DOES FIBRINOLYSIS HAVE A ROLE IN TUMOUR GROWTH AND SPREAD?

G.T.LAYER, M.PATTISON and K G.BURNAND

Department of Surgery, St Thomas' Hospital Medical School,
Lambeth Palace Road, London, SE1 7EH

Keywords: fibrinolysis, Lewis lung carcinoma, metastasis,
          plasminogen activator

INTRODUCTION

Links between coagulation and tumours have been suspected since the mid
19th century when certain thrombotic episodes were recognised as manifest-
ations of malignancy (Donati and Poggi 1980). Some tumours have been found
to have procoagulant action (O'Meara 1958) and others to have a fibrinolytic activity (Cliffton and Grossi 1955). Fibrin has been identified at
the edge of human breast (Dvorak et al 1981) and lung small cell carcinomas
(Zacharski et al 1983). The role of fibrinolysis and the fibrin envelope
has produced two polarised hypotheses. Fibrin may act as a barrier to host
defence mechanisms or serve as a framework for tumour growth and neovasc-
ularisation (Dvorak et al 1983). It may also stabilise metastases and aid
implantation into tissues (Chew and Wallace 1976). The opposite view is
that tumour has a high fibrinolytic capacity which can destroy the fibrin
barrier, facilitating invasion (Anon 1977), and is important in cell shedding, promoting metastasis (Malone et al 1979). Physiologically local alterations in plasminogen activators occur without global changes (Cederholm-
Williams 1983) and this equilibrium may exist within invasive tumours.

Drugs altering clotting and fibrinolysis have been used in animals and
man to alter the pattern of tumour growth but the results have been conflicting (Peterson 1977). Thornes (1975) claimed anticoagulants and
fibrinolytics improved survival from human cancers and White et al (1976)
found that urokinase reduced the recurrence rate of colorectal carcinoma.

We chose the Lewis lung carcinoma in the C57Black mouse to study fibrinolysis and tumour growth. Plasminogen activator has been identified in
the tissues of this tumour (Bruesch et al 1983) and Hilgard (1977) found

anticoagulants in this model reduced metastasis. In our experiments, we
used stanozolol, an anabolic steroid which enhances fibrinolysis in man,
resulting in increased fibrin degradation. A dose 60 times the human
equivalent was given weekly Its effect on mouse fibrinolysis was unknown.

MATERIALS AND METHODS

Experiment 1   Forty 8 week old female C57BlackCbi mice were randomised
into groups of 20 and were maintained at a constant temperature of 23°C,
with free access to food and water. They were weighed and examined weekly.
0.5mg stanozolol (Stromba, Sterling Research Laboratories) was administered
to one group i-m as a suspension in 0.1ml water to the right hind leg at
weekly intervals. The control group received an injection of sterile water
weekly. After 5 weeks the mice in both groups were killed for the estimation of their blood fibrinolysis. A technique for collecting 1·0ml of
blood was developed; blood from the trunk of a mouse killed by guillotine
decapitation drained into a wide-necked tube containing ice-cold citrate.
Blood escaping was collected with a citrate-rinsed glass pipette. Plasma
fibrinolytic activity was estimated by the euglobulin clot lysis time
(ECLT) as described by Marsh (1981). Fibrinogen was measured on plasma
pooled from 5 mice by Ingram's method (1952). The volume of blood obtained
from each mouse was insufficient for its estimation, necessitating pooling.

Experiment 2   Stanozolol in a 5 times higher dose (2.5mg) in 0.15ml water
was administered i-m to 9 further mice weekly for 5 weeks. They were killed
by decapitation and the blood collected for estimation of the ECLT.

Experiment 3   The Lewis lung carcinoma (3LL) was maintained in female
C57BlackCbi mice. Single cell suspensions were prepared from fragments of
fresh viable tumour. The tissue was incubated with trypsin and DNase and
then filtered into culture medium. A cell count was made with a Neubauer
chamber. The effect of stanozolol on a s-c flank inoculum of 1.3×10^5 cells
was studied in 40 mice. They were divided into 5 groups: Group 1: 2 weeks
treatment with 0.5mg stanozolol prior to tumour inoculation, then
continuing a weekly dose; Group 2: sterile water prior to tumour inoculation, then stanozolol; Group 3: sterile water throughout, before and after
tumour· Group 4: divided into mice receiving water or stanozolol alone. The
mice were weighed weekly when the size of the primary was estimated by two
perpendicular measurements using micrometer calipers. The primary tumour
weight was represented by the standard formula (National Cancer Institute):

$$\text{weight mg} = \text{length mm} \times (\text{width mm})^2/2$$

At sacrifice 5 weeks later blood was collected and the lungs removed. The
trachea was intubated with plastic tubing and the lungs insufflated with

air from a low pressure supply enabling the visible metastases to be easily counted. All blood estimations and tumour counts were performed blind.

RESULTS

Experiment 1   The weight gain in both groups was similar (41.6% drug : 38.5% water). The mice receiving weekly stanozolol had a significantly prolonged ECLT and raised fibrinogen indicating decreased blood fibrinolysis.

20 mice per group	STANOZOLOL		WATER
Mean euglobulin clot lysis time +sd	29.5+13.3		18.8+6.1
Range (min)	10-60		10-31
Significance (Mann-Whitney test)		p<0.001	
Mean pooled clot weight fibrinogen +sd	225+16		147+14
Range (mg/100ml)	216-243		135-162
Significance (Mann-Whitney test)		p=0.05	

Experiment 2   2.5mg stanozolol greatly prolonged the ECLT (160min $\pm$ 138, range 54-360) compared to the controls (p<<0.001), and the group receiving 0 5mg stanozolol (p<<0 001); supporting a dose-response relationship.

Experiment 3   Three mice in each group died at similar times from haemo-peritoneum following rupture of a too deeply placed tumour implantation. The mean primary tumour weight equivalent and the number of metastases arising in the stanozolol pretreated group (1) was significantly greater than the control group. Although the mice in group 2 had larger primaries and more metastases than group 3, the difference was not significant. The ECLT in mice receiving stanozolol was again significantly prolonged compared with controls (p<0.05) although both times were faster than before, due to poor clot precipitation The ECLT in mice with tumour was prolonged indicating quenching of fibrinolysis by the disease process.

7 mice per group	STANOZOLOL PRE- AND POST- 3LL	STANOZOLOL POST- 3LL	CONTROLS
Mean primary weight mg+sd	*5037+2131	3475+2937	*2986+1748
Range	2707-9039	1116-8930	442-4950
Significance (Mann-Whitney test) *p<0.03 compared with controls			
Mean no. metastases +sd	**28.4+13.4	23.7+11.3	**12.9+12.6
Range	14-52	11-45	0-28
Significance (Mann-Whitney test) **p<0.02 compared with controls			

DISCUSSION   The effect of stanozolol in prolonging the ECLT was unexpected, and our further experiments with other drugs (unpublished) have confirmed that the mouse fibrinolytic system responds differently to man The inhibition of blood fibrinolysis promotes increased growth and spread of the Lewis lung carcinoma, although a direct action of the drug, cannot be excluded. There was no correlation between primary weight and number of metastases, and more metastases were formed than would have been expected following the corresponding increase in size of the tumour. This implies that stanozolol had an effect both on primary growth and formation of lung metastases possibly by stabilisation of the fibrin envelope protecting the tumour and its metastatic implants. This could be tested by altering fibrinolysis on i-v artificial metastases, or by excision of the primary.

High dose stanozolol prolongs the ECLT in a dose-related manner and our pilot experiments have suggested it also increases tumour size and meta-stases when administered prior to 3LL inoculation. The quenching of the ECLT by the tumour may explain why significantly larger primaries and increased metastases occur only when the mouse is primed with drug prior to 3LL inoculation. No anabolic effects of stanozolol were seen in expt.1 with weight gain similar in both groups. Stanozolol has no corticosteroid-like action in man, and in expt.3 an immunosuppressive effect is unlikely, because in this syngeneic model no significant infiltration of host cells into 3LL metastases has been seen (Tsuruo et al 1983). Folkman and others (1983) found 71% 3LL tumour regression in mice treated with heparin and cortisone, but no effect when either was given alone. It is thus improb-able that a steroid action is responsible for 3LL tumour promotion.

It is too early to predict the effect of altered fibrinolysis on the growth and spread of a human tumour, but it is feasible that fibrinolytic enhancing agents such as stanozolol may be beneficial as adjuvant therapy.

REFERENCES
Anon, 1977, Editorial New Scientist, January 6, 15.
Bruesch, M.R., Johnson, G.L., Palackdharry, C.S., Weber, M.J. and Carl, P.
    1983, International Journal of Cancer, 32, 121.
Cederholm-Williams,S.A.,1983,British Journal of Hospital Medicine, Aug,107
Chew, E.-C. and Wallace, A.C., 1976 Cancer Research, 36, 1904.
Cliffton, E.E. and Grossi, C.E , 1955, Cancer, 8, 1146.
Donati, M.B. and Poggi, A., 1980, British Journal of Haematology, 44. 173.
Dvorak, H.F., Dickersin, G.R., Dvorak, A.M., Manseau, E.J. and Pyne, K.
    1981, Journal of the National Cancer Institute, 67, 335.
Dvorak,H.F.,Senger,D.R.and DvorakA.M.,1983,Cancer Metastasis Reviews,2,41.
Folkman, J.,Langer, R., Linhardt, R.J., Haudenschild, C. and Taylor, S.,
    1983, Science, 221,719.
Hilgard, P., 1977, British Journal of Cancer, 35, 891.
Ingram, G.I.C , 1952, Biochemical Journal, 51, 583.
Malone,J,Gervin,A,Moore,W and Keown,K,1979Journal Surgical Research,26,581
Marsh, N., 1981, Fibrinolysis, (John Wiley and Sons).
National Cancer Institute 1972. Cancer Chemotherapy Reports, III, 3(ii).
O'Meara, R.A.Q., 1958 Irish Journal of Medical Science, 396, 474.
Peterson, H -I., 1977, Cancer Treatment Reviews, 4, 213.
Thornes. R.D , 1975, Cancer, 35, 91.
Tsuruo, T., Iida, H., Tsukagoshi, S. and Ishikawa, T ,
    1983, Clinical and Experimental Metastasis, 1, 39
White, H., Griffiths, J.D and Salsbury, A.J.,
    1976, Proceedings of the Royal Society of Medicine, 69, 467.
Zacharski.L.R.,Schned,A.R. and Sorenson G.D ,1983,Cancer Research, 43,3963

ACKNOWLEDGEMENTS The authors wish to thank Prof.K.Hellmann, Dr.T.Stephens, Dr.M.Penhaligon and Sterling Research Laboratories for their generous help

INHIBITION OF METASTASIS AND CYTOTOXIC AGENT-INDUCED METASTASIS ENHANCEMENT BY LEECH SALIVARY GLAND EXTRACTS (SGE)

T.B. GASIC[1], G.J. GASIC[1], E.D. VINER[1], E.GORELIK[2], and L. MILAS[3]
[1]Pennsylvania Hospital, Philadelphia, PA; [2]Frederick Cancer Reserach Center, National Cancer Institute, Frederick, MD; [3]M. D. Anderson Hospital and Tumor Institute, Houston, TX

Keywords: Leech salivary gland extracts; metastasis enhancement

INTRODUCTION

When administered to experimental animals some chemotherapeutic drugs and ionizing radiation, can under certain experimental conditions enhance formation of metastasis from tumor cells injected intravenously (Van Putten et al. 1975; Milas & Peters 1984). The effect has been observed to occur in spontaneous metastasis formation as well (Poupon et al. 1984). Direct damage to the tissues, particularly endothelial cells of capillaries, seems to be a major mechanism for conditioning for metastasis formation, although suppression of antitumor resistance mechanisms also plays a significant role, especially in metastasis enhancement induced by chemo-therapeutic agents (Milas & Peters 1984). Although the clinical implications of these findings are still uncertain, there is a concern that these agents could promote metastatic spread, especially if they do not sterilize the primary source of circulating tumor cells. In the case of chemotherapy agents, this can occur when the administered drug is ineffective in tumor cell destruction due to intrinsic drug resistance, or when drug resistance develops during treatment. Because the induced metastasis enhancement represents potential danger, it is important to prevent or reduce it. Effective candidates are likely to be agents that are themselves antimetastatic and (or) agents that can protect tissues against the damage inflicted by the iatrogenic agents. Salivary gland extract (SGE) from leeches represents such a candidate because it is a potent antimetastatic agent (Gasic et al. 1983; 1984), and because it contains inhibitors of proteolytic enzymes (Bajkovski et al. 1984) that could inhibit or repair tissue damage. Here we report data showing SGE is effective in reducing enhancement of metastasis formation in the lungs of mice caused by cyclophosphamide (CY), cortisone, and local thoracic irradiation (LTI).

individual treatments. Here, all mice were free from pulmonary metastases (data not presented).

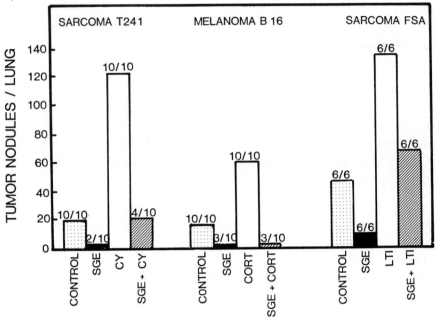

Figure 1.   Inhibition by SGE of metastasis formation and of the metastasis enhancement induced by CY, cortisone (CORT), or LTI.

DISCUSSION

Results from this study and our earlier observations (Gasic et al. 1983; 1984) show that SGE is a potent inhibitor of experimental metastases. Also, SGE was capable of reducing or abolishing the enhancement of metastasis formation induced by treatment with CY, cortisone, or LTI. The antimetastatic activity of SGE is likely to be mediated through several biological activities of SGE, which include anticoagulant and antiplatelet-aggregating activity (Gasic et al. 1983), and inhibition of proteolytic enzymes such as collagenase type IV and cathepsin B (Bajkovski et al. 1984) enzymes. By degradation of vascular basement membrane, these enzymes facilitate the exit of tumor cells into extravascular spaces and thereby ease metastasis formation. On the other hand, by preventing platelet aggregation and fibrin formation around tumor cells, anticoagulants not only reduce trapping of tumor cells in tissues, but, according to recent observations by Gorelik et al. (1984), they also make tumor cells accessible to cytotoxic NK cells. Therefore, it is likely that the antihemostatic property of SGE operates through both of these mechanims in reducing metastasis formation, and the existence of the latter mechanism is

MATERIALS AND METHODS

The antimetastatic effect of SGE was studied in an artificial metastasis assay using sarcoma T241 and melanoma B16 in C57BL/6 mice and fibrosarcoma FSA in C3Hf/Kam mice. Three doses of SGE (500-800 µg protein/injection) obtained from the Mexican leech Haementeria officinalis were given i.v. or i.p. at -2, +2, and +4 hr. relative to i.v. inoculation of tumor cells. CY, cortisone, and LTI, in doses of 200 mg/kg, 0.5 to 1 mg/kg, and 10 Gy, respectively, were administered 1 day before tumor cells. Tumor nodules in the lung were generated by injecting 5×10^4 T241 i.v., 5×10^4 B16 melanoma, or 3×10^4 FSA cells. The number of lung nodules were determined 2 weeks after FSA and 19 days after T241 sarcoma and B16 melanoma cell injection. Details of the experimental procedures have been described previously (Gasic et al. 1983; 1984). Effect of SGE on the metastasis formation in bg/+ and bg/bg mice treated and nontreated with anti-asialo GMI serum was also investigated. Anti-asialo GMI serum (Wako Chemicals USA, Inc., Dallas, TX) was inoculated i.p. 0.2 ml in dilution 1:40 1 day prior i.v. injection of tumor cells.

RESULTS

Figure 1 shows that treatment of mice with CY, cortisone, or LTI resulted in the augmentation of metastasis formation in the lungs of mice inoculated with sarcoma T241, melanoma B16, or sarcoma FSA cells. Treatment of the normal mice with SGE inhibits this lung colonization by circulating tumor cells. Also, SGE was capable of abrogating the enhancement of metastasis formation caused by treatment of tumor cell recipients with CY, cortisone, or LTI. In another study, SGE prevented CY-induced enhancement of metastases, when given within 2 hr. before and 4 hr. after CY, and even when both agents were given 4 days before tumor cells (Gasic et al. 1984).

Since a major mechanism in CY-induced enhancement of metastasis formation is suppression of NK cells (Hanna & Fidler 1980; Milas & Peters 1984), the possibility of whether SGE acted by stimulating NK cells was investigated. It was found that SGE did not affect NK cell activity either in normal or in CY-treated mice (Gasic et al. 1984). It was further found that the antimetastatic effect of SGE was more profound in mice having normal NK cell activity than in beige mice genetically deficient in NK cells function. However, when residual NK activity of beige mice was destroyed by the treatment with anti-asialo GMI serum, the antimetastatic effect of SGE was completely abrogated. In contrast, stimulation of NK reactivity of C57BL/6 mice with poly I:C and SGE treatment were more effective than

supported by the present observation that SGE antimetastatic activity was
greatly reduced in NK cell deficient mice or increased in mice having stimulated NK cell function. Thus, it is probable that SGE, through its proteolytic enzyme -inhibitory and antihemostatic properties, retains tumor
cells within the circulation where thay are more likely to be destroyed by
other mechanisms including NK cells, than once they have exited into the
extracapillary spaces.

   These mechanisms are also likely to be involved in the inhibition of metastasis enhancement caused by CY, cortisone, and LTI. However, in the experimental setting in which SGE and CY were given 4 days prior to tumor
cells, the antihemostatic effects of SGE could be less significant because
in normal mice SGE was not effective at all if given 4 days before tumor
cells (Gastic et al. 1984). There, SGE could have acted more by interfering with the damage of tissues caused by cytotoxic agents. It is possible that inhibitors of proteolytic enzymes contained in SGE neutralized
enzymes released by injured tissues that resulted in less tissue damage and
consequently in reduced probability for development of metastasis enhancement.

   In conclusion, SGE is a potent inhibitor of metastasis formation and a
potent preventor of the enhancement of metastases induced by iatrogenic
agents. The mechanism of its activity is not well understood but it includes antiplatelet-aggregating, anticoagulant, and proteolyic enzyme inhibitor
activities.

REFERENCES

Bajikovski, A.S. et al, 1984, Proceedings of the American Association for
   Cancer Research, 25, 58.
Gasic, G.J. et al, 1983, Cancer Research, 43, 1633.
Gasic G.J. et al, 1984, Cancer Research, in press.
Gorelik, E. et al, 1984, International Journal of Cancer, 33, 87.
Hanna, N. & Fidler, I.J., 1980, Cancer Invasion and Metastasis: Biologic
   and Therapeutic Aspects, (Raven Press), pp. 321.
Poupon, M.F. et al 1984, Cancer Treatment Reports, 68, 749.
van Putten, L.M. et al, 1975, International Journal of Cancer, 15, 588.

FIBRONECTIN AND CANCER METASTASIS

GILLIAN HUNT and G.V. SHERBET

Cancer Research Unit, University of Newcastle upon Tyne, Royal Victoria
Infirmary, Newcastle upon Tyne NE1 4LP

Keywords: fibronectin; rat gliomas; protease inhibitors

INTRODUCTION

The capacity of malignant tumours to invade and metastasize is probably their most important property (Carter, 1978). Primary tumours of
the nervous system, although highly invasive, rarely, if at all, metastasize to extracranial sites. Their mode of spread appears to be by direct
extension or via the cerebrospinal fluid; blood-borne or lymph borne true
metastatic dissemination has not been reported. In order to metastasize
by the haematogenous route, the tumour cell has to pass through several
stages and it is possible that the metastasis of gliomas may be restrained
at one or more points in this sequence.

In vivo, fibronectin (FN), the major high molecular weight glycoprotein present on the cell surface, is thought to play a vital role in mediating interactions between cells. In this paper, the possible link between
FN and metastatic behaviour is described. The kinetics of release of FN
from C6 rat glioma cells was compared with those of metastatic variants of
B16 murine melanoma lines F1 (low metastasis) and BL6 (high metastasis)
in the presence and absence of protease inhibitors.

MATERIALS AND METHODS

Cell culture

The melanoma lines were maintained in culture as described previously
(Sherbet, 1983).

The C6 glioma line was grown in Ham's F10 medium containing 20 mM
Hepes buffer, 15% heat-inactivated horse serum, 2.5% foetal bovine serum
(FBS) and supplemented with 1.7 mM glutamine, 0.025% w/v streptomycin
sulphate, 500 U/ml penicillin G, 60 U/ml Mycostatin and 2.5 µg/ml Fungizone.

Determination of FN

     This involved a turbidimetric assessment of its reaction with the
corresponding antiserum (Boehringer assay). The FN was then expressed as
µg fibronectin/mg total cell protein, the total protein being measured by
the Bio-Rad procedure.

Time course incubation of the cells

     Subconfluent monolayers of cells were rinsed in phosphate buffered
saline, pH 7.1 (PBS), 5 ml of pre-warmed maintenance medium [Medium 199,
without phenol red indicator (Gibco) containing 10% FBS] added and the
cells incubated at 37°C. Duplicates were performed for each time point.
The supernatant medium was then removed and the cell layer rinsed in PBS.
The cells were scraped off into 1.0 ml of solubilizing solution [0.5M
NaOH + 1% w/v mercaptoethanol] and the cell extract was stored at -20°C
until analysis.

Effect of protease inhibitors

     The above procedure was adopted, adding aprotinin or leupeptin to
the maintenance medium at 0.2 trypsin inhibitor units/ml. Trypsin inhibitor activity of the protease inhibitors was measured at 25°C, pH 8,
using benzoyl-L-arginine ethyl ester as substrate.

RESULTS

     All the cell lines studied deleted FN, although not at identical
rates [Fig. 1-3]. The BL6 and C6 cells were found to delete FN actively,
their initial rates of deletion being 0.8 and 1.7 µg FN/mg total cell
protein/minute respectively. The deletion rate in F1 was only 0.3 µg FN/
mg total cell protein/minute. On incubating the cells with aprotinin, a
broad spectrum antiprotease, the deletion of FN was significantly inhibited
in BL6 and C6 (p = 0.048 and 0.028 respectively) but not in F1.

     For BL6, the experiment was repeated using leupeptin, which speci-
fically inhibits trypsin, plasmin, papain and cathepsin B [Fig. 4]. The
deletion of FN was again significantly inhibited (p = 0.028) but overall
the effect of leupeptin was not significantly different from that of aprotinin. However, deletion of FN was prevented to a greater degree with
leupeptin than with aprotinin over the first ½ hour of incubation.

DISCUSSION

     Changes in the cell surface are considered to be an essential feature
of the transformed phenotype. Vaheri and Mosher (1978) have stated that

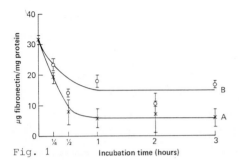

Fig. 1

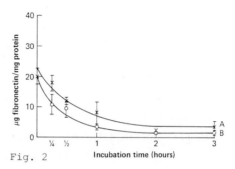

Fig. 2

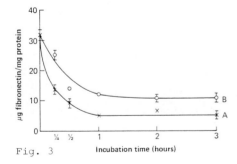

Fig. 3

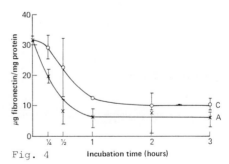

Fig. 4

Figs. 1-3. Kinetics of deletion of fibronectin and the subsequent effects of aprotinin on this deletion from BL6, F1 and C6 respectively. Fig. 4 shows the effect of leupeptin on the kinetics of deletion from BL6. A: control cells, B: aprotinin treated cells, C: leupeptin treated cells.

several transformed cell lines in vitro are deficient in cell surface FN. Confirming the work of Vaheri et al. (1976), Sherbet et al. (1982) studied the FN status of 9 human astrocytomas in culture and demonstrated that cell surface FN was considerably depleted in 7 of these cultures as compared with a normal glial cell line, although receptors for FN were still detectable on the surface of the tumour cells.

In terms of deletion of FN and the subsequent effects of aprotinin, there is a sharp contrast between the metastatic variants of B16. Both BL6 and the non-metastasizing F1 deleted FN; the rate of deletion in F1 being approximately one third of that in BL6. The C6 glioma behaved in a very similar manner to the metastasizing BL6 in this series of experiments. However, the initial rate of deletion of FN in C6 was approximately twice that in BL6. The effect of leupeptin in BL6 cells was not significantly different from that of aprotinin, suggesting that non-specific proteases may be responsible for the deletion of FN in these cells.

Deletion of FN from the cell surface may assist in the escape of tumour cells from the primary tumour; they may become less 'sticky' and more readily shed. On the other hand, lack of FN could also prevent the attachment of the released cells to the basement membrane preparatory to their penetration of the endothelium.

From these experiments, a correlation between the kinetics of FN deletion and metastatic behaviour is apparent. As the C6 behaves in a similar manner to a metastasizing cell line in vitro, it seems that factors other than FN may also contribute to the inability of gliomas to metastasize in vivo.

ACKNOWLEDGMENT

This work was supported by a research grant from the North of England Cancer Research Campaign.

REFERENCES

Carter, R.L., 1978, Investigative Cell Pathology, 1, 275.
Sherbet, G.V., 1983, Experimental Cell Biology, 51, 140.
Sherbet, G.V., Tindle, M.E. & Stidolph, S., 1982, Anticancer Research, 2, 251.
Vaheri, A. & Mosher, D.F., 1978, Biochimica et Biophysica Acta, 516, 1.
Vaheri, A., Ruoslahti, E., Westermark, B. & Ponten, J., 1976, Journal of Experimental Medicine, 143, 64.

"TRAP-DOOR" EFFECT OF THE ENDOTHELIUM - A MECHANISM OF TUMOUR CELL EXTRAVASATION ?

G. SKOLNIK[1], L. E. ERICSON[2], T. KJELLSTRÖM[1], L. REHNMAN[1] and B. RISBERG[1]

Departments of [1]Surgery I and [2]Anatomy, University of Göteborg, Sweden

Keywords: extravasation; endothelium; serotonin

INTRODUCTION

Once tumour cells released from a malignant tumour have reached the blood stream, their arrest in the microcirculation and penetration of the vascular wall are prerequisites for metastasis formation. This phase of the metastasis formation is generally referred to as tumour cell lodgement and according to previous studies it is influenced by serotonin released from platelets activated upon contact with tumour cells (Skolnik et al.1983, 1984).

Since most of the tumour cells arrested in the microvasculature are destroyed in the hostile intravascular environment, penetration of the vascular wall is necessary for their survival. Interaction between tumour cells and endothelial cells is the key event in the extravasation process, but the exact mechanisms of this interaction are far from clarified.

The use of in vitro experimental systems is considered to be a relevant model for studies on the details of a single step of metastasis formation. An in vitro model using cultured endothelial cells for studies on the extravasation process has been introduced by Kramer & Nicolson (1979).

The aim of the present study was to investigate the interaction between cultured endothelial cells from the rat and syngeneic fibrosarcoma cells and to study the effect of serotonin (5-HT) on this interaction.

MATERIAL AND METHODS

Endothelial cells from the pulmonary artery of rats of the Lister strain were cultured in monolayers and characterized with electron microscopy and factor VIII analysis as previously described by Kjellström et al.(1984). Tumour cell suspensions were prepared from a transplantable 20-methylcholantrene-induced fibrosarcoma, propagated by intramuscular transfer in syngeneic rats.

Endothelial cells of the second or third generation were grown to confluent monolayers and incubated with an equivalent number of tumour cells suspended in culture medium. Cultures were incubated for various time intervals
between 30 minutes and 24 hours. At different incubation times phase contrast
micrographs were taken and cultures were processed for electron microscopy
(TEM and SEM). Serotonin in a final concentration of 10^{-8} M alone or together
with ketanserin (a 5-HT antagonist with selective effect on 5-HT_2 receptors)
in the same concentration were added to some of the cultures.

In a set of experiments tumour cells labelled with ^{125}I-5-iodo-2-deoxy-
uridine (^{125}IUDR) were used for quantitative determinations of the number of
tumour cells remaining in the endothelial monolayer.

RESULTS

Phase contrast microscopy indicated that most of the fibrosarcoma cells
added to the endothelial monolayer attached within an hour and preferably
at the intercellular junctions of the endothelial cells.

These observations were supported by the electron microscopical findings.
In untreated cultures the tumour cells to a large extent remained on the
surface of the endothelial layer and retained a rounded shape (Fig. 1). The
tumour cells developed cytoplasmic processes which attached to the endothelial cell surface or appeared to induce a slight retraction of endothelial
cell margins, which allowed the processes to penetrate in between endothelial cells to attach to the substratum.

When serotonin (10^{-8} M) was added, retraction of endothelial cells and
formation of intercellular gaps were more prominent. Tumour cells attached
to these intercellular denuded areas. Attached tumour cells were initially
spherical but attained progressively a flattened shape. Cytoplasmic processes extending below the endothelial cells were frequent (Fig. 2), although
tumour cells completely covered by endothelial cells were rare.

When cultures were treated with both 5-HT and ketanserin, the serotonin-
induced retraction of endothelial cells was prevented and numerous rounded
tumour cells remained on the surface of the monolayer as in untreated cultures.

The results of the isotope studies supported the ultrastructural observations. After 4 hours, in cultures treated with serotonin 18% of the added
labelled tumour cells remained in the endothelial layer as compared to 11%
in untreated controls and 12% in cultures treated with both serotonin and
ketanserin.

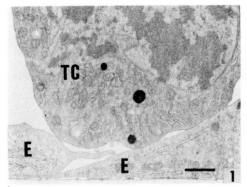
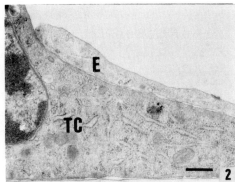

Figure 1. Control culture incubated for 2 hours with tumour cells. The tumour cell (TC) is attached to the surface of two endothelial cells (E). Bar =1 μm

Figure 2. Culture incubated with tumour cells and serotonin for 2 hours. A tumour cell (TC) is penetrating below the lateral portion of an endothelial cell (E). Bar= 0.5 μm

DISCUSSION

The multiplicity of different hypotheses on the mechanisms of tumour cell extravasation indicates the problems of interpreting in vivo observations of this process. An in vitro system, first described by Kramer & Nicolson (1979) permits more detailed studies on the interactions between tumour cells and endothelial cells. Our electron microscopic observations on tumour cell adherence to the endothelial monolayer and a subsequent slight retraction of endothelial cells are in accordance with the observations of Kramer & Nicolson (1979). The contractility of endothelial cells is, however, a controversial phenomenon (Hammersen 1980, De Clerck et al. 1981). The slight retraction observed could be an initial sign of a minor endothelial damage, as previously described by Björkerud & Bondjers (1972). An early endothelial damage caused by embolic tumour cells has been reported by Hilgard (1973) in his "minimal endothelial damage" theory as a possible mechanism of tumour cell extravasation in the microvasculature.

In previous in vivo investigations on tumour cell lodgement, serotonin antagonist treatment with ketanserin (a selective $5-HT_2$ blocking agent) was used, as $5-HT_2$ receptors are mainly located on platelets and in the vessel walls. The results of these studies demonstrated that ketanserin did not affect the initial arrest of circulating tumour cells, while it was influencing the later phase of the lodgement process, during which arrested tumour cells have to penetrate the vascular wall, thus indicating the involvement of 5-HT during this later phase (Skolnik et al.1983, 1984). On these grounds

we focused our attention on the influence of 5-HT on the interactions between tumour cells and endothelial cells. Addition of 5-HT induced endothelial cell retraction and opening of intercellular gaps, thereby facilitating
the penetration of tumour cells through the endothelial monolayer. This
ultrastructural finding was supported by the results of quantitative studies
with ^{125}IUDR-labelled tumour cells which indicated that an increased number
of labelled tumour cells were retained in the endothelial layer.

Robertson and Khairallah (1973) proposed the term "trap-door" effect to
describe the changes in the permeability of arterial endothelium to circulating macromolecules following opening and closing of interendothelial gaps
as a possible mechanism of development of initial stages of atherogenesis.
They also suggested that activated platelets may play an important role in
maintenance of abnormal vascular permeability by release of serotonin and/or
other vasoactive agents. The findings in the present study show a similarity
with the changes in morphology and permeability of arterial endothelium
described by Robertson § Khairallah (1973). Thus, the "trap-door" effect may
be a possible mechanism of the interactions between tumour cells, platelet-
released serotonin and endothelial cells leading to extravasation of tumour
cells arrested in the microvasculature.

REFERENCES
Björkerud, S. § Bondjers, G.,1972, Endothelial integrity and viability in
    the aorta of the normal rabbit and rat as evaluated with dye exclusion
    tests and interference contrast microscopy. Atherosclerosis 15, 285.
De Clerck, F., De Brabander, M., Neels, H. § Van de Velde, V., 1981, Direct
    evidence for the contractile capacity of endothelial cells. Thrombosis
    Research 23, 505.
Hammersen, F., 1980, Endothelial contraction - does it exist ? Advances in
    Microcirculation 9, 95.
Hilgard, P., 1973, The role of blood platelets in experimental metastases.
    British Journal of Cancer 28, 429.
Kjellström, T., Ahlman, H., Dahlström, A., Hansson, G.K. § Risberg, B.,1984,
    The uptake of 5-HT in endothelial cells cultured from the pulmonary arte-
    ry in rats. Acta Physiologica Scandinavica 120, 243.
Kramer, R.H. § Nicolson, G.L., 1979, Interactions of tumour cells with vas-
    cular endothelial cell monolayers: A model for metastatic invasion.
    Proceedings of the National Academy of Science, U.S.A. 76, 5704.
Robertson, A.L. § Khairallah, P.A., 1973, Arterial endothelial permeability
    and vascular disease. The "trap-door" effect. Experimental and Molecular
    Pathology 18, 241.
Skolnik, G., Ericson, L.E. § Bagge, U., 1983, The effect of thrombocytopenia
    and antiserotonin treatment on the lodgement of circulating tumour cells.
    Journal of Cancer Research and Clinical Oncology 105, 30.
Skolnik, G., Bagge, U., Dahlström, A. § Ahlman, H., 1984, The importance of
    5-HT for tumour cell lodgement in the liver. International Journal of
    Cancer 33, 519.

"CLONOGENIC" TUMOR CELL RELEASE ASSAY (CTCR ASSAY): POSSIBLE RELEVANCE TO
METASTASIS AND ITS TREATMENT

NORIO SUZUKI
Johns Hopkins Oncology Center, 600 North Wolfe Street, Baltimore, Maryland
21205, USA

Keyword: Metastasis, Tumor-cell-release, Radiation Response

INTRODUCTION

The earlier studies in the 1960's with microscopic observation of
blood-borne tumor cells did not establish the significance of blood-borne
tumor cells to the future metastatic development and prognosis of the
patients. Many recent studies, including our own, have emphasized and
dealt with the latter part of metastatic processes, i.e., processes at the
secondary sites. However, the negative results on the blood-borne tumor
cells of the patients may be due to inadequacy and limitation of the
methodologies and study designs used at that time. In the past few years,
we have been developing new methods to assay "clonogenic" tumor cell
release rate from leg tumors (CTCR assay) (Suzuki 1983a) and to determine
"clonogenic" blood-borne tumor cells using centrifugal elutriation (Suzuki
1984a). In this report we will discuss CTCR assay and its application.

METHOD

The method utilizes heavily irradiated lungs as in situ filters to
trap released tumor cells through the 22 hr incubation time prior to
preparation and "clonogenicity" assay in vitro of lung cell suspensions
(Fig. 1). The heavy irradiation of the lungs kills premetastasized tumor
cells and normal cells in the lungs. The tumor cells are identified as
colony forming cells (Fig. 2 & 3) with tumorigenicity and specific
cellular DNA content to each tumor system. Thus, this method allows us to
determine release rate of "clonogenic" tumor cells instead of incidental

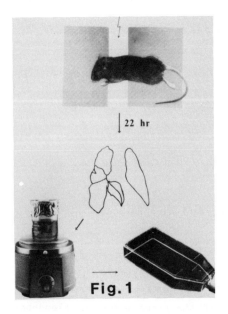

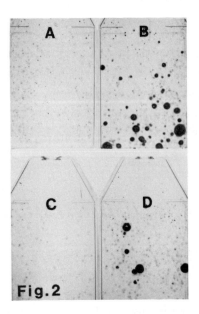

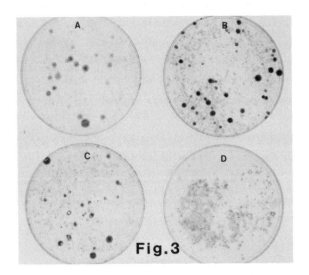

Fig. 1. Schematic presentation of CTCR assay.   Fig. 2. CTCR colonies of
FSA1231 (A, 0 hr control – no colonies; B, 22 hr with colonies) & FSA1233
(C, 0 hr control – no colonies; D, 22 hr with colonies).   Fig. 3.   CTCR
colonies (22 hr) of NFSA2ALM1 (A), KHT (B), NFSA2ALM1 in nude mice (C), &
human melanoma MeWo (D – no CTCR colonies) in nude mice.

blood-borne tumor cells (by ambiguous morphological identification used in the past). CTCR assay has been successfully applied to various tumor systems including FSA1231, FSA1233, NFSA2ALM1, NFSAI-56, NFSA2ALM1-119, KHT (all with syngeneic C3H/HeJ mice) and also, using nude mice, to NFSA2ALM1 and human melanoma MeWo (Suzuki 1983a,b; Suzuki & Kuperman submitted; Fig. 2-3 of the present study), and to determination of radiation responses of clonogenic tumor cell release (Suzuki 1984b; Suzuki & Kuperman 1984).

Table 1. CTCR rate and SLME.

Days post inject.	NFSA2ALM1	NFSA1-56	NFSA2ALM1-119
CTCR[a]			
19	28.1 $\pm$ 3.1 (16)	0.2 $\pm$ 0.2 (5)	3.6 $\pm$ 0.7 (5)
SLME[b]			
32	28.4 $\pm$ 7.2 (15)	1.1 $\pm$ 0.4 (38)	3.6 $\pm$ 0.9 (16)

a. CTCR: Clonogenic tumor cell release rate per mouse-22 hr
b. SLME: Spontaneous lung metastasis efficiency, lung nodule per mouse

Table 2. Local tumor irradiation (LTI) and metastasis.

LTI	SLME (Nodule/mouse)	Tumor size (mm^3)
Exp. 1		
Control (0 Gy)	8.3 $\pm$ 2.0 (7)	—
10 Gy - 4 Days - AMP	1.1 $\pm$ 1.0 (7) (13%)	—
Control (0 Gy)	24.1 $\pm$ 3.9 (7)	—
10 Gy - 7 Days - AMP	9.7 $\pm$ 3.7 (7) (40%)	—
Exp. 2		
Control (0 Gy)	52.6 $\pm$ 5.9 (14)	1900 $\pm$ 129
10 Gy + 10 Gy	18.5 $\pm$ 2.7 (15) (35%)	1625 $\pm$ 93 (86%)

a. AMP: Amputation of tumor bearing legs - see text

As shown in Table 1, SLME and CTCR were positively correlated with each other in NFSA system (Suzuki & Kuperman, submitted) (the tumor cell lines were established in our laboratory from a spontaneous fibrosarcoma, NFSA, of C3Hf/Bu; Ando et al, 1979). The similar positive correlation was previously observed in FSA system (Suzuki 1983b).

After 10 Gy of local tumor irradiation, CTCR was reduced to a few percent of unirradiated control during the following one or two days and gradually recovered thereafter but still remained lower after 7 days (10-30% of unirradiated control).

Dose response curves indicated that the CTCR is more sensitive than the survival of the tumor cells in the primary (the survival was determined by in vivo irradiation – in vitro clonogenicity assay): D_o = 3.8 Gy for NFSA2ALM1-CTCR curve, 3.0 Gy for FSA1231-CTCR curve, while D_o = 4.5 Gy for survival curves of these tumor cells – all irradiations were performed under Nembutal anesthesia using a ^{137}Cs irradiator.

From the data one can predict that LTI (local tumor irradiation) would reduce SLME substantially. Table 2 shows how local irradiations effectively reduce SLME. In Exp. 1 SLME was determined 14 days after AMP (amputation of tumor bearing legs) which was performed 4 days or 7 days after local tumor irradiation (10 Gy). In Exp. 2, two 10 Gy irradiations were carried out on day 12 and 19, and SLME was determined on day 33 after tumor cell inoculation in the leg (no AMP). In these experiments SLME was reduced to 15–40% of unirradiated control as expected from the CTCR radiation response.

As a conclusion, CTCR assay may be useful to determine the role of "clonogenic" tumor cell release in metastasis and to obtain basic data useful for prevention and control of metastasis.

REFERENCES

Ando, K., Hunter, N., & Peters, L.J., 1979, Immunologically nonspecific enhancement of artificial lung metastases in tumor-bearing mice. Cancer Immunology & Immunotherapy, 6, 151.

Suzuki, N., 1983a, New method to quantitate clonogenic tumor cells in the blood circulation of mice. Cancer Research, 43, 5451.

Suzuki, N., 1983b, Variant selection and blood-borne "clonogenic" tumor cell release from NFSA2ALM1 tumors, British Journal of Cancer, 48, 827

Suzuki, N., 1984a, Centrifugal elutriation and characterization of tumor cells from venous blood of tumor-bearing mice: possible relevance to metastasis, Cancer Research, 44, 3505.

Suzuki, N., 1984b, Radiation response of "clonogenic" tumor cell release from NFSA2ALM1 tumors, Radiation Research, 98, 649.

Suzuki, N., and Kuperman, S., 1984, Radiation response of "clonogenic" tumor-cell-release (CTCR) from FSA1231 tumors, Abstract of the 26th Annual Scientific Meeting of the American Society for Therapeutic Radiology and Oncology, October 7-12, 1984.

Suzuki, N., and Kuperman, S., submitted, A new metastasis system derived from a mouse fibrosarcoma (NFSA) of spontaneous origin: possible importance of "clonogenic" tumor-cell-release, British Journal of Cancer.

TUMOUR METASTASIS AND CELL DEFORMABILITY.

1. ASSESSMENT BY NUCLEPORE FILTRATION

G.D. SHANTZ[1], F.J. NORDT[2], T. OCHALEK[3], and M.M. BURGER[1]

[1]Dept. of Biochem., Biocenter, University of Basel, Switzerland

[2]Dept. of Preclin. Research, Sandoz Ltd., Basel, Switzerland

[3]Institute of Mol. Biol., Jagellonian University, Krakow, Poland

Keywords: B16 Melanoma / Metastasis / Deformability / Pressure Filtration

INTRODUCTION

The ability of tumour cells to deform may enable them to escape from the primary tumour, extravasate and invade host tissue. The purpose of these studies was to develop appropriate methodology for assessing the passive deformability of tumour cells of low and high metastatic potential. Passive, in contrast to active, deformability is defined as the capacity of tumour cells to deform in response to mechanical forces, e.g. pressure.

In the past, capillary techniques have been used to measure the deformability of one or only a portion of one cell (Weiss 1976). In contrast, with Nuclepore filtration techniques (Sato et al. 1977, Khato et al. 1979, Erkell et al. 1982), the deformability of an entire population of heterogeneous tumour cells may be studied. However, cell filterability is influenced by a variety of biological and technological factors (Nordt 1983). Thus, in order to be interpretable, Nuclepore filtration techniques must fulfil certain criteria, namely: 1) what goes in must come out, i.e., a high percentage of cells must be able to be recovered in the filtrate; 2) cellular aggregation should be minimized by choosing conditions which permit relatively short filtration times; 3) cell viability should be high and not lost upon filtration; 4) cell size distribution should not be influenced by filtration; 5) it is necessary to exclude that differences in cell to filter and cell to cell adhesion of different cell lines are responsible for differences in filterability. In order to fulfil these criteria, certain experimental parameters such as cell to pore ratio, filtration pressure and cell culture conditions were first standardized.

Treatment of Metastasis

METHODS

Table 1. Origin of Melanoma lines and their metastatic potential.

Melanoma line	Origin	Metastatic potential (%)[a]
F1A	Clone of B16-F1	28
NR4	Filter migration selectant of B16-F1	79
a5b1/a	Wheat germ agglutinin-resistant line of B16-F1	36
a5b1/x	Ricin-resistant revertant of a5b1/a	83

Mean cell diameter was similar for F1A, NR4 (17.0μm) and a5b1/a & x(18.6μm)
[a]Evaluated after amputation of the primary tumour (Tao & Burger 1982).

  Melanoma cell lines (Table 1) were grown on petri dishes in Eagle's
MEM with 10% H.I. FCS plus supplements and serially transferred by removal
with EDTA. For cell filtration tests, cells were removed with PBS $Ca^{++}Mg^{++}$
free PBS, resuspended in filtration medium (FM = growth medium – FCS,
+ 0.01 M hepes buffer and filtered through a Nalgene 0.2 μm filter) during
constant exposure to 95% O_2 and 5% CO_2. 1 ml aliquots of tumour cell suspensions were filtered at constant pressure through an area of 19.6 mm^2 of
Nuclepore filters held in place by a custom made plastic holder. The time
for passage of the suspension through the filter was recorded. Cell viab-
ilities were determined by trypan blue dye exclusion. Cell size distributions were determined with a Coulter counter.

RESULTS AND DISCUSSION
  Filtration experiments were first designed to determine if a significant
percentage of the lowest metastatic line could pass through the filter
within a short time period i.e., 1-2 min. To avoid cell aggregation, low
cell to pore ratios (0.5) were first tried. However, even when the pressure
was relatively low (5 cm H_2O), medium was lost quickly (20.4 sec.) through
open pores before all cells could pass through the filter. Raising the cell
to pore ratio (to 40) blocked medium loss, but required a certain minimum
pressure (50 cm H_2O) before a significant percentage (92.4%) of F1A cells
could be forced through the restrictive pores within a short time period
(114.2 ± 6.1 sec.).

Culture conditions also influenced tumour cell filterability. E.g., F1A cells derived from cultures which were either too sparse (2 day 40% confluent) or too overcrowded (3 day over-confluent "starving" cultures) gave filtration times which were significantly longer (1367.5 ± 46.7 sec.) or shorter (38.5 ± 3.9 sec.) than 2 minutes. Thus, for comparison of filterabilities, tumour cells were always derived from similar culture conditions i.e., from 2 day healthy subconfluent cultures where filtration times for the lowest metastatic lines were routinely in the range of 1-2 minutes.

After standardization of these experimental parameters, a significant difference in tumour cell filterability between low and high metastatic melanoma cells could be observed. For instance, the highly metastatic NR4 and a5b1/x lines were 4 and 2 times more filterable respectively than their low metastatic counterparts. (Table 2). Viability of all 4 tumour lines was not significally reduced upon filtration. In addition, the cell size distribution of each tumour line was similar before and after filtration (Shantz et al. 1984).

Table 2. Filterability of melanoma cells of low and high metastatic potential.

Tumour line	Cells filtered (%)	Cell viability (%)	Filtration time (sec) (%)
F1A	91.9 ± 4.3	83.5 ± 3.4	107.0 ± 15.4
NR4	87.8 ± 4.3	82.2 ± 2.2	26.0 ± 8.8
a5b1/a	78.5 ± 5.5	73.1 ± 1.8	170.7 ± 31.0
a5b1/x	84.8 ± 4.0	78.3 ± 4.2	91.6 ± 13.3

Each value represents the mean of triplicate determinations from 2 experiments; cell to pore ratio =40; for F1A/NR4 and a5b1/a & x, pore diam. = 10 and 12 μm and pressure = 50 and 30 cm H_2O respectively.

These differences in tumour cell filterability could not be explained by their adhesive properties, either by cell to filter or by cell to cell adhesion. E.g., when filters were exposed to tumour cell suspensions for 6 min. and subsequently dipped gently into filtration medium, no cells remained on the filter. Thus, cell to filter adhesion did not occur within this time period. This is in accordance with earlier studies (Tullberg & Burger 1984) in which positive charges had to be introduced onto filters before the negatively charged malanoma cells could adhere to the surface.

Further examination of the medium into which the filters were dipped revealed some cell to cell adhesion. This was slight, but similar for the a5b1 lines. In contrast, the low metastatic F1A line showed the presence of small loosely adherent cell aggregates whereas the NR4 line remained as single cells, even over a period of 20 min. Thus, the possibility remained that the higher degree of aggregation of the low metastatic F1A line could account for its lower degree of filterability. However, when such cells were filtered in media in which they could not aggregate ($Ca^{++}Mg^{++}$ free PBS) a 3.6 fold difference in cell filterability between F1A and NR4 remained (Shantz et al. 1984). Thus, it appears unlikely that adhesive properties account for differences in filterabilty of F1A and NR4 melanoma cells. We conclude, therefore, that these differences in filterability reflect differences in cellular deformability.

This communication provides the first evidence that deformability of tumour cells dervived from solid tissue may be related to their metastatic potential. The capacity of such cells to deform passively was not associated with microtubule structure (data not shown), Rather, the deformability of these cells appears to be dependent on the integrity of actin micro-filaments (Shantz et al. 1984). It should be cautioned however, that these results reflect only one aspect of the more complex process of cellular deformability which occurs in vivo. Furthermore, the situation described here is not applicable to all types of tumour systems as exemplified by certain lymphomas (Shantz & Schirrmacher 1979) in which preliminary studies suggest that the more highly metastatic cells are less deformable.

REFERENCES

Erkell, L.J., Ryd, W., & Hagmar, B., 1982, Invasion & Metastasis, 2, 260.
Khato, J., Sato, H., Suzuki, M., & Sato, H., 1979, Tohoku Journal of Experimental Medicine, 128, 273.
Nordt, F.J., 1983, Annals of The New York Accademy of Sciences, 416, 651.
Sato, H., Khato, J., Sato, T., & Suzuki, M., 1977, Gann Monographs on Cancer Research, 20, 3.
Schirrmacher, V. & Shantz, G., 1979, In: Function and Structure of the Immune System, 769. Ed. W. Ruchholtz & H.K. Muller-Hermelink Plenum N.Y.
Shantz, G. & Schirrmacher, V., 1979, Tumor Metastasis and cell-mediated immunity in a model system in DBA/2 mice. 3. Induction and specificity of syngeneic sytotoxic T cells. In: Cell Biology and Immunology of leucocyte function, 725. Ed. M.R. Quaestal, Academic Press, New York.
Shantz, G., Ochalek, T., Nordt, F., Tullberg, K., Burger, M.M., 1984, Tumor metastasis and cell deformability. 2. Correlation between tumor cell filterability and metastatic potential (In preparation).
Tao, T.W., & Burger, M.M., 1982, International Journal of Cancer, 29, 425.
Tullberg, K.T., & Burger, M.M., 1984, Invasion & Metastasis (in the press).
Weiss, L., 1976, Cell deformability. Some general considerations. In: Fundamental aspects of metastasis, 305. Ed. L. Weiss, North-Holland, Amsterdam.

MEMBRANE PERMEABILITY CHANGES INDUCED BY THE ANTITUMOUR LYMPHOKINE
LEUKOREGULIN

S.C. BARNETT and C.H. EVANS
National Cancer Institute, N.I.H., Bethesda, Maryland, 20205, USA

Keyword: Leukoregulin, flow cytometry, membrane permeability

INTRODUCTION

Lymphokines can modify many aspects of tumour development including
prevention of carcinogenesis, elimination of preneoplastic cells and
suppression as well as erradication of tumorigenic cells (see review of
Evans, 1983). The anticancer activities associated with lymphotoxin (Evans
and DiPaolo, 1981) recently have been demonstrated to be properties of a
new lymphokine that is biochemically distinct from lymphotoxin (Ransom and
Evans, 1983). This new anticancer lymphokine has been termed leukoregulin
to denote its leukocyte origin and ability to regulate tumour cell growth.
(Cleveland et al., 1984). In this study cell perturbations were examined to
analyse leukoregulin's mode of action. Tumour cell surface conformation
and plasma membrane permeability changes in human erythroleukaemia K562
cells were measured by forward light scatter and fluorescein diacetate
fluorochromasia respectively with a FACS IV flow cytometer. Cell membrane
effects were detectable as early as 5 minutes with a maximum achieved 2
hours after leukoregulin target cell exposure. Flow cytometric examination
of a variety of molecular probes affecting membrane permeability, ionic
channels and fluxes revealed that leukoregulin dramatically alters membrane
ion fluxes. Membrane probes affecting calcium ion flux but not sodium or
potassium flux enhanced leukoregulin's action and the calcium ionophore
A23187 had permeability altering kinetics similar to leukoregulin. Thus,
leukoregulin can rapidly alter membrane permeability and calcium ions may
be an important mediator in leukoregulin's anticancer activity.

METHODS

Leukoregulin Production

Leukoregulin was isolated from phytohemagglutinin stimulated human peripheral blood mononuclear leukocytes (Evans, 1984). Lymphokine was concentrated 50 fold by diafiltration versus phosphate buffered saline-0.1% polyethelene glycol (PEG) (Ransom et al., 1982) and fractionated by isoelectric focusing (Ransom and Evans, 1983) in a pH 4-6 gradient. Leukoregulin from the pI 4.5-6.0 lymphokines was then isolated on a Toyasoda G3000 SWG HPLC column. The samples were isocratically eluted with 0.02 M sodium phosphate-0.01% PEG, pH 7.4. Using this procedure greater than 50% of the original activity was recovered possessing a pI of 5.0 and MWavg of 50,000.

Measurement of Membrane Permeability Changes

K562 cells (Ransom and Evans, 1982) were treated with leukoregulin for two hours and then with 6.25μg fluoroscein diacetate/10^6 cells/ml RPMI 1640 medium for 5 minutes. Using this method one unit of leukoregulin produces a 50% decrease in 488nm light scatter and fluorescence resulting from retained intracellular fluorescein measured in a FACS flow cytometer cell sorter.

K562 cells were also treated with a variety of membrane active chemicals prior to the addition of leukoregulin (Table 1). The FDA fluorochromasia of these cells were compared with cells treated with leukoregulin.

Table 1. Membrane probes and their mode of action.

Probe	Mode of action	Reference
Calcium ionophore (A23187)	Increases permeability to Ca^{++}	Reed and Lardy, 1972.
Oubain	Inhibits Na^+/K^+ pump, enhances intracellular mobilisation of Ca^{++}	Lamb and MacKinnon, 1971.
Amphotericin B	Increases permeability to various ions, increases Na^+ transport	Yorio and Benoit, 1983.
Calmodulin	Binds Ca^{++}	Cheung, 1970.
Nifedipine } Verapamil }	Ca^{++} channel blockers	Naylor and Poole-Wilson, 1981.
Amiloride	Inhibits Na^+ transport	Sariban-Sohraby et al., 1984.
Diphenylhydantoin	Increases Na^+ transport and stimulates Na^+/K^+ pump	Lewin and Black, 1971.
Sodium ionophore (Monensin)	Increases permeability to Na^+	Haney and Hoehn, 1967.
Potassium ionophore (Valinomycin)	Increases permeability to K^+	Van Heeswick et al., 1984.

RESULTS

Comparison of Membrane Probes with Leukoregulin

Leukoregulin at 0.25-30.0 units/ml alone, induced a 10-90% increase in membrane permeability of K562 cells. The membrane probes at 10^{-5}-10^{-9} M, except for calcium ionophore, by themselves did not alter K562 membrane permeability.

Calcium ionophore, oubain and amphotericin B, however, enhanced leukoregulin's activity whilst only calmodulin produced a small inhibitory effect on membrane permeability. The Ca^{++} channel blockers and membrane probes that affected the flux of Na^+ or K^+ had no effect on leukoregulin's mode of action. Thus, increasing the permeability of K562 cells to Ca^{++}, and/or mobilizing intracellular calcium stores may affect leukoregulin activity. Calcium ionophore alone also induced permeability changes in K562 cells, and there was no change in this effect when the Ca^{++} channel blockers were present. When leukoregulin and the calcium ionophore were incubated together with the K562 cells, the observed permeability changes induced were from 16-91% greater than expected, indicating a synergistic mode of action. Therefore, the ionophore and leukoregulin may alter membrane permeability via a similar mechanism. Calmodulin is known to bind Ca^{++}, so its inhibitory effect on leukoregulin may be solely due to the removal of Ca^{++} at the cell surface, thus decreasing Ca^{++} available for transmembrane and intracellular transport.

Kinetics of Leukoregulin and Calcium Ionophore Action

The kinetics of leukoregulin and the calcium ionophore on the permeability changes of the K562 cells were closely comparable. Permeability changes induced by each were detectable as early as 2-5 minutes after incubation with K562 cells. The only difference was that after 2 hours the leukoregulin effect plateaued whilst the ionophore evoked further changes in membrane permeability.

CONCLUSION

Membrane probes that affected calcium ion flux but not sodium or potassium ion flux also affected the mode of action of leukoregulin, a lymphokine which exhibits several anticancer actions. The calcium ionophore A23187 had kinetics similar to leukoregulin in terms of inducing permeability changes in K562 cells. In addition the effects of the ionophore were synergistic with leukoregulin when both were incubated with the K562 cells. Thus the antitumour and anticarcinogenic action of leukoregulin may be mediated via an alteration in Ca^{++} flux resulting in an increase in intracellular calcium.

REFERENCES

Cheung, W.Y., 1970, Biochemical and Biophysical Communications, 38, 533-538.
Cleveland L. et al., 1984, Federation Proceedings, 43, 1981.
Evans C.H. and DiPaolo J.A., 1981, International Journal of Cancer, 127, 45-49.

Evans C.H., 1983, Journal of National Cancer Institute, 71, 253-257.
Evans C.H., 1984, Journal of Immunological Methods, 67, 13-20.
Haney M.E. and Hoehn M.M., 1967, Antimicrobal Agents in Chemotherapy, 349.
Lamb J.F. and MacKinnon M.G.A., 1971, Physiology, 213, 665-657.
Lewin E. and Black V., 1971, Neurology, 21, 647-657.
Naylor W.G. and Poole-Wilson P.H., 1981, Basic Research in Cardiology, 26, 1-15.
Ransom J.H. and Evans C.H., 1982, International Journal of Cancer, 29, 451-458.
Ransom J.H. et al., 1982, Cellular Immunology, 67, 1-13.
Ransom J.H. and Evans C.H., 1983, Cancer Research, 32, 5222-5227.
Reed P.N. and Lardy H.A., 1972, Journal of Biological Chemistry, 247, 6970-6977.
Sariban-Sohraby S. et al., 1984, Nature, 308, 80-82.
Van Heeswick M.P.E. et al., 1984, Journal of Membrane Biology, 79, 19-31.

THE EFFECTS OF THE PYRIMIDO-PYRIMIDINE DERIVATIVE RX-RA85 ON TUMOUR CELL GROWTH IN VITRO AND IN VIVO

Rosemarie B. LICHTNER, Gillian HUTCHINSON and Kurt HELLMANN

Cancer Chemotherapy Department, Imperial Cancer Research Fund,

PO Box 123, London, WC2A 3PX, UK

Keyword: RX-RA85, B16, 3LL, YML lymphoma

INTRODUCTION

Metastasis is a complex phenomenon involving detachment of cells from the primary tumour, invasion into blood vessels transport in the circulation, arrest in the microvasculature and finally extravasation into normal tissue followed by growth into a secondary tumour. During their transport in the circulation, tumour cells are believed to be capable of interacting with host platelets, lymphocytes and vascular endothelium. Blood platelet-tumour cell interaction has been considered important in the lodgement step. Platelet aggregation is controlled by the internal calcium concentration which is controlled by cAMP dependent kinases. The PDE inhibitor dipyridamole and its derivative RA233 have been shown to inhibit platelet aggregation in vitro and tumour cell induced platelet aggregation in vivo (Gastpar, 1972). They are able to reduce tumour cell adhesion to the vessel wall (Gastpar, 1972) and to increase circulation time of i.v.-injected tumour cells (Ambrus et al., 1978). Investigations into the effect of RA233 on experimental and spontaneous metastasis in animal tumours however gave conflicting results which may be due to the short half-life of RA233 in vivo. We therefore tested the effects of the much more potent (x 10^4 - measured on platelet PDE) and longer lasting dipyridamole derivative RX-RA85 on tumour cell growth in vitro and in vivo.

METHODS

The effect of treatment of Lewis lung (3LL) and B16 cells with RX-RA85 on colony formation in vitro was tested as described elsewhere (Li and Hellmann, 1983). For tumour cell transplantation non-necrotic tumour tissue was chopped finely and 0.1 ml tumour mash injected s.c. L1210 and S180

Tumour (inoculation site)	Treatment schedule	Primary tumour growth	Lung metastases number	Extrapulmonary tumour growth	Median survival time
S180 mouse ascites (i.p.)	Control	–	–	–	–
	RX-RA 85[a]	reduced	–	–	–
	RX-RA 85[b]	slightly increased	–	–	–
L1210 mouse leukemia (s.c.)	Control	–	–	–	–
	RX-RA 85[a]	–	–	–	unchanged
	RX-RA 85[b]	–	–	–	unchanged
Y ML hamster lymphoma (s.c.)	Control	–	–	–	–
	RX-RA 85[b]	unchanged	unchanged	unchanged	unchanged
Lewis lung carcinoma (s.c.)	Control	–	–	–	–
	RX-RA 85[a]	unchanged	increased	–	–
B16 melanoma (s.c.) removal of primary	Control	–	–	–	–
	RX-RA 85[b]	unchanged	–	unchanged	unchanged

Table 1. Growth of some animal tumours in primary and metastatic sites after treatment of animals with 8 mg/kg RX-RA25 i.p. daily (a) or 100 mg/l RX-RA85 in the drinking water (~ 20 mg/kg/day) (b).

ascites were injected as single cell suspensions. B16 cells were harvested
from tissue culture plates by detaching them with 2mM EDTA and injected after
3 washings i.v. into mice. RX-RA85 was solubilized with minimum amounts of
hydrochloric acid and diluted with distilled water.

RESULTS

   RX-RA85 has an inhibitory effect on tumour cell growth in vitro. If
B16 or 3LL cells are exposed to RX-RA85 either for 24 hr or continuously the
EC_{50} is between 1-3 μg/ml (data not shown). Daily i.p. injection of 8 mg/kg
RX-RA85 into mice bearing S180 ascites inhibited tumour growth (Table 1).
Administering RX-RA85 continuously in the drinking water (~20 mg/kg/day)
failed to inhibit growth of S180 ascites, L1210 mouse leukemia or growth and
metastasis of YML hamster lymphoma and B16 melanoma (Table 1). Administering
8 mg/kg daily i.p. to 3LL bearing mice resulted in an increase of lung
metastases with no apparent effect on primary tumour growth (Table 1). Injecting B16 cells i.v. into mice treated 1-2 hrs before with 20 mg/kg RX-RA85
i.v. resulted in decrease of lung colony number with an increase of extrapulmonary tumours (Table 2). On the other hand, oral administration of 20
mg/kg RX-RA85 1 hr before i.v.-injection of B16 cells had no effect on lung
or extrapulmonary tumour colony numbers (Table 2).

Time between administration of RX-RA85 and i.v.-injection of B16 cells (hrs.)	Lung nodule number	Extrapulmonary tumour growth
Control	-	-
1[a]	decreased	increased
2[a]	decreased	slightly increased
Control	-	-
1.5[a]	decreased	increased
Control	-	-
1[b]	unchanged	unchanged

Table 2. Tumour growth in C57BL/mice given i.v.-injection of 2 x
10^5 B16 cells. Mice were treated i.v. with 20 mg/kg RX-RA85 (a) or
orally with 20 mg/kg RX-RA85 (b) at the indicated times prior to
tumour cell injection.

CONCLUSION

   This study shows that RX-RA85 inhibits tumour cell growth in vitro
and ascites tumour growth in vivo if the drug is given i.p. Oral administration of RX-RA85 in dosages where platelet functions are inhibited are

unable to decrease spontaneous or experimental metastasis formation in the
animal tumours tested.   On the contrary spontaneous metastasis of 3LL
bearing mice is increased.   It could be that oral administration of RX-RA85
results in blood levels sufficient to inhibit platelet function, but not
tumour cell growth.   On the other hand it might be that a direct effect
of i.v. administered RX-RA85 on i.v. injected B16 tumour cells could be responsible for the decreased lung colony formation in experimental metastasis
with concomitant increase in extrapulmonary tumours.

Our results confirm the findings by others that antiplatelet and antimetastatic actions of drugs are not necessarily linked (Atherton et al.,
1975; Hilgard et al., 1976; Mussoni et al., 1978).   Furthermore platelet
aggregating ability and metastatic potential do not appear to be connected
at least for some tumour lines (Estrada and Nicolson, 1984).

REFERENCES

Ambrus, J.L., Ambrus, C.M., and Gastpar, H., 1978, Journal of Medicine,
    9, 183-186.
Atherton, A., Busfield, D., and Hellmann, K., 1975, Cancer Research, 35,
    953-957.
Estrada, J., and Nicolson, G.L., 1984, International Journal of Cancer, 34,
    101-105.
Gastpar, H., 1972, Acta Medica Scandinavica Supplementum 525, 269-271.
Hilgard, P., Heller, H., and Schmidt, C.G., 1976, Zeitschrift fuer Krebs-
    forschung und Klinische Onkologie, 86, 243-250.
Li, X.-T., and Hellmann, K., 1983, Clinical and Experimental Metastasis,
    1, 181-190.
Mussoni, L., Poggi, A., De Gaetano, G., and Donati, M.B., 1978, British
    Journal of Cancer, 37, 126-129.

INTERACTIONS OF INDOMETHACIN AND NATURAL CYTOTOXIC EFFECTOR CELLS IN THE
INHIBITION OF METASTASIS

A.M. FULTON AND G.H. HEPPNER
Michigan Cancer Foundation, 110 E. Warren, Detroit, MI, U.S.A.

Keyword: Prostaglandins, Indomethacin, Metastasis

INTRODUCTION

   Prostaglandins are a group of related lipids synthesized from
arachidonic acid via the cyclooxygenase enzyme pathway. They are normal
products of most or all mammalian cells and have numerous biologic
functions. They have been implicated as regulators of cell replication,
differentiation and host tumor interactions. Some prostaglandins are
produced in abnormally high amounts by tumor cells and that excess
prostaglandin production may be advantageous to the tumor cell. Plescia
et al. (1975) and Strausser and Humes (1975) first showed that the
prostaglandin inhibitors indomethacin and aspirin could inhibit the growth
of murine fibrosarcomas. It was first proposed by Plescia that
tumor-associated prostaglandins could be immunosuppressive and thus,
perhaps, allow tumor cells to avoid immune destruction.

   The metastatic process is a complex phenomenon that requires the
successful completion of many steps e.g., intravasation, transport, and
entry into new parenchyma. Each of these steps depends upon different
cellular functions and it can be expected that the most successful (most
metastatic) tumor cells have acquired phenotypes which allow them to do
these things better than other cells. Excess prostaglandin synthesis
might increase a tumor cell's ability to metastasize at a number of
possible steps. Tumor-associated thromboxane might induce platelet-tumor
emboli which may aid in the vascular dissemination and trapping of
metastatic cells (Honn, 1983). The ability of the E prostaglandins to
suppress many immune functions including Natural Killer (NK) activity,
might provide a selective survival advantage for tumor cells. NK cells
appear to be important in controlling metastatic dissemination (Hanna &

Fidler, 1980) and their function is inhibited by PGE (Droller, et al., 1978).

Bennett et al. (1977) first reported that human breast tumors that had metastasized to the bone had higher levels of PGE-like material than non-bone seeking tumors. Our system of mouse mammary adenocarcinomas, which possess a wide range of biologic phenotypes, including a varying ability to metastasize, provides an excellent model with which to examine the biologic role of tumor-associated prostaglandins in tumor growth and metastasis.

RESULTS

To first study the biologic role of prostaglandins in primary tumor growth we determined the effect of indomethacin on the growth of subcutaneously transplanted tumors in vivo and in vitro. These results can be summarized as follows: (1) Oral indomethacin or piroxicam leads to the complete regression of the poorly metastatic, highly immunogenic, low PGE tumor 410, whereas two highly metastatic, high PGE tumors are partially inhibited, with a few complete regressions, and significantly slower growth rates (Fulton, 1984a). (2) Indomethacin inhibits the synthesis of PGE in vitro and is not cytotoxic to tumor cells. In fact, indomethacin stimulates tumor cell replication in vitro (Fulton, 1984b). (3) In situ levels of PGE in a series of murine mammary lesions ranging from preneoplastic hyperplastic alveolar nodules to highly metastatic primary tumors are positively correlated with metastatic ability (Fulton, 1981). (4) In situ PGE levels are products of tumor cells and tumor-associated macrophages (TAM). TAM from different tumors are heterogeneous in their levels of PGE (Mahoney et al., 1983).

To determine if prostaglandins affect the metastatic behavior of mammary tumors, tumors were transplanted subcutaneously and mice received oral indomethacin or vehicle control. To prevent death from the primary tumor before lung metastases were visible, tumors were removed, on an individual basis, when they had reached a predetermined size and mice were sacrificed, necropsied and examined for metastases three weeks later. Using the highly metastatic, high PGE, highly immunogenic tumor 410.4, tumors in control mice achieved an average diameter of 15 mm 45 days post-transplantation whereas tumors in indomethacin-treated mice reached the same size at 53 days, on average. Upon autopsy, all mice in both groups had at least one visible lung metastasis but the mean number of lung metastases in drug treated mice was significantly reduced, 32.8 compared to 53.9.   Subcutaneous growth of the poorly immunogenic, high PGE tumor 66, which is metastatic in most mice but produces few lung colonies per mouse, was not inhibited.   Indomethacin-treated mice, however, had an average of 1.4 lung metastases versus 3.5 and 4.1 for untreated and vehicle-treated controls, respectively.

   In an initial attempt to determine if the inhibitory effects of indomethacin are related to NK cell function, we tested our tumor lines for susceptibility to killing by natural killer-natural cytotoxic cells. In 18 hour assays with poly I:C activated spleen effector cells and ^{3}H-proline labelled target cells, we found that the two nonmetastatic lines 410 and 168 were susceptible to killing with cytotoxicities of 25% and 32% at an effector to target ratio of 200:1.   The metastatic lines 410.4 and 66 were more resistant to killing with cytotoxicities of 5% and 4%.   If target cells were preincubated for 24 h in the presence of indomethacin (1 uM) the susceptibility of all targets was increased.   The lipoxygenase inhibitor nordihydroguaiaretic acid (NDGA) had no effect on cytotoxicity except at the very highest concentrations in which case it was also directly toxic to target cells.

CONCLUSIONS

   We have shown that levels of PGE in situ are positively correlated with the metastatic potential of a number of murine mammary adenocarcinomas. The subcutaneous growth of these transplantable tumors is markedly inhibited by the oral administration of the cyclooxygenase inhibitors indomethacin and piroxicam.   Oral indomethacin, at non-toxic doses, consistently reduces the number of spontaneous metastases of two highly metastatic tumors.

   We have initiated studies to determine the mechanisms of this indomethacin-mediated effect.   We are studying the possible interactions of NK cells and immunosuppressive prostaglandins.   We find that two metastatic tumor lines are more resistant to killing by natural cytotoxic cells than are two low metastatic lines.   When any of these targets are precultured in the presence of indomethacin, their susceptibility to killing increases.   The presence of the lipoxygenase inhibitor, NDGA, at noncytotoxic concentrations, has no effect on tumor target susceptibility.

Although these effects of indomethacin are consistent and reproducible, they are only seen at the highest doses of indomethacin and, even at this concentration, tumor cell susceptibility never approaches 100% killing. Therefore, further experimentation is necessary to determine if the tumor-inhibitory effects of indomethacin seen *in vivo* are mediated, at least in part, through enhancement of natural cytotoxic defense mechanisms.

REFERENCES

Bennett, A., Charlier, E., McDonald, A., Simpson, J. & Stamford, I., 1977, Lancet, ii, 624.

Droller, M., Schneider, M., & Perlmann, P., 1978, Cellular Immunology, 39, 165.

Fulton, A., 1981, Proceedings of the American Association for Cancer Research, 22, 61.

Fulton, A., 1984a, Cancer Research, 44, 2416.

Fulton, A., 1984b, International Journal of Cancer, 33, 375.

Hanna, N., & Fidler, I., 1980, Journal National Cancer Institute (USA), 65, 801.

Honn, K., 1983, Clinical and Experimental Metastasis, 1, 103.

Mahoney, K., Fulton, A., & Heppner, G., 1983, Journal of Immunology, 131, 2079.

Plescia, O., Smith, A., & Grinwich, K., 1975, Proceedings of the National Academy of Science (USA), 72, 1848.

Strausser, H., & Humes, J., 1975, International Journal of Cancer, 15, 724.

ORGAN-SPECIFIC EFFECTS ON METASTATIC TUMOUR GROWTH:

STUDIES INVOLVING TRANSPLANTATION TECHNIQUES

E. HORAK, D.L. DARLING and D. TARIN

Nuffield Department of Pathology, (University of Oxford), John Radcliffe

Hospital, Oxford OX3 9DU

Keywords: Metastasis - Organ distribution - In vitro invasion -

         Microenvironment

INTRODUCTION

Earlier investigations in this laboratory have shown that approximately 30% of autochthonous mammary tumours in C3H/A^{vy} mice metastasise spontaneously (Price et al. 1982), and that the secondary deposits occur almost exclusively in the lungs. Also, when disaggregated cells from these mammary tumours are inoculated intravenously, a similar pattern of preferential pulmonary colonisation is noted (Tarin & Price 1979). Studies with labelled tumour cells (Juacaba et al. 1983) demonstrated that they reached all organs within 15 minutes of intravascular inoculation and that the dose of cells arriving in each site is not directly related to the development of colonies. These observations suggest that the microenvironment in the sites of lodgement influences metastasis formation.

Further studies (Horak et al. 1984) indicated that normal organs contain diffusible factors which can encourage or suppress the survival and adhesion of tumour cells in vitro and the findings agreed with the organ distribution of mammary tumour deposits observed in vivo. The present study was therefore undertaken to test whether a direct link can be demonstrated between these in vitro and in vivo phenomena. The method used was the implantation of organ fragments which had already been shown, by co-culture with mammary tumour cells, to have effects on tumour cells in vitro. The results support the interpretation that the organ-specific effects observed in vitro influence the growth and survival of disseminated tumour cells in vivo.

MATERIALS AND METHODS

Naturally-occurring mammary carcinomas of C3H/A^{vy} mice were used for all experiments. This report describes the findings with the first 25 tumours studied. Normal lungs and livers were obtained from tumour-free animals of the same strain, chopped into 1 mm^3 cubes with scalpel blades, and placed in culture (20 fragments per flask) in a little fresh medium. The cultures were then seeded with 2 x 10^6 living tumour cells, suspended in 2 ml Eagle's minimal essential medium, containing 10% foetal calf serum, l-glutamine and antibiotics. The normal tissue fragments and tumour cells were then co-incubated for 96 hours at 37°C and 5% CO_2, at the end of which time the organ fragments were collected with a pipette and washed in fresh medium. Groups of 6 fragments were implanted into each of 3 syngeneic animals, subcutaneously into the flank. Implant-bearing animals were killed and autopsied after 3 months, or sooner if they developed tumours larger than 2 cm in diameter, or became ill. At autopsy the sites of implantation and all internal organs were examined and, if macroscopic tumours or metastases were found, histological examination was performed to confirm mammary origin.

The types of results observed and the terms used for categorising the primary tumours studied according to their behaviour in these experiments are explained in Diagram 1 below.

DEFINITION OF TERMS USED

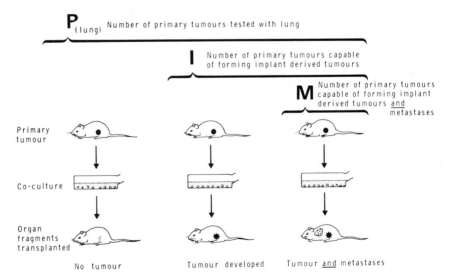

RESULTS

The re-implantation of organ fragments after co-culture with tumour cells showed that the cells which attach to them or invade them can sometimes form tumours, and even metastasise spontaneously in the new host. Table 1 shows that such implant-derived tumours (IDTs) formed much more frequently from re-implanted lung fragments than from those of liver which is known to be a rare site for spontaneous or induced metastases of natural murine tumours (Price et al. 1982; Juacaba et al. 1983).

Spontaneous metastases from IDTs originated only from lung-implants and were found only in the lungs of the hosts. However, primary tumours capable of forming IDTs were more frequently metastatic in their new hosts (54%) than the overall (unselected) population of primary tumours in their original hosts (31%) [Table 2].

Table 1. Frequency of tumour formation (I/P)
from implanted organ fragments.

Invaded organ	Lung	Liver
I/P	13/25 (52%)	2/13 (15%)

Table 2. Frequency of metastases.

	From I$_{(lung)}$	From I$_{(liver)}$
M/I	7/13 (54%)	1/2
Spontaneous metastasis in undisturbed animals	8/25 (32%)	

CONCLUSIONS

Some IDTs form metastases spontaneously. The higher incidence of metastases among primary tumours that can form IDT than in the original tumour population indicates that the organs "select" a population with higher metastatic/invasive capability.

We provisionally consider that this process of cell selection is influenced both by the organs and by the intrinsic properties of the tumour cells. Thus, with lung, which is a "favoured" site of metastases, 52% of the primary tumours were capable of forming IDTs (which is evidence of intrinsic growth potential; whilst only 15% of the same primary tumours did

so with the liver fragments, which provides evidence of a host-organ
mediated effect.

   These findings provide a direct link between the preferential organ
distribution of murine mammary tumour metastases observed in vivo, and the
organ-specific effects on mammary tumour cell survival and attachment
in vitro described elsewhere (Horak et al. 1984). They therefore support
the interpretation that normal host organs could by mechanisms similar to
those observed in vitro, modulate the survival and growth of metastasis-
competent tumour cells arresting within them.

REFERENCES

Horak, E., Darling, D.L. & Tarin, D., 1984 (this volume).
Juacaba, S.F., Jones, L.D. & Tarin, D., 1983, Invasion Metastasis, 3, 208.
Price, J.E., Carr, D., Jones, L.D., Messer, P. & Tarin, D., 1982, Invasion
    Metastasis, 2, 77.
Tarin, D. & Price, J.E., 1979, British Journal of Cancer, 39, 740.

KARYOTYPIC DIVERSITY BETWEEN NON METASTATIC AND METASTATIC HAMSTER TUMOURS
OF CLONAL ORIGIN

DAVID M. TEALE, ROBERT C. REES, JOHN LAWRY AND CHRISTOPHER W. POTTER
Department of Virology, University of Sheffield, Sheffield S10 2RX

Keywords: ploidy, heterogeneity, metastasis

INTRODUCTION

Cells isolated from metastatic foci have been shown to differ from
their original primary tumour with respect to NK susceptibility (Brooks
et al, 1981); immunogenicity (Schirrmacher, 1979); cell biochemistry
(Chatterjee and Kim, 1978); surface antigens (Fogel et al, 1979) and
karyotype (Rabotti, 1959). The source of this cellular diversity is believed to be a consequence of genetic variability within the primary
neoplasm (Nowell, 1976) and indeed non-random genetic changes have been
associated with several human and experimental tumours (Rowley, 1981).

The formation of metastatic deposits is therefore believed to be a
non-random event relying on the intrinsic properties of the cell types
resident within, and dissociating from, the primary tumour.

Metastatic deposits from a HSV-2 induced hamster fibrosarcoma have
previously been shown to differ in several properties (Walker et al, 1982)
including NK susceptibility (Teale et al, 1983) and immunogenicity
(Teale et al, 1984). In the present communication the ploidy of the
parent (HSV-2-333-2-26) tumour and its in vitro and in vivo derived clones
is described together with their metastatic profile. The evidence provided
suggests that the primary neoplasm is genetically homogeneous and that
cellular diversity may arise post-dissemination.

METHODS

Tumours

The HSV-2-333-2-26 cell line (parent) was originally obtained by
in vitro transformation of hamster embryo fibroblasts with inactivated
HSV-2: this cell line was kindly provided by Dr. F. Rapp, Department of

Microbiology, Pennsylvania State University, Hershey, PA,USA. The
in vivo derived clones, met A - G, were derived from lung foci in hamsters
whose primary parent load had previously been resected. Following in vivo
passage, in vitro cultures were established.

The in vitro derived clones were derived by two methods: clones 1-6
were derived by soft agar cloning, whilst S4A, S7A & S7B, S8B and S9D &
S9E were obtained by limiting dilutions isolation.

Metastatic Potential of the Tumour Lines

Tumour cells (10^4 cells in 0.1 ml) from in vitro cultures were
injected s.c. into groups of hamsters, and tumours resected approximately
three weeks later (10-15 mm, mean tumour diameter). Animals showing
symptoms of respiratory distress were sacrificed and examined for metastatic disease. Experiments were terminated 12 weeks post-resection and a post-
mortem examination performed.

Cell Cycle Analysis

Tumour cells (10^6 cells in 0.1 ml) from in vitro cultures were
incubated with 50 µl triton X-100 for 1 min. at room temperature. To this
0.4 ml of mithromycin and ethidium bromide (1:1 ratio) was added,
incubated at room temperature for 5 min. and read at 475 nm Laser using
a Fluorescent Activated Cell Sorter (F.A.C.S.).

RESULTS

The genetic content of all hamster cell lines was assessed as
previously described, using a fluorescent DNA stain and analysis on a
F.A.C.S. The results, shown in Table 1, indicate normal diploid hamster
kidney cells and PBLs to have a G1 peak at channel number 45 and a G2
peak at channel number 90. In contrast, the parent(HSV-2-333-2-26) cell
line was shown to have a G1 peak at channel 70 and a G2 peak at channel
number 140, indicating the cell line to be tetraploid. The ploidy of the
16 cloned hamster cell lines was assessed in a similar manner, and as
shown in Table 1, varied between diploid and polyploid populations.

The results of tumour resection expts (Table 1) indicate a correlation between ploidy and metastatic potential. Thus, highly metastatic
cell lines were consistently diploid whilst weakly or non-metastatic cell
lines were of a higher ploidy. Investigating the HSV-2-333-2-26 cell
line further, and using the scroll on the F.A.C.S., it was found that no
diploid cells were present within the parent population (see Fig.1a).

Table 1.   Metastatic potential and ploidy of the parent (HSV-2-333-2-26) cell line and its in vivo and in vitro cloned sublines.

Clone	FACS Channel No. G1	G2	Metastatic potential.	Clone	FACS Channel No. G1	G2	Metastatic potential.
Met A	54	117	++++	Parent	76	138	+
Met B	47	100	++++	Met C	63	115	++
Met E	50	92	++++	Met D	72	132	+
Met F	48	90	++++	Met G	114	200	+
Cl.1	52	104	++++	S8B	78	122	-
Cl.3	48	98	++++	S9D	90	178	-
Cl.6	48	96	++++	S9E	82	160	-
S4A	45	92	++++	PBLs	45	92	
S7A	49	102	++++	Kidney cells	46	90	
S7B	46	82	++++				

Metastatic potential assessed as highly metastatic (++++), metastatic (+++), weakly metastatic (++), sometimes metastatic (+) and non-metastatic (-).

In a further experiment, diploid (Met B) tumour cells were cultured with parent tumour cells at varying concentrations (10%, 1.0%, 0.1% and 0.01%). As few as 0.01% Met B tumour cells were detectable by the described method (results not given) and as shown in Figs 2c and d this population increases in number on subsequent culture.

Figure 1.   Cell cycle analysis of (a) a pure parent population. (b) parent population plus 0.01% Met B, day 0 in culture. (c) parent population plus 0.01% Met B, day 23 in culture. (d) parent population plus 0.01% Met B, day 30 in culture.

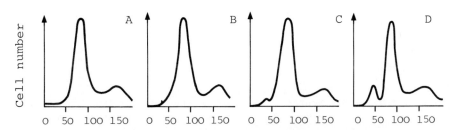

Fluorescence Intensity (Channel No.)

CONCLUSION
     Rabotti (1959) described the ploidy of 4 human breast adeno-carcinomas and showed the cells from the primary tumour to be mainly diploid whilst those from the axillary lymph node and kidney metastases were of a higher ploidy. The present communication extends this work to an HSV-2 induced hamster fibrosarcoma and its in vivo isolated cells and in vitro derived clones, verifying the finding that primary and metastatic cells can vary in their DNA content.
     The HSV-2-333-2-26 parent tumour appears to be polyploid and weakly or non-metastatic. Diploid cells, however, were isolated from in vivo lung foci and in vitro derived clones, which were highly metastatic

in tumour resection experiments. In contrast, polyploid cells were also
isolated which were non- or weakly metastatic and may have arisen in vivo
by random metastasis. The phenotypic characteristics were stable on
in vivo and in vitro passage.

The heterogeneity of the cell population resident within the primary
tumour is now recognised (Fidler and Hart, 1981; Di Renzo et al, 1983)
and Nowell (1979) has hypothesized that acquired genetic variability is
responsible for this diversification. In the present study however,
highly adapted metastatic diploid clones were isolated from the parent
tumour where no diploid cells were detectable. In addition, small
numbers of diploid cells, when added to the parent population were
shown to increase in number upon culture, indicating that if
'specialised' diploid cells were present then they would possess the
ability to grow into a detectable population.

The HSV-2-333-2-26 parent tumour therefore appears to be genetically
homogeneous in this regard, suggesting that genetic variability is
acquired post-dissemination.

REFERENCES.

Brooks, C. G., 1981, International Journal of Cancer, 28, 191.
Chatterjee, S.K. & Kim, V. 1978, Journal of the National Cancer Institute,
     61, 151.
Di Renzo, H.F. & Bretti, S. 1983. International Journal of Cancer, 30, 751.
Fidler, I.J. & Hart, I.R. 1981, European Journal of Cancer and Clinical
     Oncology, 17, 487.
Fogel, M., Gorelick, E., Segal, S. 1979. Journal of the National Cancer
     Institute, 62, 585.
Nowell, P.C., 1979, Science, 23.
Rabotti, G. 1959, Nature (London), 183, 1276.
Rowley, J.D., 1981, Nonrandom chromosome changes in human leukaemia.
     In: Genes, chromosomes and neoplasia; F. E. Arrighi, Potu,U, Roa, and
     Elton Stubblefield (Eds). (Raven Press) New York, p273.
Schirrmacher, V., Bosslet, K., Shantz, G., Glaver, K., Hubsch, D., 1979,
     International Journal of Cancer, 23, 45.
Teale, D.M., Rees, R.C., Clark,A., Potter, C.W. 1983,
     Cancer Letters, 19, 221.
Teale, D.M., Rees, R.C., Clark, A., Potter, C.W. 1984,
     International Journal of Cancer, 33, 701.
Walker, J.R., Rees, R.C., Teale, D.M., Potter, C.W., 1982,
     European Journal of Cancer and Clinical Oncology, 18, 1017.

ACKNOWLEDGMENTS.
     The authors wish to thank Mrs. C. Mullan for preparation of this
manuscript.

EXPRESSION OF AN EXTRA GLYCOPROTEIN IN POLYMORPHONUCLEAR CELLS ISOLATED FROM CANCER BEARERS

W.-S. CHAN, A.J.E. GREEN, C.M. PAGE and G.A. TURNER
Department of Clinical Biochemistry and Metabolic Medicine, Medical
School, University of Newcastle upon Tyne. NE2 4HH

Key words: Polymorphonuclear cells : Proteins : Lectins

INTRODUCTION

The primary function of polymorphonuclear cells (PMN) is to engulf and
kill invading micro-organisms. It is well known, however, that PMN can
infiltrate many types of animal and human tumours and exhibit changes in
properties related to the presence of malignancy, such as; cytotoxicity
against the tumour cells (Katano & Torisu, 1982); suppression of tumour
metastasis (Glaves, 1983); decreased resistance to invading micro-organisms
(Gandossini et al., 1981), and a reduction in migration and chemotaxis
(Corberand et al., 1982; Ward & Berenberg, 1974). Furthermore, we have
demonstrated marked PMN infiltration into a subcutaneous (s.c.) hamster
lymphosarcoma and its liver metastasis, which was not seen in a non-
metastatic lymphosarcoma (unpublished observation). These findings suggest
that changes in biochemical properties of PMN may occur during direct or
indirect interaction with tumour cells and these may be important in
influencing metastasis. In this study we compare the protein and glycoprotein components of PMN isolated from the normal and short-term inflammatory hosts, and the tumour bearers.

METHODS

Metastatic lymphosarcomas (Chan et al., 1984) were routinely
transplanted in Syrian cream hamsters (WO/CR strain; Wrights of Essex) by
s.c. injection, major metastases being found in the liver.

PMN were prepared from normal peripheral blood by centrifugation at
400g for 15 min. The leucocyte-enriched buffy coat obtained was washed
twice with phosphate buffer saline Ca- and Mg-free (PBS 'A'). This

preparation was further purified by separation on Lymphoprep (Bøyum, 1964) followed by a Percoll continuous density gradients (Chan et al., in press). Purified PMN were then washed with PBS 'A'.

PMN were also prepared from hosts in which a short-term inflammatory response had been generated by i.p. injection of 0.8% Oyster glycogen (Chan et al., 1984) and after 4 hours peritoneal cells were harvested. Purified preparations were obtained by using the Percoll technique.

PMN from the peripheral blood of tumour bearers were also obtained by using the Lymphoprep technique. It was found that PMN from tumour-bearers had a lower density than PMN from normal blood.

The PMN from s.c. tumours and their metastases were prepared as follows: Tumour tissue was disaggregated in collagenase as previously described (Chan et al., 1984). The resultant cell suspension containing ~20% PMN was separated into subpopulations by velocity sedimentation at unit gravity (Wells, 1982) in the CelSep apparatus. The PMN and tumour cell-enriched populations were obtained by pooling cell fractions.

The purity of PMN preparations always exceeded 85%, as determined by differential counts on Giemsa/May Grunwald stained cytocentrifuged preparations.

In other experiments, membranes were isolated from s.c. tumour tissue which had marked PMN infiltration using a two-phase polymer (Polyethylene glycol 6000 and Dextran T500) method (Chan et al., 1984).

Purified PMN from the peripheral blood of tumour bearers were treated with trypsin by incubating with 0.25% enzyme solution in PBS 'A' at 37°C for 30 min with gentle shaking. Cells were washed and pelleted.

Normal cells, tissues and thioglycollate-induced macrophages were prepared as described by Chan et al., (1984, in press).

Cell and tissue proteins were extracted with 0.5% Triton X-100. The extracts were electrophoresed in SDS-slab gels. Separated proteins were stained with Coomassie blue and glycoproteins were labelled using ^{125}I – wheat germ agglutinin (WGA) and ^{125}I-Concanavalin A (Con A), the lectin binding being detected by autoradiography. Details of these methods have been previously described (Chan et al., 1984, in press).

RESULTS

Fig 1 illustrates representative Coomassie blue stained electrophoretic patterns and corresponding Con A autoradiographs of PMN extracts. No consistent differences in either Coomassie blue staining or Con A binding

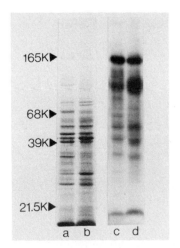 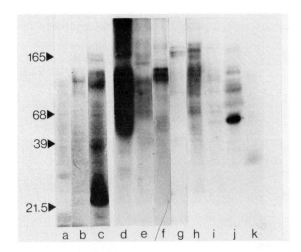

Fig 1.(left) Electrophoretic patterns of PMN extracts prepared from
(a,c) glycogen-induced cells and (b,d) peripheral blood of tumour bearers.
Tracks a and b show Coomassie blue staining and tracks c and d show the
Con A binding patterns.

Fig 2.(right) Autoradiographs of WGA-binding to separated extracts of
(a) normal peripheral blood PMN, (b) glycogen-induced PMN and (c) peripheral blood PMN of tumour bearers, (d) thioglycollate-induced macrophages,
(e) non-activated macrophages, (f) kidney, (g) lung, (h) spleen cells, (i)
liver, (j) serum and (k) erythrocytes.

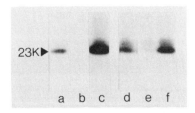 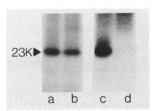

Fig 3.(left)Autoradiographs of WGA-binding pattern of 23Kd region of
s.c. tumour cell suspension (a-c) and liver metastases (d-f) separated by
unit gravity sedimentation; a,d, unfractionated tumour cells; b,e, tumour
cell-enriched fractions; c,f, PMN-enriched fractions.

Fig 4.(right) Autoradiographs of WGA-binding pattern of the 23Kd region
of tumour cell before (a) and after (b) trypsin treatment and of tumour
tissue (c) and membrane (d) isolated from this tissue.

were observed with PMN extracts prepared from normal peripheral blood, glycogen-induced cells, tumour-bearers' peripheral blood , s.c. tumour and liver metastases.

With WGA labelling, all PMN extracts prepared from tumour bearers showed a strong band at 23K dalton that was not seen in the PMN extracts from the non-tumour bearers (Fig 2 a,b,c,; fig 3 c,f). This 23Kd glycoprotein was undetected in extracts of many normal cell types and tissues (Fig 2 d-k).

Fig 3 shows the WGA-binding patterns of extracts from sub-populations of tumour cell suspensions. The 23Kd glycoprotein is not expressed by the tumour cell-enriched fraction but it is strongly expressed in the PMN-enriched fraction.

Fig 4 shows that this protein was not removed by mild trypsin treatment of the cells and it is also absent in membrane preparations, suggesting that it is not a membrane associated component.

DISCUSSION

In these studies we have clearly shown that this 23Kd WGA-binding protein, previously found in a hamster lymphosarcoma and its metastases (Chan et al., 1984), is due to infiltrating PMN. It is not expressed in normal and inflammatory PMN nor in many other types of cells and tissues. As yet we do not know its biochemical function in cancer. It may be involved in a PMN-mediated tumour cytotoxicity mechanism, or may be reflection of the process of PMN infiltration or relate to some other interaction between PMN and tumour cells.

REFERENCES

Bøyum, S., 1964, Nature, 204, 793.
Chan, W.-S., Jackson, A. and Turner, G.A., 1984, British Journal of Cancer 49,181.
Chan, W.-S., Jackson, A. and Turner, G.A., 1984, Invasion and Metastasis (in press).
Corberand, J., Benchekroum, S., Nguyen, F., Laharrague, P. and Pris, J., 1982, Cancer Research, 42, 1595.
Gandossini, M., Souhami, R.L., Babbage, J., Addison, I.E., Johnson, A.L. and Bercubaum, M.C., 1981, British Journal of Cancer, 44, 863.
Glaves, D., 1983, Invasion and Metastasis, 3, 160.
Katano, M., Torisu, M., 1982, Cancer, 50, 62.
Ward, P.A. and Berenberg, J.L., 1974, The New England Journal of Medicine, 290,76.
Wells, J.R., 1982, A new approach to the separation of cells at unit gravity. In Cell Separation Methods and Selected Applications Vol.1, edited by T.G. Pretlow II and T.P. Pretlow, P.169.

THE KIDNEY INVASION TEST (KIT) : MACROSCOPIC QUANTIFICATION OF MALIGNANT
INVASION IN VIVO

W. DISTELMANS, R. VAN GINCKEL, W. VANHERCK and M. DE BRABANDER
Laboratory of Oncology, Division of Cellular Biology and Chemotherapy,
Department of Life Sciences, Janssen Pharmaceutica Research Laboratories,
2340 Beerse, Belgium

Keywords: kidney invasion test, microtubule inhibitors; MO_4 fibrosarcoma

INTRODUCTION

It has been demonstrated in vitro with microtubule inhibitors that a
difference can be made between growth inhibitory and antiinvasive properties of antineoplastic drugs (Mareel & De Brabander, 1978). We have been
able to confirm these findings in vivo by means of an assay which allows
a rapid macroscopic evaluation of compounds with potential antiinvasive
properties.

MATERIAL AND METHODS

Using the "subrenal capsule implantation" technique (Bogden et al.,
1978), 1 mm^3 fragments of MO_4 fibrosarcomas were inserted beneath the
kidney capsule of syngeneic or allogeneic mice (fig. 1). The 2 main diameters of the tumour were evaluated in situ under a microscope and
measured in ocular micrometer units (10 OMU = 1 mm). Tumour size was expressed as the average of the 2 diameters. On day 7, mice were killed and
the tumour size was measured again (fig. 2). Hemisection of the kidney
through the middle of the tumour towards the pelvis showed a semicircular
invasion of the MO_4 fragment into the renal parenchyma (fig. 3). The
degree of invasion was macroscopically assessed by proportioning the
length of the invasive front (I) to the total tumour thickness (T) (fig.
4). One of the hemisections was fixed and prepared for histological
study. The effect of the microtubule inhibitor tubulozole (Van Ginckel
et al., 1984) was compared with etoposide. Both drugs were injected intraperitoneally Q2D, days 1, 3, 5.

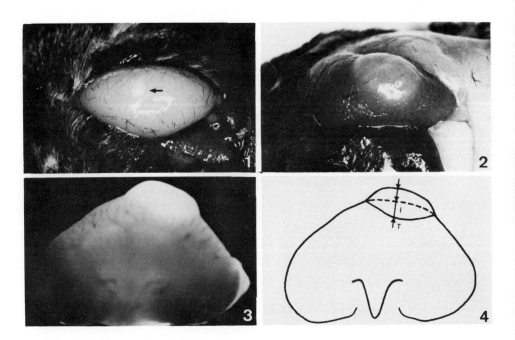

RESULTS (table 1)

Table 1. Evaluation of growth and invasion of MO_4 fragments in male Swiss
Albino mice on day 7 post implantation.
Tubulozole vs. etoposide ip Q2D, days 1, 3, 5. Six animals per
concentration.

agent	dose (mg.kg⁻¹)	TS_i	TS_f	△TS (%)	T	I/T	invasion rate (I/T x 100)	N	D
controls	—	12.5	38.0	204	14.5	11/14.5	76		
		9.0	39.0	333	14.5	11/14.5	76		
		12.0	42.5	254	16.0	12/16	75		
		12.5	38.0	204	15.0	10.5/15	70		
		12.0*		229*	15.0*		75.5*	1	1
tubulozole	80	10.5*		100*	5.5*		50*	3	
	40	14.0		139	8.5		45.5	2	
	20	13.5		150	13		53.5	1	2
etoposide	10	13.0		43	6.5		73		4
	5	12.5		108	6		75		1
	2.5	11.0		185	8		68	2	

TS_i : initial tumour size
TS_f : final tumour size
TS% : tumour growth (%): (TS_f-TS_i/TS_i) x 100
T : total tumour thickness

I : invasion
N : necrotic MO_4 fragment
D : dead animal
* : median

Macroscopic evaluation

Growth inhibition

Both drugs exerted a dose dependent inhibition of tumour growth. (ΔTS% and T).

Invasion

Invasion rate of controls · 75.5 %

Though the 80 mg.kg^{-1} tubulozole and 5 mg.kg^{-1} etoposide schedule produced a similar growth inhibition (ΔTS% and T), only tubulozole protected against infiltration of the renal parenchyma (invasion rate resp. 50 % and 75 %). This tendency was also noticed at other concentrations. The reproducibility of these results was checked in a second matched experiment, which revealed remarkable consistency (data not shown). In both replicates, only tubulozole was found to exert a significant inhibition of invasion, whereas etoposide did not show any affect (2 tailed Mann-Whitney U test).

Histologic examination of invasion

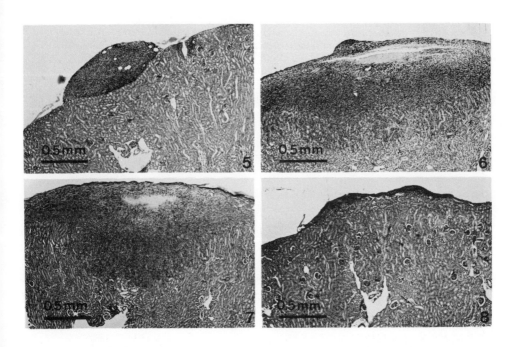

Figure 5 : "DAY 0".
          Clean interface between the MO_4 tumour and the renal parenchyma.
Figure 6 : "DAY 7" CONTROL.
          Remarkable invasion of both strands and solitary "islands" of
          MO_4 cells into the parenchyma. Focal destruction of kidney
          tissue. Median invasion rate : 67 % (3 slides).
Figure 7 : "DAY 7" 5 mg.kg^{-1} ETOPOSIDE.
          Invasive front is undistinguishable from control tumours.
          Median invasion rate : 64 % (7 slides).
Figure 8 : "DAY 7" 80 and 40 mg.kg^{-1} TUBULOZOLE.
          Complete "DAY 0" - like interface (found in 4/14 slides).
          Median invasion rate : 20 % (80 mg.kg^{-1}; 3 slides)
                                 14 % (40 mg.kg^{-1}; 11 slides).

CONCLUSION

    Microtubule inhibitors which are inhibitory for invasion of MO_4 cells
in vitro, maintain this effect in vivo.

    Quantitative discrimination can be made macroscopically between anti-
invasive compounds and invasion permissive drugs.

    This in vivo assay for invasion might be an important tool in the
rapid selection of such compounds.

REFERENCES

Bogden, A.E., Kelton, D.E., Cobb, W.R. and Esber, H.J., 1978, A rapid
    screening method for testing chemotherapeutic agents against human
    tumor xenografts. In Houchens and Overjerd, The use of athymic (nude)
    mice in cancer research, pp. 231-250 (Gustav Fischer, New York).
Mareel, M.M. and De Brabander, M.J., 1978, Effect of microtubule inhibi-
    tors on malignant invasion in vitro. The Journal of the National
    Cancer Institute, 61 : 787.
Van Ginckel, R., De Brabander, M., Vanherck, W. and Heeres, J., 1984, The
    effects of tubulozole, a new synthetic microtubule inhibitor on experi-
    mental neoplasms. European Journal of Cancer and Clinical Oncology,
    20, 99.

MODULATION BY TISSUE ENVIRONMENT OF HUMAN TUMOUR GROWTH AND EXPRESSION OF FIBRINOLYTIC ACTIVITY[1]

J.F. CAJOT[2], J.E. TESTA[3], B. SORDAT[3] and F. BACHMANN[2]
[1]Supported in part by the Swiss Cancer League, grant no. FOR. 252, AK. 83(4) and the Swiss Science Foundation, grant no. 3.406.83
[2]Central Haematology Laboratory, University of Lausanne, Medical School, 1011 Lausanne, Switzerland
[3]The Swiss Institute for Experimental Cancer Research, 1066 Epalinges, Switzerland

Keyword: fibrinolysis, plasminogen activators, invasion

INTRODUCTION

Invasive human primary colon carcinomas transplanted as subcutaneous (SC) xenografts into the nude mouse exhibit an expansive pseudo-benign growth pattern. In contrast, when implanted into the gut (GI) of the animal, a typical invasive growth behaviour is observed (Wang et al. 1984). Since plasminogen activators (PA) have been associated with the invasive properties of tumours, we investigated a possible modulatory effect of the host tissue environment on tumour PA expression.

We report here on the characterization and quantitation of PA activity present in extracts of human primary colon carcinomas as well as SC and GI xenografts into nude mice.

METHODS

Collection of tumours

Primary colon carcinomas were obtained shortly after surgical excision. Suspensions of these and of established colon carcinoma cell lines Co 112 and Co 115 were implanted SC or GI into nude mice as previously described (Wang et al. 1984).

Tissue extraction of PAs

One gramme of tumour tissue was homogenized in 5 ml 0.5 M NaSCN for 20 min at 4 $^{\circ}$C. After centrifugation at 6000g, and 4 $^{\circ}$C, supernatants were stored in aliquots at −70 $^{\circ}$C until use.

Zymographic revelation of extracted PAs

Mr determination and semiquantitative analysis of PAs were performed by sodium dodecyl sulfate polyacrylamide gel electrophoresis (SDS-PAGE) followed by transfer of the polyacrylamide gels onto plasminogen-rich, fibrin-agarose underlays (Granelli-Piperno & Reich 1978).

Quantitation of PA activity

Total PA-mediated fibrinolytic activities (FA) of tumour extracts were assayed using the ^{125}I-fibrin plate assay (Unkeless et al. 1973). Urokinase (u-PA) and tissue-activator (t-PA) related activities were similarly measured and are defined as the observed decrease in FA in the presence of antibodies against human u-PA or human t-PA.

RESULTS

Colon carcinoma xenografts in the SC space showed a locally expansive growth. Invasion was minimal and the tumour cell mass was generally circumscribed by multiple layers of stromal fibrocytic cells (Figure 1a). In contrast, using the gut-implantation route, colon xenografts expressed a marked macro- and microinvasive behaviour. Both Co 112 and Co 115 tumour cell lines (Wang et al. 1984) as well as tumour cells obtained from early-passage SC xenografts of primary carcinomas were capable of infiltrating the various layers of the mouse colonic walls (Figure 1b).

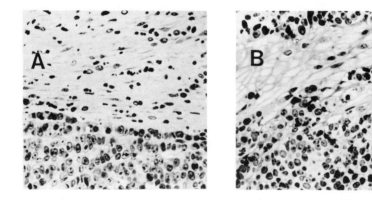

Figure 1.   Photographs showing a SC (a) versus a GI (b) xenograft.

Extracts of four human primary colon carcinomas obtained shortly
after surgical excision and of their respective SC xenografts in nude
mice were assayed for PA activity on ^{125}I-fibrin plates. Primary
tumour extracts yielded approximately equal amounts of u-PA and t-PA
related activities (Figure 2, upper columns). An 8-fold decrease in
total FA was observed in the SC xenograft compared to that of the
primary colon carcinomas (Figure 2, lower columns).

In addition, we have analyzed semiquantitatively by zymographic
revelation PA expression in human colon carcinoma cell lines Co 112
and Co 115 xenografted either SC or GI in nude mice. Co 112 SC
xenograft extracts showed mostly human u-PA activity (54 kilodaltons
(kD)) with traces of murine PA activity (t-PA, 75 kD; u-PA, 48 kD)
(Figure 3, lanes 1-3). Co 112 GI xenografts exhibited significantly
higher human u-PA activity (Figure 3, lanes 4-6). Co 115 SC xenograft
extracts did not exhibit PA activity of human, and only traces of
murine, origin (Figure 3, lanes 7-9). Gut-implanted Co 115 tumours
revealed, besides murine PA activity, human t-PA activity (68 kD)
(Figure 3, lanes 10-12).

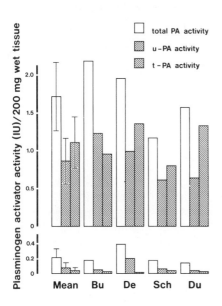
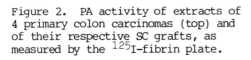
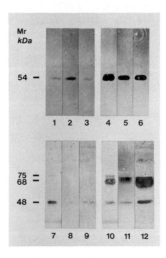

Figure 2. PA activity of extracts of
4 primary colon carcinomas (top) and
of their respective SC grafts, as
measured by the ^{125}I-fibrin plate.

Figure 3. Zymograms of SC and
GI xenograft extracts.
Lanes 1-3:   Co 112 SC grafts.
Lanes 4-6:   Co 112 GI grafts.
Lanes 7-9:   Co 115 SC grafts.
Lanes 10-12:   Co 115 GI grafts.

CONCLUSIONS

Invasive human primary colon carcinomas passaged as SC xenografts
in nude mice exhibit a pseudo-benign growth pattern accompanied by
an 8-fold decrease in PA activity relative to the primary tumour.
Two colon carcinoma cell lines derived from invasive primary tumours
also exhibit non-invasive growth patterns and low human PA expression
when inoculated SC in nude mice. However, when these cell lines are
inoculated into the gut wall, the resulting tumours are highly
invasive and human PA activities are markedly increased. These
results demonstrate a modulatory effect on tumoral PA expression by
host tissue environment, and suggest in this particular experimental
system, that fibrinolysis may play a role in tumour invasion.

REFERENCES

Granelli-Piperno, A. & Reich, E., 1978, Journal of Experimental
    Medecine, 148, 223.
Markus, G., 1984, Seminars in Thrombosis and Hemostasis, 10, 61.
Unkeless, J.C., Tobia, A., Ossowski, L., Quigley, J.P., Rifkin, D.B.
    & Reich, E., 1973, Journal of Experimental Medecine, 137, 85.
Wang, W.R., Sordat, B., Piguet, D. & Sordat, M., 1984, Human colon
    tumors in nude mice: implantation site and expression of the
    invasive phenotype. In Immune-Deficient Animals 4th Int. Workshop,
    edited by B. Sordat (Karger), p.239.

ULTRASTUCTURAL STUDIES OF INVASION IN VITRO

P. AULENBACHER[1], H.-O. WERLING[1], S. PAKU[2] and N. PAWELETZ[1]

[1]Institute of Cell and Tumor Biology, German Cancer Research Center,
 D-6900 Heidelberg, FRG
[2]Permanent address: Semmelweis University, Budapest, Hungaria

Keywords: Ultrastructure; invasion

INTRODUCTION

It is extremely difficult to study invasion phenomena in situ since the organism is too complex. Therefore, the classical way of investigating these phenomena is the establishment of appropriate models (Poste, 1982).

In addition to two- and three-dimensional tissue culture models (Gerstberger & Paweletz, 1981; Nicolson, 1982; Benke et al., 1984), organ cultures have been used to mimic the environment and conditions within the intact organism (Mareel, 1983).

Our model to study invasion phenomena fulfils some important criteria for tumour models: two tumour cell variants with different metastatic capacities are confronted with small pieces of the aortic wall of adult rats in a syngeneic system. This system may also be used for immunocyto-chemical or pharmaceutical studies, and provides the possibility to quantify the results.

MATERIALS AND METHODS

BDX-rats were used as donors of the aortas. The animals were anaesthe-sized, the thorax was opened and the aorta was taken out. It was cut into small tube-like pieces of approximately 0.5 cm and washed in Hanks' balanced salt solution. The tubes were opened and cultivated innerside up in petri dishes with RPMI-medium supplemented with 10% FCS. These pieces were confronted by dripping tumour cell variants on them for 30, 60 and 120 min. They were then fixed and processed for transmission and scanning electron microscopy.

Our rat tumour cells were the two variants AS and ASML derived from a sarcoma of the BDX-rat, as obtained from Matzku (Matzku et al., 1983).These

tumour cells spontaneously metastasize to the lung via the lymphatic
pathway. Very few metastases are formed from the AS Variant, but the ASML
cells are highly metastatic.

Both variants are kept in RPMI-medium supplemented with 10% FCS under
normal conditions. Aggregates from AS-cells were used according to the
Moscona-technique and confronted in the same way as single cells. We used
the aggregates after a 72h aggregation.

RESULTS

Controls of the aortic wall had never been in contact with tumour cells
and showed no significant alterations after 2h of observation. Preparative
damages were infrequent but the cutting process sometimes altered the edges
of the pieces by causing retractions of the endothelial cells.

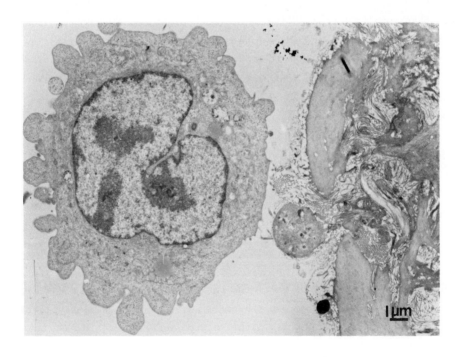

Figure 1. ASML-cell on top of the fibrous matrix.

ASML-cells which were confronted with the aortic endothelium exhibited
only a very weak adhesiveness to the endothelial cells. There was almost no
alteration of their spherical shape during the whole confrontation period.
In regions where the endothelial cells had disappeared from the underlying

fibrous matrix, the tumour cells tended to adhere much better, but they also remained spherical (Figure 1).

The AS-cells behaved in a completely different manner. They adhered firmly to the endothelial cells and started to spread by developing a mouse-like shape. During this spreading process the tumour cells began to undermine the endothelial cells, which then became detached (Figure 2) and were destroy-ed. Some tumour cells penetrated the endothelial layer in the regions where the endothelial cells had partially withdrawn. This is interpreted as the first stage of extravasation. We did not observe a penetration of the fibrous matrix, even after a prolonged period of confrontation.

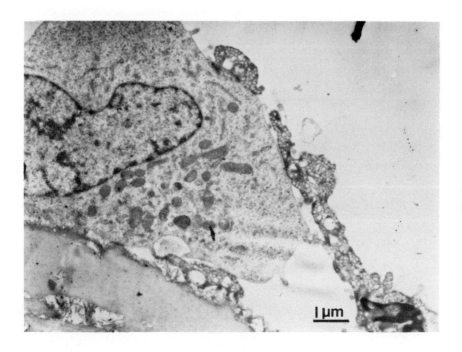

Figure 2. AS-cell detaching an endothelial cell.

We observed a loosening of the contacts between the tumour cells soon after confrontation of 72h old AS-aggregates with the aortic wall. The basic cells which were in close proximity to the endothelium began to separate from the bulk of the aggregate forming a base. These separating cells then began to penetrate the endothelium and became flattened. The partially flattened cells at the base of the aggregate behaved like single cells.

DISCUSSION

The data indicate large differences in the in vitro and in vivo growth characteristics of these two tumour cell variants. The AS variant which is weakly metastatic in vivo invades actively in vitro and destroys the endothelial cell layer. These cells are firmly attached to all offered substrates and they spread widely. The in vivo highly metastatic ASML variant appears extremely inactive in all in vitro tests (Benke et al., 1984; Paweletz et al., 1984) and is strongly inflexible. On the other hand, the cytogenetic analysis (Werling et al., 1984) of these two variants strongly indicates that ASML-cells are more malignant than those of the AS variant. This difference between in vivo and in vitro behavior might be explained by the environmental conditions. In the in vitro experiments, all functions of the blood coagulating system, all host reactions ranging from natural defense to the specific immunological defense mechanisms and the activities of other blood cells (like platelets) are completely lacking, Also, we do not know what physiological conditions are necessary for the tumour cells to become active. It also remains unclear how the in vivo environment induces the ASML cells into a spontaneous metastatic process.

In summary, the ASML variant which is highly metastatic in vivo appears inactive in vitro without signs of invasion. The low metastatic AS variant in vivo exhibits invasive activities in vitro. Thus, we conclude that results obtained in vitro cannot directly be correlated to in vivo situations.

REFERENCES

Benke, R., Werling, H.O. & Paweletz, N., 1984, Anticancer Research, in press.
Gerstberger, R. & Paweletz, N., 1981, European Journal of Cell Biology, 26, 136.
Mareel, M., 1983, Cancer Metastasis Reviews, 2, 201.
Matzku, S., Komitowski, D., Mildenberger, M. & Zoller, M., 1983, Invasion and Metastasis, 3, 109.
Nicolson, G., 1982, Journal of Histochemistry and Cytochemistry, 30, 214.
Paweletz, N., Werling, H.O., Aulenbacher, P. & Spiess, E., 1984, Scanning Electron Microscopy II, 183.
Poste, G., 1982, Methods and models for studying tumor invasion. In Tumor Invasion and Metastasis, edited by L.A. Liotta & I. Hart.

INVASION OF HIGH AND LOW METASTATIC MURINE TUMOUR CELLS IN TWO IN VITRO
QUANTITATIVE ASSAYS

C. A. WALLER, M. BRAUN and V. SCHIRRMACHER
Institute for Immunology & Genetics, German Cancer Research Centre,
Heidelberg, FRG

Keywords: invasion; lymphoma; brain microspheres

INTRODUCTION

Tumour cell invasion is an important step in the metastatic cascade
during which cells travel from the primary tumour to distant sites, there
to form secondaries. The investigation of invasion in vitro poses problems,
as any system designed to measure invasiveness must be both representative
of the situation in vivo and at the same time reproducible, controllable
and quantitative.

We have studied invasion using the Eb/ESb mouse lymphoma system,
comprising 4 related lines of varying metastatic capacity. Previous work
using non-quantitative assays showed that there were profound differences
in behaviour between Eb (low metastatic) and ESb (high metastatic) lines
when the cells were confronted in vitro with mouse lung tissue or bovine
vascular endothelial cells and their extracellular matrix (Lohmann-Matthes
et al. 1980, Vlodavsky, Schirrmacher et al. 1983, Vlodavsky, Fuks et al.
1983). We have now extended these studies, using two quantitative assays,
to two new sublines ESb-M and Eb-Fl, of low and high metastatic capacity,
respectively.

Tumour cells and assays

Eb is a low metastatic methylcholanthrene induced lymphoma of DBA/2
mice. ESb is a spontaneous variant thereof, arising during i.p. passage,
which is highly metastatic. Both these lines grow in suspension in vitro.
ESb-M is a low metastatic line derived from ESb in vitro by selection for
plastic adherence. Eb-Fl is a fusion between Eb and a bone marrow macrophage. It is highly metastatic and partially adherent. Tumour cells were
routinely cultured in RPMI 1640 + 5% FCS. For invasion studies they were
prelabelled with ^{75}Se-methionine.

INVASION ASSAYS

Brain microsphere assay

   Brains from newborn DBA/2 mice were pushed through 200 um nylon mesh,
the washed cell suspension was then placed in rotation culture for 10 - 14
days at 70 r. p. m. The resultant 400 - 500 um spheres were then pipetted,
500 per well in 500 ul of RPMI 1640/10% FCS, into 12 well plates. 2×10^5
labelled tumour cells were then added in a further 500 ul RPMI/FCS, and
cultured at 70 r.p. m. for 24 hours. After this time the cells and microspheres were vigorously mixed with a pipette, the microspheres allowed to
settle, and 0,5 ml medium with the still suspended cells removed to one 72
x 12 mm tube (Tube a). The remaining 0,5 ml containing cells and all the
microspheres was removed to a second tube (b) and the well was washed out
with two 0,5 ml aliquots of PBS, which were added to b. Tube a was then
centrifuged and 0,2 ml of the supernatant removed to a 3rd tube (c). All 3
tubes were then counted in a gamma counter and the % of cell bound counts
residing in the microspheres calculated as follows:

b-(1.5 x c) = counts in half the "non invaded cells" = NI
a-(2,5 x c) = counts in remaining half "non invaded cells" plus counts of
               "invaded" cells present in the microspheres = I

% cell bound counts present in the microspheres= $\dfrac{I - NI}{I + NI}$ x 100

Spontaneous release of radiaoctivity at 24 hrs was 25 - 40%.

Boyden chamber endothelial assay

   Bovine vascular endothelial cells were grown to confluence on 5 um pore
Millipore filters, and then cultured a further 10 days in ascorbic
acid/dextran containing Dulbecco's MEM to encourage secretion of extracellular matrix. Replicate 13 mm circles were punched out using a cork
borer, and mounted in blind well chemotaxis chambers, thus dividing the
chambers in two. The lower compartment contained 0,2 ml RPMI + FCS, and in
some cases, either 10^{-7} FMLP (n-formyl-methionyl-leucyl-phenylalanine) or
C5a (zymosan treated mouse serum) as chemoattractant. The upper compartment
contained 0,7 ml RPMI/FCS with 5×10^4 labelled tumour cells. The chambers
were incubated for 24 hours, then the contents of the upper compartment,
the filter, and the contents of the lower compartment were removed to
separate tubes for gamma counting. After allowing for background release,
the % of cell-bound counts residing in the filter, and the lower chamber,
was calculated.

RESULTS

Brain microsphere assay

The percent of cell-bound gamma counts, representing the number of invading tumour cells, found in the microspheres after 24 hours co-culture, is shown below.

Tumour cell line	% cell-bound counts in microspheres. Mean ± S. E.
Eb	15.3 ± 3
ESb	53.3 ± 8
Eb-Fl	66.0 ± 5
ESb-M	56.3 ± 8

The clear quantitative difference in invasive capacity between Eb and ESb had been previously observed. (Schirrmacher et al. 1982). Eb-Fl, a fusion product between the low-metastatic Eb and a bone marrow macrophage, is highly metastatic in vivo, and very invasive in vitro. However ESb-M, derived from ESb by selection for adhesion to plastic, is as invasive as its parent line, yet in vivo forms few or no metastases.

Boyden chamber endothelial assay

The invasive capacity of the four tumour lines, as measured by their ability to adhere to and penetrate endothelial cell layers plus secreted extracellular matrix is shown below. In the absence of any chemotactic factor, small numbers of all four types of tumour cells were found in the lower chambers. Eb cells were least "invasive" in this respect, only 0.4% of the cell bound counts being found in the lower compartment after 24 hours, while 4, 7, and 10 times as many ESb, Eb-Fl and ESb-M cells (1,6%, 3% and 4%) were found to have crossed the filter. The addition of chemotactic factors to the lower chamber did not seem to have any consistent effect on the numbers of tumour cells able to traverse the endothelial/ECM barrier. However, more Eb, ESb and ESb-M cells were found associated with the filter when 10^{-7} M FMLP was present, and significantly more of all the four tumour line cells were found in the filters when 1:10 zymosan treated serum was present.

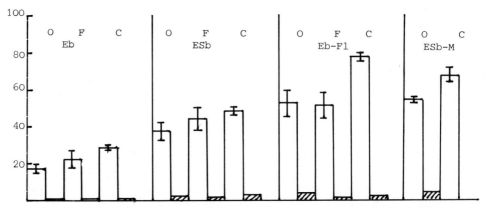

% of cell-bound counts in the filter, and in lower compartment after 24 hours. O - no chemoattractant, F = 10^{-7} FMLP, C = zymozan treated serum.

DISCUSSION

These two assay systems give essentially the same results when used to measure the invasive capacity of the four tumour lines. The poorly meta-static line Eb showed little ability to penetrate brain microspheres and correspondingly low affinity for endothelial cell monolayers. However small numbers of these tumour cells could act in an invasive manner in both assays, and these cells may be a metastatic subpopulation responsible for the low but reproducible level of metastasis seen in vivo.

The highly metastatic lines ESb and Eb-Fl were also both very invasive in vitro, however a similar level of invasiveness was recorded for ESb-M, which metastasises very poorly in vivo. The ability to invade, therefore, while a prerequisite for metastasis, is not in itself sufficient.

REFERENCES

Lohmann-Matthes, M., Schleich, A., Shantz, G. & Schirrmacher V., 1980, Tumor metastases and cell-mediated immunity in a model system in DBA/2 mice: VII interaction of metastasizing and non metastasizing tumours with normal tissue in vitro. Journal of the National Cancer Institute, 64, 1413.

Schirrmacher, V., Waller, C. A. & Vlodavsky, I., 1982, In vitro invasion of lymphomas with different metastatic capacity. In B and T cell Tumours, Biological and Clinical aspects. UCLA Symposium on Molecular and Cellular Biology, Vol. XXIV, edited by E. Vitetta & C. F. Fox ((Academic Press), p. 307.

Vlodavsky, I., Fuks, Z., Bar-Nev, M., Ariav,Y. & Schirrmacher, V., 1983, Lymphoma cell mediated degradation of sulfated proteoglycans in the subendothelial extracellular matrix: Relationship to tumour cell metastasis. Cancer Research, 43, 2704.

Vlodavsky, I., Schirrmacher, V., Ariav,Y. & Fuks, Z., 1983, Lymphoma cell interaction with cultured vascular endothelial cells and with the subendothelial basal lamina: Attachment, invasion and morphological appearance. Invasion and Metastasis, 3, 81.

TEMPERATURE-DEPENDENCE OF PNKT-4B FROG RENAL CARCINOMA CELL INVASION IN VITRO

M. MAREEL[1], E. BRUYNEEL[1], K. TWEEDELL[2], R. McKINNELL[3] and D. TARIN[4]

[1]Laboratory of Experimental Cancerology, Department of Radiotherapy and Nuclear Medicine, University Hospital, De Pintelaan 185, B-9000 Gent, Belgium

[2]Department of Biology, University of Notre Dame, Notre Dame, Indiana 46556, U.S.A.

[3]Department of Genetics and Cell Biology, University of Minnesota, Saint Paul, Minnesota 55108-1095, U.S.A.

[4]Nuffield Department of Pathology, John Radcliffe Hospital, University of Oxford, Oxford OX3 9DU, U.K.

Keyword : Lucké carcinoma; temperature-dependent invasion

INTRODUCTION

The Lucké renal adenocarcinoma of the leopard frog, Rana pipiens, is a herpesvirus-induced tumour exhibiting temperature-dependent metastatic behaviour (Lucké & Schlumberger 1949). This temperature-dependent aspect of spontaneous metastasis has been exploited in studies of the mechanisms of metastasis (review by McKinnell & Tarin 1984). The specific objective of the present work was to ascertain if invasion by this tumour is similarly affected by temperature.

Mareel et al. (1984) reported that malignant M04 mouse fibroblastic cells invaded embryonic chick heart in vitro at 30.5° or higher but failed to do so at 29° or lower. Investigation of the relevance of this observation for metastasis is hampered by the difficulty of keeping endothermic animals at different well-controlled body temperatures. Therefore, we adapted the in vitro invasion assay (Mareel et al. 1979) for frog tissue culture. Fragments of tadpole heart were confronted with PNKT-4B frog carcinoma cells (Tweedell 1978) in organ culture and analysed histologically after various periods of incubation at 7°, 20°, and 28°. The PNKT-4B cells invaded tadpole heart at 28° but not at 20° or at 7°.

MATERIALS AND METHODS

The PNKT-4B cell line, derived from a pronephric carcinoma (Tweedell 1978), was maintained at 20° in Leibovitz L-15 medium (Leibovitz 1963 : with 359.0 instead of 190.0 mg Na_2HPO_4/litre) plus 2 parts distilled water and 1 part foetal calf serum supplemented with L-glutamine (0.05% w/v), penicillin (250 units/ml) and fungizone (2 µg/ml).

Tadpole heart fragments, ca. 0.4 mm diameter, were confronted with PNKT-4B fragments removed from confluent cultures and preincubated at 20° or at 28° following a modification of the chick heart invasion assay (Mareel et al. 1979). After

24h individual confronting pairs were transferred into 5 ml Erlenmeyer flasks with 1.5 ml fluid culture medium for further incubation on a shaker at 28° (after preincubation at 28°) and at 20° or at 7° (after preincubation at 20°). The culture medium was refreshed every 4 days.

After 1, 4, 8 and 14 days triplicate cultures were fixed and embedded in paraffin as described elsewhere (Mareel et al. 1981). Whole confronting pairs were serially sectioned and stained with hematoxylin and eosin. The interaction between the PNKT-4B cells and the heart tissue was analysed semi-quantitatively according to a grading system modified from that used in the chick heart assay (Bracke et al. 1984) : Grade II, when the PNKT-4B cells were found at the periphery of the heart tissue; Grade III, when the PNKT-4B cells had occupied and/or replaced less than half of the heart tissue; Grade IV, when PNKT-4B cells had occupied and/or replaced more than half of the heart tissue. Tadpole heart fragments were cultured alone and processed as described for confronting pairs. All experiments were repeated once within an interval of 1 year. The number of cultures subjected to histological examination was 57.

RESULTS

At 28° (Figure 1d) PNKT-4B cells progressively occupied and replaced the heart tissue. At 20° (Figure 1c) PNKT-4B cells surrounded the heart fragment. Although the frontier between the confronting partners was irregular in some cultures no evidence for progressive occupation was found. At 7° (Figure 1b) the bulk of PNKT-4B cells remained at the site of attachment to the heart tissue for the whole period of incubation. Blocked metaphases (Levan 1954) were suspected in PNKT-4B cells (Figure 1b). Tadpole heart, cultured alone at 20° or at 28° retained its normal structure throughout incubation (Figure 1a). A semi-quantitative evaluation of the interaction between PNKT-4B cells and heart tissue based on the histology of serial sections is given in Table 1. PNKT-4B cells were easily recognized through their large nucleoli and basophilic cytoplasm.

DISCUSSION

These experiments show that PNKT-4B frog carcinoma cells are invasive in vitro at 28° but not at 20° nor at 7°.

The arguments for interpreting the histological analysis   as relevant for invasiveness or non-invasiveness of the PNKT-4B cells derive from comparison with the behaviour of cells of endothermic animals confronted with chick heart fragments in a similar organ culture assay (for reviews see Mareel 1982 and 1983). In the latter assay, non-invasive cells or invasive cells in presence of anti-invasive agents

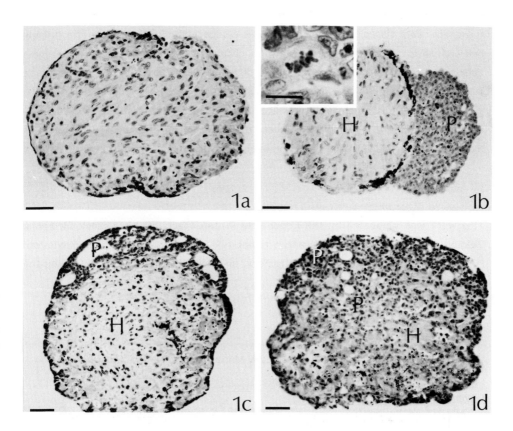

Figure 1. Light micrographs of 8 μm-thick-sections from a tadpole heart fragment (a) and from confrontations between PNKT-4B cells (P) and heart fragments (H) (b, c and d) cultured during 14 days at 7º (b), at 20º (a and c) and at 28º (d). Staining with hematoxylin-eosin. Scale bars = 50 μm (inset : 10 μm).

Table 1. Semi-quantitative evaluation of the interaction between PNKT-4B cells and tadpole heart fragments in organ culture.

Temperature	Grading after			
	1 day	4 days	7 to 8 days	14 days
7º	N.D.	$II^*(3)$	$II^*(3)$	$II^*(6)$
20º	$II^{**}(4)$	$II^{**}(6)$	$II^{**}(6)$	$II^{**}(10)$
28º	$II^{**}(3)$	$II^{**}(5)$	$III(5)$	$IV(6)$

Number of cultures between brackets.
N.D. = not done.
Grade II with ($**$) or without ($*$) surrounding of the heart tissue by PNKT-4B cells.
Invasion (which occurs only at 28º) is indicated by Grades III and IV.

surrounded the chick heart fragments in a fashion similar to the way PNKT-4B cells surrounded the tadpole heart fragments at 20°. Invasive cells occupied and replaced the chick heart tissue in the way PNKT-4B cells occupied and replaced the tadpole heart tissue at 28°. Similar results were obtained with MO4 mouse fibrosarcoma cells which invaded the chick heart at 30.5° or higher but not at 29° or lower (Mareel et al. 1984).

The present observations with PNKT-4B cells suggest that temperature-dependent variations in invasion contribute to temperature-dependent variations in metastasis observed with the Lucké tumours in vivo.

ACKNOWLEDGEMENTS

This work was supported by the Fonds voor Wetenschappelijk Onderzoek, Brussels, Belgium (20093) and NATO Research Grant N° 438/84. We thank J. Roels van Kerckvoorde for preparing the illustrations, and G. Matthys-De Smet for typing the manuscript.

REFERENCES

Bracke, M.E., Van Cauwenberge, R.M.-L. & Mareel, M.M., 1984, Clinical and Experimental Metastasis, 2, 161.
Leibovitz, A., 1963, American Journal of Hygiene, 78, 1973.
Levan, A., 1954, Hereditas, 40, 1.
Lucké, B. & Schlumberger, H., 1949, Journal of Experimental Medicine, 89, 269.
Mareel, M.M., 1982, The use of embryo organ cultures to study invasion in vitro. In Tumor Invasion and Metastasis, edited by L.A. Liotta & I.R. Hart (Martinus Nijhoff Publishers), p.207.
Mareel, M.M., 1983, Cancer Metastasis Reviews, 2, 201.
Mareel, M.M., Bruyneel, E.A., Dragonetti, C.H. & De Bruyne, G.K., 1984, Clinical and Experimental Metastasis, 2, 107.
Mareel, M.M., De Bruyne, G.K., Vandesande, F. & Dragonetti, C., 1981, Invasion and Metastasis, 1, 195.
Mareel, M.M., Kint, J. & Meyvisch, C., 1979, Virchows Archiv B Cell Pathology, 30, 95.
McKinnell, R.G. & Tarin, D., 1984, Cancer Metastasis Reviews, (in the press).
Tweedell, K.S., 1978, Pronephric tumor cell lines from herpes virus transformed cells. In Oncogenesis and herpes viruses, edited by G. de-Thé, W. Henle & F. Rapp (3rd Inter Symp, Inter Agen Res Cancer, Lyon), p.609.

INHIBITORY EFFECT OF DIFFERENT FLAVONOIDS ON THE INVASION OF MALIGNANT MO4 CELLS INTO EMBRYONIC CHICK HEART IN VITRO[*]

M. BRACKE[1], R. VAN CAUWENBERGE[2] and M. MAREEL[2]

[1]On leave from the Laboratory of Histology, State University of Ghent, Belgium

[2]Laboratory of Experimental Cancerology, Department of Radiotherapy and Nuclear Medicine, University Hospital, De Pintelaan 185, B-9000 Ghent, Belgium

[*]This work was supported by the Fonds van de Sportvereniging tegen de Kanker, (Brussels, Belgium), and by the Intern Krediet (216/519) van de Onderzoeksraad van de RUG (Ghent, Belgium).

Keywords : Invasion, flavonoids, (+)-catechin, warfarin

INTRODUCTION

An anti-invasive effect of the flavonoid (+)-catechin has recently been shown in vitro (Bracke et al. 1984). This molecule completely inhibits invasion at concentrations that allow proliferation of the malignant cells. One explanation for this effect is offered by the observation that (+)-catechin protects collagen against breakdown by mammalian collagenases (Kuttan et al. 1981). If collagenases play a role in invasion (Woolley et al. 1980), (+)-catechin might hinder invasion of malignant cells by modifying the extracellular matrix of the host tissue. We describe here the effect of different flavonoids and of warfarin on invasion of MO_4 cells in vitro. The purpose was to find a relationship between structure and activity of these structurally related molecules.

MATERIALS AND METHODS

Assay for invasion

Aggregates of MO_4-cells were confronted with precultured heart fragments (PHF) in vitro, as described by Mareel et al. (1979). MO_4-cells are virally transformed neonatal C_3H/He mouse cells (Billiau et al. 1973), which are invasive in vivo (Meyvisch & Mareel 1982) and in vitro (Mareel et al. 1979). Embryonic chick heart fragments were precultured in the presence of different concentrations of flavonoids for 4 days. After a confrontation period of 4 days in the presence of the same concentration of the drug the cultures were fixed in Bouin-Hollande's solution. Serial 8 μm-thick paraffin sections were stained with hematoxylin-eosin or with an antiserum that selectively reveals chick heart antigens (Mareel et al. 1981).

The volume of each confronting culture after 4 days of incubation was calculated from measurements of the largest and the smallest diameter (Attia & Weiss 1966).

Different grades of morphological interaction between MO_4-cells and PHF can be

Treatment of Metastasis

indicated by I to IV, as described by Bracke et al. (1984). Grades I and II are encountered when invasion is absent, while grades III and IV are typical of invasion.

Drugs

The following flavonoids were tested : (+)-catechin, quercetin (both from Sigma) Saint-Louis, Mo), (-)-epicatechin (Baker, Deventer, The Netherlands), rutin (Fluka, Buchs, Switzerland), troxerutin (Zyma, Galen, Switzerland), delphinidin chloride (ICN, New York, N.Y.), (-)-catechin (gift from M.-F. Maignan, Zyma, Nyon, Switzerland), 3-methyl quercetin (gift from D. Vanden Berghe, U.I.A., Antwerp, Belgium), warfarin (Coumadine, Sarva, Brussels, Belgium). Warfarin is structurally related to the flavonoids, but does not belong to this group of molecules.

Figure 1 shows the structures of these molecules. The number of experiments and the concentrations of the drugs are indicated in table I.

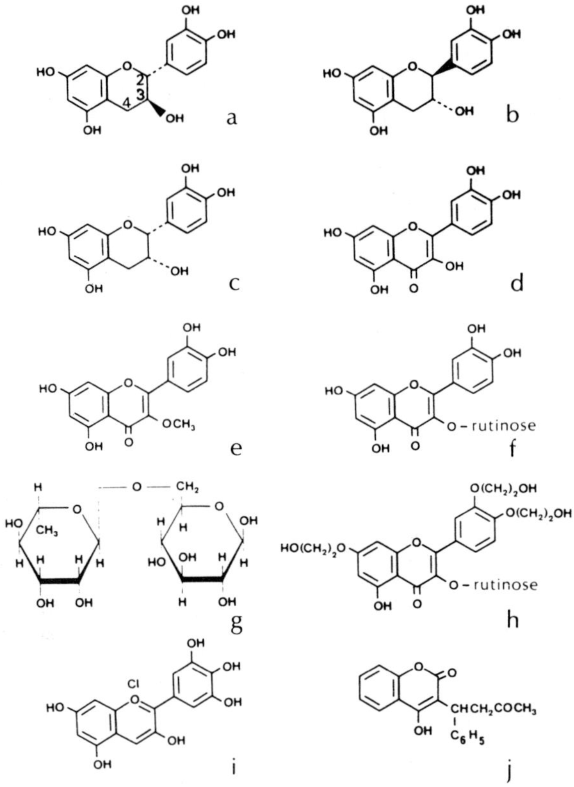

Figure 1. Dotted line - wedge presentations of the structure of 8 flavonoids [a = (+)-catechin, b = (-)-catechin, c = (-)-epicatechin, d = quercetin, e = 3-methyl quercetin, f = rutin, g = rutinose, h = troxerutin, i = delphinidin chloride] and warfarin (j).

RESULTS

Table I summarizes the results with the flavonoids and warfarin. Untreated confronting cultures always show grade IV.

Table 1. Semiquantitative evaluation of the interaction of MO_4 cells with PHF in the presence of different flavonoids and warfarin in vitro.

MOLECULE	CONCENTRATION mM	GRADE OF INTERACTION[a] I	II	III	IV
(+)-CATECHIN	0.10				■■■
	0.25	■	■■	■	
	0.50	■■	■		
	0.75	■■	■		
	1.00				T[b]
(-)-CATECHIN	0.10			■■	■
	0.50			■■	
	1.00				T
(-)-EPICATECHIN	0.10		■	■	■■
	0.50		■■	■	
	1.00				T
RUTIN	0.10			■	■■■
	0.50		■	■	■
	1.00				T
TROXERUTIN	0.10				
	0.50	■		■■	■■
	1.00			■■	
QUERCETIN	0.10			■	■■
	0.50		■		
	1.00		■		T
3-METHYL QUERCETIN	0.003			■■	■
	0.03			■■	■
	0.32				T
DELPHINIDIN CHLORIDE	0.10			■■	■
	0.50		■	■	■■
	1.00				T
WARFARIN	0.10				■■
	0.19				■■
	0.32				■■

[a]Every black square represents one culture
[b]In cultures indicated with "T" the morphology of the cells was altered to such an extent that toxicity was assumed (pycnosis and acidophilic cytoplasm).

A reproducible and complete inhibition of invasion (grade I) could only be gained after treatment with (+)-catechin. Grade I was also observed once with troxerutin. Grade II was the most frequent interaction in cultures treated with 0.50 mM (-)-epicatechin and 0.50 mM quercetin, but was also observed with 0.50 mM rutin and 0.50 mM delphinidin chloride.

The increase of the volume of confronting pairs after 4 days was less pronounced in treated than in untreated cultures. However, cultures treated with troxerutin had the same volume as untreated ones. With warfarin the volumes of the confronting cultures were greater than in controls.

DISCUSSION

Compared to other flavonoids (+)-catechin yields the most reproducible and complete inhibition of invasion in vitro. Its enantiomer (-)-catechin, however, does not inhibit invasion at all. Both molecules differ from each other by the spatial position of the hydroxyl group at C3 and the dihydroxyphenyl group at C2. (-)-Epicatechin shows an anti-invasive activity which is intermediate between (+)- and (-)-catechin. In (-)-epicatechin the dihydroxyphenyl group at C2 is in the same position as in (+)-catechin, while the hydroxyl group at C3 is as in (-)-catechin. Both (+)-catechin and (-)-epicatechin lack a ketone function at C4, which is present in other, less active flavonoids (rutin, troxerutin, quercetin and 3-methyl quercetin). The absence of any anti-invasive activity of warfarin may be due to the absence of a substituted phenyl group at C_2.

Our results with different flavonoids and warfarin suggest that the anti-invasive activity is depending on the position of the dihydroxyphenyl group at C2 on the one hand, and on the absence of a ketone function at C4 on the other hand.

REFERENCES
Attia, M. & Weiss, D., 1966, Cancer Research, 26, 1787.
Billiau, A., Sobis, H., Eyssen, H. & Van den Berghe, H., 1973, Archiv für die gesamte
    Virusforschung, 43, 345.
Bracke, M., Van Cauwenberge, R. & Mareel, M., 1984, Clinical and Experimental
    Metastasis, 2, 161.
Kuttan, R., Donelly, P. & Di Ferrante, N., 1981, Experientia, 37, 221.
Mareel, M., Kint, J. & Meyvisch, C., 1979, Virchows Archiv (Cell Pathology), 30, 95.
Mareel. M.. De Bruyne, G., Vandesande, F. & Dragonetti, C., Invasion and Metastasis,
    1, 195.
Meyvisch, C. & Mareel, M., 1982, Invasion and Metastasis, 2, 51.
Woolley, D., Tetlow, L., Mooney, C. & Evanson, J., 1980, Human collagenase and its
    extracellular inhibitors in relation to tumor invasiveness. In Proteinases and Tumor
    Invasion, edited by P. Sträuli et al. (Raven Press), p.97.

DIFFERENT HUMAN PLATELET-TUMOR CELL INTERACTIONS ACCORDING TO THE TUMOR CELL LINES

A. CAMEZ[1,2], F. CALVO[2], M.C. BRYCKAERT[1], E. CORVAZIER[1], J. MACLOUF[1] and G. TOBELEM[1]

[1]U. 150 INSERM, Hôpital Lariboisière, 2 rue Ambroise Paré, 75010 Paris
[2]Département d'hématologie, Hôpital Saint Louis, Place du Docteur Fournier, 75010 Paris, France

Keywords: tumor-cells, platelet aggregation

INTRODUCTION

The interaction between platelets and tumor cells may influence the development of metastasis as shown by Gasic (1977).

We studied two different human carcinoma cell lines which had opposite activity on human heparinized platelet rich plasma (PRP).

MATERIAL AND METHODS

Aggregation studies

Human mammary carcinoma cell lines, MCF_7 and MDA-MB 231, as described by Cailleau (1974) and Soule (1973) were used.

PRP's were obtained from normal volunteers, from an afibrinogenemic platient, and from a type I thrombasthenic patient, using heparin (5 U/ml) as anticoagulant.

Platelet aggregation was measured turbidimetrically as previously described by Gasic (1977).

6 KETO PGF 1 ∝ was measured by radio-immuno-assay (RIA) (Maclouf, 1976).

RESULTS AND DISCUSSION

The MCF_7 cell line induced platelet aggregation in all the PRP's obtained from 7 normal volunteers. The aggregating activity, which appeared without lag phase, was dependent on the tumor cell concentration and needed cells to be alive. It was independent of the degree of confluency when cells were harvested at different points in the growth phase. The aggregating activity was associated to the pellet obtained by sedimentation at 800 g for 5 minutes, but not present in the supernatant medium in which cells had been incubated, nor in the buffer in which they had been resuspended. This suggests that a close interaction between tumor cells and platelets was needed.

It was totally inhibited by creatine-phosphate creatine-phosphokinase (CP-CPK), apyrase and prostaglandin E_1 (PGE_1), suggesting the aggregation to be ADP mediated (fig. 1).

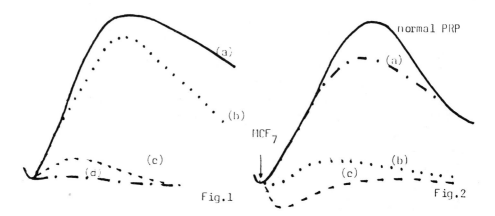

Fig.1   Fig.2

Figure 1. MCF_7 induced platelet aggregation (a), inhibition by CP-CPK (c), PGE_1, apyrase (d) no inhibition by Hirudin (b).

Figure 2. No aggregating activity in a type I thrombasthenic patient PRP (c), nor in an afibrinogenemic patient PRP (b). Aggregating activity restored in this latter PRP by addition of fibrinogen (a).

No aggregating activity was observed either in a type I thrombasthenic patient PRP, or in an afribinogenemic patient PRP; but the addition of fibrinogen in this latter PRP restored the aggregating activity. Therefore platelet membrane glycoprotein GP IIb, IIIa and plasmatic fibrinogen are necessary for MCF_7 induced platelet aggregation to occur (fig. 2).

The other cell line, MDA MB 231 did not induce platelet aggregation in all the PRP's from 6 normal volunteers and even inhibited both ADP and arachidonic acid induced platelet aggregation (fig. 3).

The inhibiting activity was independent of the tumor cell concentration and of the degree of confluency when cells were harvested at different points in the growth phase.

It was present in the buffer in which cells had been resuspended. It could be related to the generation of prostacyclin (PGI_2) by the tumor cells, since, by RIA, an increased level of 6 keto $PGF_1\alpha$ was found in the culture medium (fig. 4).

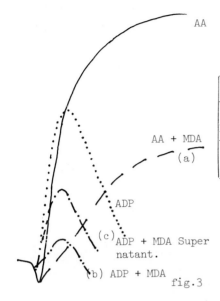

day	1rst	3rd	7th
MDA. MB 231	110	185	45
MCF7	-	-	30

fig.4

fig.3

Figure 3. MDA inhibiting activity of arachidonic acid (AA) (a), and ADP (b) induced platelet aggregation. MDA supernatant inhibiting activity.

Figure 4. Measurement of 6 keto $PGF_1\alpha$ in MDA cell culture medium (pg/ml).

Our results confirm that different responses can be observed with different cell lines. The physiopathological role of these different interactions needs to be specified.

REFERENCES

Cailleau, R. et al. 1974, Journal of the National Cancer Institute 53, 661.
Gasic, G.J. et al, 1977, Laboratory Investigation, 36, 413.
Maclouf, J. et al, 1976, Biochemica et biophysica Acta 431, 139.
Soule, M.D. et al, 1973, Journal of the National Cancer Institute, 51, 1409.

ACKNOWLEDGEMENT

This work was supported by INSERM and by a grant from ARC (Association pour le developpement de la Recherche sur le Cancer, Villejuif, France)

CHARACTERISATION OF PLASMINOGEN ACTIVATORS SECRETED BY HUMAN MALIGNANT CELLS

S.A. CEDERHOLM-WILLIAMS, S. HOULBROOK, N.W. PORTER, J.M. MARSHALL and H. CHISSIC

Nuffield Department of Obstetrics and Gynaecology, John Radcliffe Hospital, Oxford OX3 9DU, UK

Keywords: Plasminogen Activator Zymograms

INTRODUCTION

Plasminogen activators are highly specific serine proteases found in trace quantities in most non-malignant human tissues. The increased levels of proteolytic activity exhibited by malignant tissues and expressed in cell culture is largely due to the action of these enzymes. Recent rapid advances in the study of plasminogen activators has resulted in the complete characterisation of these enzymes and it is evident that the major specific plasminogen activating enzymes are the products of two separate genes (Cederholm-Williams 1984). Urokinase (u-PA) is found both as a single chain inactive proenzyme (mol.wt 54,000) and as a double chain active enzyme of identical molecular weight. An active degraded form of u-PA (mol.wt 32,000) may be found in certain tissues. The other major plasminogen activating enzyme is tissue plasminogen activator (t-PA) which can be obtained from non-malignant tissues as both single or double chain active enzyme of molecular weight 65-70,000.

Plasminogen activators are secreted by cultured malignant cells in variable quantities and can exhibit a wide range of molecular weights (25-120,000). This present communication describes a very powerful technique for characterising plasminogen activators and shows that the multiple forms of these enzymes secreted by malignant cells in culture are derivatives of either u-PA or t-PA.

METHODS

Biopsy samples of malignant tissues were grown as explants or were disaggregated with trypsin-EDTA, and cultured in DMEM supplemented with 10% calf serum, penecillin and strepto-mycin and buffered with 10mmol/l HEPES. Once cultures (both mixed or single cells) had obtained confluence (25 cm²) they were maintained in serum free medium for 24h and conditioned media analysed.

Plasminogen activator assay was performed on fibrin-agar plates prepared as follows:

Bovine fibrinogen (Sigma Chemicals) dissolved in 0.15mol/l NaCl and depleted of plasminogen by treatment with Sepharose-lysine is diluted to a final concentration of 2mg/ml clottable protein and stored at -20°C. Agarose (Sigma Chemicals) 20mg/ml in Tris-0.1mol/l, NaCl-0.15 mol/l, CaCl-4mmol/l buffer pH7.4 is rapidly melted in a microwave oven and cooled to 50°C, mixed with an equal volume of fibrinogen 2mg/ml with added human lysyl-plasminogen to a final concentration of 10-20µg/ml. Specific IgG fraction may be added at this stage. Fibrin polymerisation is initiated by the addition of bovine thrombin (Diagen Diagnostics, Thame) to a final concentration of 0.25 units/ml. The mixture is thoroughly mixed and allowed to set/clot in petri dishes or on polyester sheets (Gelbond) for at least 60 minutes. These plates or films can be stored at 4°C for up to 7 days before use. Wells (2.5mm) are cut in the gel and samples (10µl) or standards (urokinase 0.5-100 units/ml) added. The fibrin-agar plates are then incubated at 37°C for 17-24h in a humidified chamber. Activity is determined by measuring the product of the diameters of the lysis areas measured at right angles to each other and the $logD^2$ related to log concentration of the lysis areas produced by the dilutions of standard (log units). In the absence of added human plasminogen no or only slight lysis is induced by plasminogen activators.

Plasminogen activator typing is determined by adding to the gels or sample specific rabbit IgG fractions against human urinary u-PA or human uterine t-PA. These antibodies completely abolish the activities of their respective antigens but show no cross reactivity with respect to activity inhibition. Reduction of activity induced by a specific IgG fraction represents the proportion of this enzyme in a particular sample. Antibodies to u-PA and uterine t-PA have been prepared in this laboratory.

Plasminogen Activator Zymography: plasminogen activators in tissue culture media or in standard samples are first separated according to molecular weight by electrophoresis in polyacrylamide gel gradients (10-15%) containing SDS using a Protean 600 slab gel system (BioRad Ltd., Watford).

Running gel: A linear gradient of polyacrylamide is cast by mixing the following two solutions (A + B) with a three channel pump (Pharmacia Ltd., Milton Keynes). Solution A (12ml) consists of a final concentration of 10% and solution B contains a final concentration of 15% polyacrylamide, composed as follows: **Solution A:** Tris-Cl, pH8.6, 1.5mol/l, 3.0ml; acrylamide/bis 45%:1.2%, 2.7ml; H_2O, 5.8ml; sodium dodecyl sulphate, 10%, 0.1ml; TEMED, 0.025ml; riboflavin, 0.01%, 0.35ml.   **Solution B:** Tris-Cl, pH8.6, 1.5mol/l, 3.0ml; acrylamide/bis 45%:1.2%, 4.0ml; sodium dodecyl sulphate, 20%, 0.1ml; glycerol, 75%, 1.2ml; TEMED, 0.025ml; riboflavin, 0.01%, 0.35ml; water, 3.3ml. The solutions are mixed as a linear gradient, poured into a gel casting frame (1.5mm) and polymerised with flourescent light.

Stacking gel: is prepared by mixing Tris-Cl pH8.6, 0.5mol/l, 5.0ml; acrylamide/bis 45%: 1.2%, 1.3ml; sodium dodecyl sulphate, 10%, 0.2ml; TEMED, 0.05ml; ammonium persulphate, 10%, 0.4ml; water, 13.2ml. The stacking gel is allowed to polymerise on top of the running gel and contains the sample well combs.

Sample buffer: samples are mixed with equal volumes of sample buffer (Tris-Cl, pH8.6, 0.5mol/l, 2.5ml; glycerol, 75%, 2.5ml; SDS, 10%, 5.0ml; water, 10ml). The samples are not boiled nor reduced.

Electrophoresis: samples (10-50µl) are applied to each well and carefully overlayed with running buffer. Each sample is diluted to contain approximately 1IU/ml plasminogen activator activity. Molecular weight standards (Pharmacia Ltd., Milton Keynes) containing bromophenol blue are also run with the samples. Electrophoresis is performed using an **electrode buffer** (Tris-0.018mol/l; glycine-0.096mol/l; SDS-1g/l, adjusted to pH8.6) in both upper and lower chambers. Electrophoresis is carried out at 10-20mA per gel until the samples have entered the running gel (indicated by the bromophenol blue), then at 50mA/gel until the dye reaches the bottom of the running gel.

Following removal from the electrophoresis apparatus the polyacrylamide gel may be cut into sections for protein staining or autoradiography and for zymography.

Zymography: following electrophoresis the gel is soaked in Triton X-100, 500ml, 2.5% and agitated for 2h to remove SDS. The gel is then overlayed with a fibrin-agar film (on Gelbond) and incubated at 22°C overnight. This gel may contain specific IgG fractions for plasminogen activator discrimination. The fibrin-agar overlay is removed and photographed, or dried and stained with amido-black-0.1%. Plasminogen activator activity is evident as clear lysis zones corresponding to the electrophoresis bands. Comparison with the fixed and stained polyacrylamide gel strips containing the molecular weight standards indicates the approximate molecular weight (+5000) of the enzymes.

RESULTS

Figure 1 is a representative polyacrylamide gel electrophoresis zymogram showing purified plasminogen activators and results obtained from conditioned media from malignant and non-malignant cells. Figure 2 shows the identical electrophoretogram overlayed with fibrin-agar gel containing rabbit IgG fraction against u-PA and t-PA.

Lane 2 (Fig. 1) shows purified u-PA (mol.wt 54,000) obtained from the urine of healthy adults, and Lane 1 (Fig. 1) shows u-PA that has been proteolytically degraded to yield the lower molecular weight (31,000) derivative. Lane 3 (Fig. 1) shows t-PA isolated from non-malignant human uterus (mol.wt 65,000-67,000). Two forms of t-PA of similar molecular weight are frequently observed, and occasionally form of molecular weight of 42,000.

Lane 4 (Fig. 1) shows plasminogen activator from the culture media of a human malignant melanoma and Lane 5 (Fig. 1) shows the pattern obtained from the media of non-malignant embryonic cells. **Each of these plasminogen activator forms have been found in media from different malignant cell cultures, either singly or in all combinations.**

Figure 2 shows the same gel except that the u-PA and t-PA have been inhibited. All the different molecular weight forms so far identified have been susceptible to antibodies against u-PA or t-PA.

Variable quantities of plasminogen activators (0-12IU/ml) have been detected in different cultures. Culture media in which no activity can be detected by the fibrin-agar plate assay often have a preponderance of the higher molecular weight forms (>100,000) which may be reactivated inhibitor complexes.

DISCUSSION

Though the malignant cell cultures so far examined exhibit a wide range of molecular weight forms of plasminogen activator only u-PA and t-PA antigens have been detected. It is concluded that generally malignant cells in culture secrete only derivatives of the normally expressed plasminogen activators and no distinct 'malignant' plasminogen activator exists. The zymographic technique described is a very powerful tool particularly when used in conjunction with Western and Southern blotting techniques.

ACKNOWLEDGEMENTS

This work is supported by grants from the Cancer Research Campaign and British Heart Foundation.

REFERENCE

Cederholm-Williams, S.A., 1984. Molecular Biology of Plasminogen Activators and Recombinant DNA Progress. BioEssays, 1, 168-173.

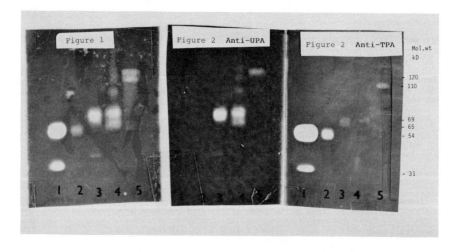

Figures showing zymographic analysis of plasminogen activators.

EXTRACELLULAR HYALURONIDASE-SENSITIVE COATS PRODUCED BY
TUMOR CELLS AND THEIR RELEVANCE TO METASTASIS

W.H. McBRIDE
Department of Radiation Oncology, University of California,
Los Angeles 90024

Keyword: hyaluronate, coats, metastasis, glycosaminoglycans

INTRODUCTION

The nature of the extracellular matrix a cell produces appears to reflect
its differentiation stage, its proliferative age and functional status. At
the same time it can influence these processes. For example, glycosaminoglycans (GAGs), which are major components of matrices, have been shown to
affect cell proliferation, differentiation, adhesion, recognition and
mobility (Toole 1981). It would be surprising therefore if GAG production
by tumor cells was not important in the processes of tumor growth and
metastasis.

The question we have asked is whether a tumor cell's ability to elaborate
a pericellular hyaluronate coat confers upon it a selective advantage when
it comes to run the gauntlet leading to metastasis formation. Many tumor
cells and normal cells elaborate translucent pericellular coats several um
thick soon after isolation from a cell mass (Clarris & Fraser 1967; McBride
& Bard 1981). They do so within a few hours of _in vitro_ culture and
presumably do the same _in vivo_. On the basis of enzyme sensitivity the coat
can be said to be a hyaluronate gel although the presence of other sub-
stances within the gel cannot be excluded. Hyaluronate is shed from the
pericellular coat into the surrounding medium and is continuously replaced.
In vitro these coats exclude particles such as red cells, bacteria and
carbon which is a convenient means of detection. They cannot be seen by
conventional microscopy but if specimens are freeze-dried they can be
detected by scanning electron microscopy (Bard et al. 1983). The coats
have been shown to protect cells against the attentions of cytotoxic lymphocytes (McBride & Bard 1981) and viruses (Clarris et al. 1976). In addition,
others have shown that hyaluronate can be important in cell aggregation
(Underhill & Toole 1981), movement, proliferation and differentiation

(Toole 1981), processes which are relevant in tumor growth and metastasis, and differences between normal cells and cancer cells with respect to hyaluronate metabolism (Nigam et al. 1982) may account for differences in their behavior.

For these reasons, we investigated the contribution coat formation makes to a cell's ability to metastasise. In our previous studies we were struck by the heterogeneity in coat production within tumor cell populations. In this report, by cloning tumor cells, we show that this heterogeneity is not genetically imposed but that cells lacking the ability to produce coats are inefficient in forming artificial metastases suggesting that the phenotypic production of hyaluronate by a tumor cell may protect it during the trauma of the metastatic process.

MATERIALS AND METHODS

Tumor cells and cloning

Tumor cells were obtained from a methylcholanthrene-induced fibrosarcoma (Fsa) maintained in vivo (McBride & Bard 1981). Cells were plated in RPMI 1640 with 10% fetal calf serum (Gibco) and after 7 days were cloned in 0.3% semi-solid agar. Uncloned cells were maintained in bulk culture. The ability of single cells to elaborate coats was tested by adding sheep red cells to tumor cells previously incubated for 16 hr in 96 well plates (McBride & Bard 1981). After 10 min the presence of a translucent halo excluding red cells around the tumor cell was taken as demonstrating coat production. Some uncloned 24 hr old cultures were mutagenised with 0.3 ul/ml ethylmethane sulfonate (Sigma) for 18 hr at 37°C. These cells were also cloned after 7 days growth.

Scanning electron microscopy (SEM)

The procedures used have been described (Bard et al. 1983).

RESULTS AND DISCUSSION

Hyaluronidase-sensitive coats around cells can be visualised by adding particles such as red cells which are excluded from entering a translucent zone around cells. Alternatively, they can be seen by SEM provided the cells are fixed carefully, frozen rapidly and freeze-dried. Alcohol causes them to collapse. Fig 1 shows the size of these coats as obtained by SEM. Fsa cells plated 24 hr previously are approximately 12 um in diameter if they are processed by critical point drying. If freeze-dried they are 22 um including extracellular material. This is removed by hyaluronidase

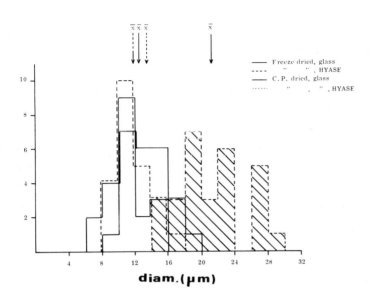

Fig 1. Histograms showing cell diameter of critical point dried and freeze-dried Fsa cells with and without prior hyaluronidase treatment (1 iu/ml).

treatment to give cells averaging 13.5 um. A 4-5 um coat extending beyond the cell surface agrees with previous estimates (McBride & Bard 1981).

Not all cells in a culture produce coats. The percentage varies but rarely goes above 75%. To establish whether this heterogeneity was genetic, 98 Fsa clones were established. All of these contained a percentage of positive cells showing that the variability observed in coat production is not genetically determined. Attempts were made to establish cell lines that were unable to form coats by cloning of mutagenised cells. Four were found out of 130 clones. To investigate whether coat production could protect cells during the metastatic process 10^5 cells from each of these 4 negative clones and 31 others were injected iv into syngeneic mice. The clones gave rise to a wide spread of tumor colony numbers in the lung (0-136), far greater than the uncloned population (28-50), suggesting hetero-geneity in the original population. Of the 4 negative clones, 3 gave no lung colonies, one gave 22, suggesting that inability to elaborate coats left cells more vulnerable to hazards inherent in the metastatic process. The clone that gave rise to 22 colonies reverted to coat production before it could be retested. The 3 negative clones gave no colonies in a sub-sequent experiment but then reverted to coat production showing that they were unstable. These reverted clones formed colonies on reinjection.

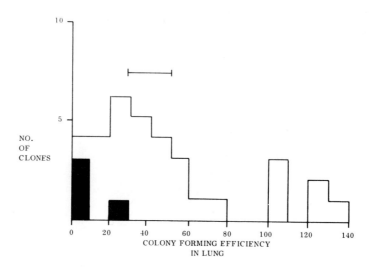

Fig 2. Lung colony forming efficiency of Fsa clones. Clones unable to form
coats are in black. The bar is the range of colonies from uncloned, bulk-
cultured Fsa. 6 mice minimum per group.

   The process of metastasis is a complex series of steps and to successfully complete the series, cells must have many attributes and utilize many
different functions. The experiments reported here suggest that the ability
to secrete hyaluronate might protect a cell during the metastatic process.
It could do this by forming an insulating layer around the cell which could
protect against potentially lethal attack by host cells or fluids as can
happen *in vitro* (McBride & Bard 1981). Alternatively it could aid cell
movement and invasion enabling the tumor cell to more readily establish
itself.

REFERENCES

Bard, J.B.L., McBride, W.H. & Ross, A.R., 1983, Journal of Cell Science,
     62, 371.
Clarris, B.J. & Fraser, J.R.E., 1967, Nature, 214, 1159.
Clarris, B.J., Fraser, J.R.E. & Rodda, S.J., 1974, Annals Rheumatic
     Diseases, 33, 260.
McBride, W.H. & Bard, J.B.L., 1981, Journal of Experimental Medicine,
     149, 507.
Nigam, V.N., Brailovsky, C.A. & Bonaventure, J., 1982, Glycosaminoglycans
     and proteoglycans in neoplastic tissues and their role in tumor growth
     and metastasis. In Glycosaminoglycans and Proteoglycans in
     Physiological and Pathological Processes of Body Systems, edited by
     R.S. Varma & R. Varma (S. Karger), p. 356.
Toole, B.P., 1981, Glycosaminoglycans in morphogenesis. In Cell Biology
     of Extracellular Matrix, edited by E. Hay (Plenum Press), chapter 9.
Underhill, C.B. & Toole, B.P., 1981, Experimental Cell Research, 131, 419.

H-2 EXPRESSION, IMMUNOGENICITY AND METASTATIC PROPERTIES OF BL6 MELANOMA CELLS TREATED WITH MNNG

E. GORELIK

National Cancer Institute-Frederick Cancer Research Facility, Frederick, Maryland 21701

Keywords: H-2 expression; MNNG

INTRODUCTION

A large body of experimental data accumulated over the past 5 years indicates that treatment of various tumor cells with the mutagen $\underline{N}$-methyl-$\underline{N}$'-nitro-nitrosoguanidine (MNNG) results in a substantial increase in the immunogenicity of treated tumor cells (Boon 1983). Immunogenic variants of the MNNG-treated tumor cells were unable to grow in immunocompetent mice, but developed progressively growing tumors in immunosuppressed mice or athymic nude mice (Boon 1983).

In the present study we investigated the effect of MNNG treatment on the immunogenic and metastatic properties of BL6 melanoma cells. Since H-2 antigens may play an important role in the immunogenicity of tumor cells (Festenstein and Schmidt 1981) as well as in their metastatic ability (De Baetselier et al. 1980; Gorelik et al. 1982a), we also investigated the H-2 antigen expression in MNNG-treated and nontreated melanoma cells.

METHODS

The studies were performed using B16 melanoma and its cell variants. MNNG treatment was performed using BL6 melanoma cells. These tumor cells were selected by Dr. Hart from the B16F10 melanoma subline based on their ability to penetrate the mouse bladder wall. Melanoma cells that underwent six rounds of selection by bladder penetration were termed the bladder 6 (BL6) melanoma subline. These melanoma cells express high invasive properties and a high ability to develop spontaneous pulmonary metastases (Hart 1981).

BL6 melanoma cells (1×10^6/ml) were incubated with 3.3 µg/ml of MNNG (Sigma Chemical Co., St. Louis, Mo.) at 37°C for 1 hr. After washing, the surviving tumor cells were expanded. MNNG treatments of the BL6 melanoma cells were repeated at 1-month intervals. Melanoma cells treated with MNNG 1, 2 or 3 times were designated as BL6T1, BL6T2, and BL6T3, respectively.

Tumorigenic and immunogenic properties of tumor cells were tested by i.f.p. inoculation into syngeneic immunocompetent or immunosuppressed (irradiated 550R) C57BL/6 mice. Tumor growth of these cells was also assessed in athymic nude mice. Metastatic properties of the tumor cells were tested by their ability to develop spontaneous metastases after surgical excision of the local i.f.p. tumors or experimental metastases after i.v. inoculation of the tested melanoma cells.

H-2 antigen expression was investigated using flow cytometry analysis and monoclonal antibodies kindly provided by Dr. D. Sachs (Immunology Branch, NCI, NIH, Bethesda, Md.). The following monoclonal antibodies were utilized: anti-H-2K^b (hybridoma line 28-13-3S), anti-H-2D^b (hybridoma 28-11-5S), anti-Ia^b, detecting private specificity Ia.20 (hybridoma 25-5-16S) and public specificity Ia.8 (hybridoma 28-16-8S) (Sachs et al. 1980). Immunofluorescence staining was performed according to Mathieson et al. 1980).

RESULTS AND DISCUSSION

The data presented in Table 1 indicate that the low metastatic melanoma lines B16 and B16F1 had higher levels of H-2 expression than the high metastatic subline B16F10 or BL6 melanoma cells. Melanoma sublines selected on the high metastatic ability completely lost their H-2K^b antigens and express low level of H-2D^b antigens (Table 1).

It is of interest that MNNG treatment caused a dramatic increase in the expression of both H-2K^b and H-2D^b antigens (Table 1). None of the tested melanoma sublines treated or untreated with MNNG expressed serologically detectable class II MHC antigens.

When MNNG-treated and untreated BL6 melanoma cells (5×10^4) were inoculated i.f.p. into C57BL/6 mice (12 mice per group), tumor growth was observed in 100% of mice inoculated with BL6 melanoma cells, 80% of mice transplanted with BL6T1 cells, and 30-32% of mice injected with BL6T2 or BL6T3 cells. However, when BL6T2 or BL6T3 cells were inoculated into irradiated (550R) C57BL/6 mice or nude mice, progressively growing tumors

Table 1. H-2 antigen expression on the cell surface of B16 melanoma
cell variants.

Tumor	Characteristics	% positive cells	
		$H-2K^b$	$H-2D^b$
B16	Initial population	31.6[a]	26.9
B16F1[b]	Low metastatic subline	20.6	24.5
B16F10[b]	Selected on high lung colonization	3.5	9.1
B16F10BL6[c]	Selected on high invasiveness	1.2	10.1
BL6T1	One treatment with MNNG	50.2	79.2
BL6T2	Two treatments with MNNG	47.4	76.5
BL6T3	Three treatments with MNNG	46.7	76.9

[a]Using monoclonal antibodies and flow cytometry analysis, the expression of
 $H-2K^b$ and $H-2D^b$ antigens on the cell surface of B16 melanoma cell variants
 was investigated.
[b]Melanoma lines selected by Dr. J. Fidler.
[c]Melanoma line selected by Dr. I. Hart.

developed in all mice. C57BL/6 mice that rejected the first inoculum of
BL6T2 melanoma cells were also resistant to the consequent injections of
increased doses $(0.5-1 \times 10^6)$ of the same tumor cells.

In order to assess the metastatic properties of the selected sublines,
C57BL/6 mice were inoculated i.v. with 5×10^4 tumor cells (Table 2).
In mice inoculated with BL6T1 and especially BL6T2 cells, the number of
metastatic foci in the lungs was substantially lower than in mice inoculated
with the original BL6 melanoma cells. All BL6 pulmonary metastases were
black, whereas after inoculation of BL6T1 cells some of the nodules in the
lungs were black and some were white. All BL6T2 pulmonary metastases were
amelanotic. The observed differences in the number of metastatic foci can
hardly be attributed to retardation of their growth and development of
visible tumor nodules. In vitro, the proliferative activity of BL6T2 cells
was higher than B16 melanoma cells (data not shown).

In the next experiment, C57BL/6 mice received 1.2×10^5 tumor cells and
harvesting of the lungs was postponed up to 25 days after tumor cell inoculation when mice inoculated with BL6 melanoma cells started to die. All lung
surfaces of these mice were covered with black tumor masses. In the same
time period mice inoculated with BL6T2 cells had only 10 metastatic nodules
and substantial differences in the total weight of lungs with metastases
(Table 2).

Table 2. Metastasis formation after i.v. inoculation of tumor cells.

Experiment number	Tumor line	Median number of lung metastases (range)	Weight (mg) of lungs with metastases (range)
1	BL6	53 (10–106)	ND
	BL6T1	7 (1–104)	ND
	BL6T2	1 (0–3)	ND
2	BL6	confluent growth	715 (533–955)
	BL6T2	10 (6–21)	274 (204–560)

C57BL/6 mice were inoculated i.v. with 5×10^4 (Exp. 1) or 1.2×10^5 (Exp. 2) tumor cells. The numbers of tumor nodules in the lungs were counted 16 (Exp. 1) or 25 (Exp. 2) days after tumor cell inoculation. Nine mice per group.

In order to assess the ability of BL6T2 cells to develop spontaneous pulmonary metastases, C57BL/6 mice were inoculated i.f.p. with increased doses (3×10^5) of BL6T2 tumor cells in order to overcome the resistance of the recipients to these tumor cells. Amelanotic local tumors appeared in 60% of C57BL/6 mice and in 100% of nude mice inoculated with BL6T2 tumor cells (Table 3). All mice inoculated with BL6 melanoma cells developed progressively growing black tumors. When local tumors reached a size of 8–9 mm in diameter, half the mice received i.p. 0.2 ml of anti-asialo GM_1 serum (dilution 1:30), which depressed the NK reactivity of the mice and increased metastasis formation (Gorelik et al. 1982b). Five days later, tumors 10–11 mm in diameter were removed. The number of metastatic foci in the lungs was determined 25 days later. Postoperative pulmonary metastases did not appear in 83% of the mice from which BL6T2 tumors were excised. No increase in the number of metastases or percent of mice with metastases was found when BL6T2-bearing mice were pretreated with anti-asialo GM_1 serum. It seems that inhibition of metastasis formation was due mostly to T cell-mediated immunity, since in nude mice BL6T2 and BL6 tumors were similar in their ability to develop spontaneous metastases. Depression of NK activity in nude mice increased the formation of metastasis by both BL6T2 and BL6 tumors (Table 3).

Thus, these data indicate that treatment of B16 melanoma cells with MNNG resulted in the dramatic increase of class I antigen of H-2 complex and immunogenicity of the treated tumor cells. A decrease in the metastatic ability of treated BL6T2 cells was associated with their ability to elicit host immune responses. Although antitumor immune response failed to destroy

Table 3. Development of postoperative BL6 and BL6T2 metastases
in C57BL/6 and nude mice.

Mice[a]	Tumor	% of mice with tumor	Anti-asialo GM$_1$ serum treatment	Median no. of post-operative metastases (range)	% of mice with metastases
C57BL/6	BL6	100	−	4 (0–16)	83
	BL6	100	+	11 (3–25)[b]	100
	BL6T2	60	−	0 (0–1)	17
	BL6T2	60	+	0 (0–2)	17
Nude	BL6	100	−	7 (3–14)	100
	BL6	100	+	15 (4–29)	100
	BL6T2	100	−	3 (0–9)	78
	BL6T2	100	+	19 (2–confluent)[b]	100

[a]C57BL/6 or nude mice were inoculated i.f.p. with 3 x 10^5 BL6 or BL6T2
tumor cells. When tumors reached 8–9 mm in diameter some mice received
i.p. 0.2 ml of anti-asialo GM$_1$ serum (dilution 1:30). Local tumors 10–11
mm in diameter were removed. Mice were killed 25 days after tumor
excision and numbers of metastases in the lungs were counted.
[b]Significantly different (p < 0.05) from mice untreated with anti-asialo
GM$_1$ serum according to Mann–Whitney U test.

local tumor mass in mice inoculated with increased doses of BL6T2 cells,

this immune response can be rather efficient in the elimination of

solitary metastatic cells. This conclusion is supported by the fact that

immunization of mice bearing BL6 melanoma with the immunogenic tumor cell

variants did not influence local tumor growth, but inhibited growth of

postoperative tumor metastases (to be published).

REFERENCES

Boon, T., 1983, Advances in Cancer Research, 39, 121.
De Baetselier, P., Katsav, S., Gorelik, E., Feldman, M. & Segal, S., 1980,
    Nature, 288, 179.
Festenstein, H. & Schmidt, W., 1981, Immunological Review, 60, 85.
Gorelik, E., Fogel, M., De Baetselier, P., Katazv, S., Feldman, M. & Segal,
    S., 1982a, Immunobiological diversity of metastatic cells. In Cancer
    Invasion and Metastasis, edited by L. Liotta and I. Hart (Martinus
    Nijhoff), p. 134.
Gorelik, E., Wiltrout, R., Okumura, K., Habu, S. & Herberman, R., 1982b,
    International Journal of Cancer, 30, 107.
Hart, I., 1981, Cancer Biology Reviews, 2, 29.
Mathieson, B., Sharrow, S., Bottomly, K. & Fowlkes, B., 1980, Journal of
    Immunology, 125, 2127.
Sachs, D., Mayer, N. & Ozato, K., 1981, Hybridoma antibodies directed
    toward murine H-2 and Ia antigens. In Monoclonal Antibodies and T Cell
    Hybridomas, edited by G. Hammerling, et al. (Elsevier/North-Holland),
    p. 96.

DIFFERENT HOMING PATTERNS OF ISOLATED LYMPHOMA CELLS; RELATIONSHIP WITH CELL SURFACE MORPHOLOGY AND CHROMOSOMAL ABERRATIONS

A.W.T. KONINGS[1], B. de JONG[2] and C.E. HULSTAERT[3]
[1]Department of Radiopathology, [2]Department of Medical Genetics and [3]Centre for Medical Electron Microscopy, University of Groningen, Groningen, The Netherlands

Keyword: Lymphoma; homing patterns; karyotype

INTRODUCTION

Cancer cells exhibit an "organ pattern" for localization of metastatic growth. Many years ago, clinical observations led Paget (1889) to propose the "seed and soil" hypothesis, which states that certain cancer cells will grow readily in certain tissues but not in others. The mechanisms of selection at the level of tumor cell/organ cell interactions are of great importance and not known. The surface of tumor cells will probably play an important role in the homing pattern of different cancers.

This communication reports on a change in the homing pattern characteristics of a population of tumor cells during their growth in culture. The tumor cells were obtained from the blood of lymphoma bearing C57BL mice. The high-grade malignant lymphoma arose spontaneously in the C57BL mouse several years ago and has been transplanted weekly, by intraperitoneal injection of 10^6 tumor cells obtained from the spleen. At different stages of the in vitro growth of the tumor cells, cytogenetic as well as morphological studies have been performed.

RESULTS

The initial proliferation of the tumor cells appeared to occur predominantly in the spleen, both after intravenous (i.v.) and intraperitoneal (i.p.) injection. This murine tumor was characterized as a B cell lymphoma according to the working proposals published by Krueger and Meyer (1982); monoclonal surface- and intracellular-immunoglobulins were present. The animals die in 8 ± 1 days after inoculation of 10^6 neoplastic spleen cells. At the seventh day after tumor transplantation blood cells were mixed with saline (1:1) and the lymphoma cells were isolated on isopaque ficoll. After

washing, the cells (mainly lymphocytes and lymphoma cells) were cultured in
RPMI 1640 medium supplemented with 2 g/liter $NaHCO_3$, 10% fetal calf serum,
50 µg/ml streptomycin and 50 IU/ml penicillin. During the first weeks in
culture the characteristics of the cells with respect to homing patterns
and karyotype did not differ from the freshly isolated tumor cells from the
blood or the spleen. The clonogenic ability of this cell population on soft
agar was less than 0.1% (see figure 1). When injected (i.v. or i.p.) in the

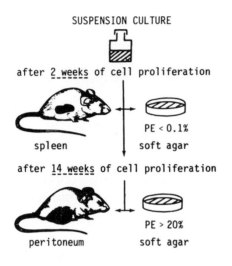

Figure 1. Characteristics of the early and late stages of a cell culture originating from lymphoma cells isolated from blood.

mouse, these cells caused a massive enlargement of the spleen and to a
lesser extent of the liver, with no peritoneal tumor growth or ascites

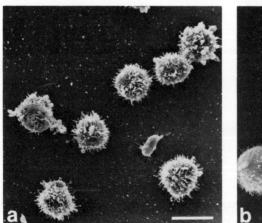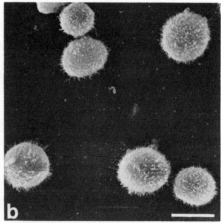

Figure 2. Scanning electron micrograph (SEM) of cells obtained from an early (2 weeks) stage (a) and from a late (3 months) stage (b) of cell culturing. Bar: 10 µm.

production. Cytogenetic studies indicated that many cells had 41 or 42 chromosomes with mostly one or two structurally abnormal ones.

After about 3 months of cell culturing an increase in cellular volume had taken place and the clonogenic ability of the cells was much higher (>20%). After i.p. injection of these cells, no cell proliferation in the spleen could be observed; the homing pattern of these cells was character- ized by a peritoneal growth as ascites cells.

Scanning electron microscopy (SEM) showed that the cells which pre- ferred to home to the spleen (2 weeks cell culture) were characterized by a rough surface with stubby microvilli, blebs and ruffles (figure 2, a), while the cells which liked to stay and proliferate in the peritoneal cavity (3 months culture) showed thinner microvilli, which were abundantly present (figure 2, b).

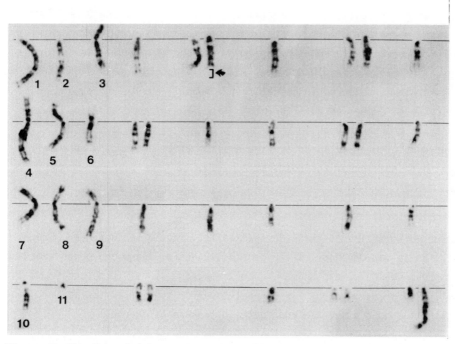

Figure 3. The G-banded karyotype of a cell obtained from a late (3 months) stage of cell culturing. The total number of chromosomes is 37 with 11 non- random and 1 random (arrow) abnormal ones.

The number of chromosomes of the latter cell population was decreased (37-39) and a number of 11 nonrandom chromosomal aberrations, mainly trans- locations, was observed. An example of a G-banded karyotype obtained from a cell of the population with the peritoneal homing characteristics is shown in figure 3. These cells have no B cell character (IgM, λ).

DISCUSSION

The experimental results show that a population of tumor cells in culture may change drastically with respect to genotype, surface morphology and homing characteristics. It seems that the cells which like to home in the spleen of the mouse are smaller, contain fewer fine microvilli and have a less abnormal karyotype than the ascites-growing cells.

It is not clear at the moment whether the tumor cells which prefer to home in the peritoneal cavity were already present as a minor subpopulation of the original cells harvested from the blood or whether these cells have been formed via genotypic changes during the in vitro culturing. There are indications that the ascites-type cells are already present as a very small minority during the first weeks of cell culturing. It may be that selective pressure during the in vitro growth of the original tumor population has led to a dominance of the ascites-type cells, because environmental conditions were unfavourable for continuous proliferation of the B cell lymphomas originally present.

It cannot be excluded however, that cytogenetic changes have occurred during the first weeks in culture. Tumor cell populations are genetically less stable as compared to normal cells (Nowell, 1983). Phenotypic instability (e.g. expressed as alterations in cell surface properties) due to genotypic changes may be an important property of malignant cells. This might enable tumor cells to survive environmental pressures, eventually leading to killing of the host.

ACKNOWLEDGEMENTS

The authors like to thank Jelleke Dokter, Ingrid van der Meer, Freark Dijk, Aukje van der Meer, Willy Lemstra, Engbert Blaauw and Josée Wagenaar for the invaluable help and their contributions to this project; Dr. J.W. Smit (Div. of Haematology) is acknowledged for the identification of immunoglobulins on the surface and in the cytoplasm of the cells.

REFERENCES

Krueger, G.R. & Meyer, E.M., 1983, Classification of malignant lymphomas of the mouse using morphological, immunological and cytochemical methods; a working proposal, Journal of Cancer Research and Clinical Oncology, 104, 41.
Nowell, P.C., 1983, Tumor progression and clonal evolution: The role of genetic instability, Chromosome Mutation and Neoplasia, edited by J. German (New York, Alan R. Liss Inc.), p. 413.
Paget, S., 1889, The distribution of secondary growth in cancer of the breast, Lancet, 1, 571.

REDUCED LEVELS OF WGA – BINDING PROTEINS IN METASTATIC NODULES: A SITE-
MODULATED PHENOMENA

GRAHAM A. TURNER AND WAI-SHUN CHAN
    Department of Clinical Biochemistry and Metabolic Medicine, The Medical
School, University of Newcastle, Newcastle upon Tyne, NE2 4HH

Keyword: Lectin : Membrane : Metastases : Protein

INTRODUCTION

It is generally agreed that the properties of the tumour cell surface
are important in metastasis (Turner, 1982; Weiss and Ward, 1983; Nicolson,
1984), but the precise nature of the changes involved are difficult to
discover. Current thinking would suggest that if metastatic cells possess
important structural changes in their cell surface, these are more non-
specific than originally anticipated. Recently, we found that the lectin,
wheat germ agglutinin (WGA), detected a number of different membrane
glycosylated protein species that were much reduced when the tumour cells
were growing as liver metastases (Chan et al., 1982). Furthermore, similar
changes could be induced if the tumour was directly injected into the liver
(Chan et al., 1984). The present studies were undertaken to extend these
observations by using other lectins; a different metastatic model; tumour
tissue from various implantation sites; and purified tumour cell subpopulations.

METHODS

Metastatic (ML) and non-metastatic lymphosarcomas (NML) were raised
subcutaneously (sc) in Syrian hamsters (WO/CR strain); the former line
resulted in liver metastases, whereas the latter line did not metastasize
(Guy et al., 1980). Lewis lung carcinomas (LL) were raised sc in C57 Bl6
mice; this line metastasizes to the lungs (Turner and Weiss, 1981). In
some experiments with the ML and NML, tumour tissue were transplanted into
sites other than the sc using standard surgical procedures. Purified
suspensions of ML cells were prepared using collagenase (Chan et al., 1984).
Tumour cell suspensions (3×10^8) were separated on the basis of cell size

by subjecting them to sedimentation under unit gravity on a shallow
gradient (1 to 4%) of Ficoll using the CelSep apparatus. The composition
of cell preparations were determined by microscopic examination of Giemsa/
May Grunwald-stained cytocentrifuge preparations. Glycoproteins were
extracted from chopped tissue or single cells by using Triton X100. These
were separated by electrophoresis on SDS polyacrylamide gradient (7.5% to
20%) gels. The separated components were detected by their Coomassie blue
staining and by their binding to ^{125}I-WGA or other lectin (Con A, RCA-60,
Gorse), as indicated by autoradiography. All separations were calibrated
with molecular weight markers, and some autoradiographs were quantitated by
scanning on a laser densitometer. All techniques have been previously
described in detail (Chan et al., 1984; Chan et al., in press).

RESULTS

    Fig 1 compares the electrophoretic patterns of extracts of sc and
metastatic tumour tissue as shown by protein staining and lectin-binding.
WGA was the only reagent that detected a difference in composition between
the two types of tumour extract. This difference was detected with both
the ML and LL tumour lines.

    Fig 2 compares the WGA binding for ML tumours implanted into different
sites (sc, muscle, liver, kidney and spleen). Measurements were made by
scanning the autoradiographs. For each experiment, the WGA binding is
expressed as a ratio of the binding to an extract of sc tumour. The binding
varied according to the site in which the ML tumour was growing. Extracts
from liver and spleen showed low WGA binding, whereas those from muscle and
sc gave high binding. In similar experiments with the NML no variation in
WGA binding with the site of tumour growth could be detected. (data not
shown).

    Fig 3 shows typical results for the WGA binding to extracts from five
pooled cell fraction obtained after subjecting a tumour cell suspension to
fractionation by cell size. Fraction 'a' contained mainly macrophages
whereas fraction 'e' contained mainly polymorphs. The tumour cells are
contained in fractions 'b' to 'd' with the majority in 'c'. It can be seen
that the majority of the WGA binding is associated with the presence of
tumour cells. There is a band at 23K daltons that is related to the
polymorph content of the fraction, but the WGA binding and macrophage content
are not closely associated.

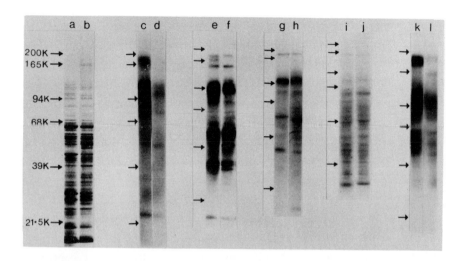

Figure 1.   Electrophoretic patterns of Triton X100 extracts of sc (a,c,e,g, i,k, and metastatic (b,d,f,h,j,l) tumour as detected by Coomassie blue (a & b); WGA (c & d); Con A (e & f); RCA-60 (g & h); Gorse (i & j); WGA (k & l).   Tracks a-j ML tumour; tracks k & l LL tumour.

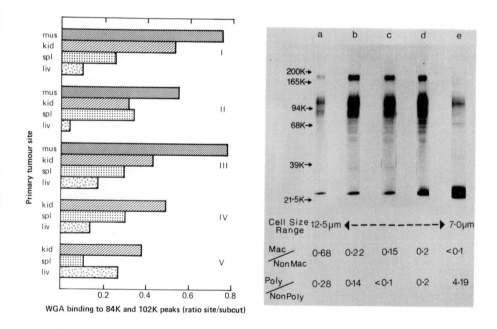

Figure 2 (left).   WGA-binding to the electrophorotic peaks of extracts from ML tumour growing in different sites.   Figure 3 (right) WGA patterns for ML cell fractions from the CelSep.

DISCUSSION

Our present findings suggest that the WGA-binding proteins we have detected involve a certain class of surface macromolecules that vary with the site of tumour implantation and arise mainly from the tumour cell population. At this stage it is difficult to precisely identify the nature of the binding sites concerned, because our results could be explained by binding to sialic acid as well as N-acetylglucosamine groupings. Interestingly, other studies have suggested that sialic acid may play an important role in metastasis by selectively masking certain sugar sequences (Altevogt et al., 1983).

It seems possible that the changes we have found could be part of a general mechanism involving metastatic cells, because we obtained similar results for two metastatic lines, but the WGA-binding of a non-metastatic line did not vary. Also, a reduction in WGA binding by some glycoproteins from lung metastases has been reported by Steck and Nicolson (1983).

The reason for the tumour having different surface properties when growing in different sites in unknown. As the site of tumour cell implantation can affect local growth and spread (Keller, 1981; Schirrmacher et al., 1982; Turner et al., 1984) it might be speculated that there could be association between this factor and the changes we have observed. Many factors allow the metastatic cell to adapt and survive, but the ability of the tumour to modulate its properties according to the site of growth may be a critical feature for continued successful spread, and one to bear in mind in developing future therapeutic strategies.

REFERENCES

Altevogt, P., Fogel, M., Cheingsong-Popov, R., Dennis, J., Robinson, P. and Schirrmacher, V., 1983, Cancer Research, 43, 5138.
Chan, W-S., Jackson, A. and Turner, G.A., 1982, British Journal Cancer, 46, 474.
Chan, W-S., Jackson, A. and Turner, G.A., 1984, British Journal Cancer, 49, 181.
Chan, W-S, Jackson, A. and Turner, G.A., 1984, Invasion and Metastasis (in press).
Guy, D., Latner, A.L, Sherbet, G.V., and Turner, G.A., 1980, British Journal Cancer, 42, 915.
Keller, R., 1981, Invasion and Metastasis, 1, 136.
Nicolson, G.L., 1984, Experimental Cell Research 150, 3.
Schirrmacher, V., Fogel, M., Russmann, E., Bosslet, K., Altevogt, P. and Beck, L., 1982, Cancer Metastasis Reviews, 1, 241.
Steck, P.S. and Nicolson, G.L., 1983, Experimental Cell Research, 147, 255.
Turner, G.A. and Weiss, L., 1981, Cancer Research, 41, 2576.
Turner, G.A., Chan, W-S., Jackson, A., 1984, British Journal Cancer (In press).
Weiss, L. and Ward, P.M., 1983, Cancer Metastasis Reviews, 2, 11.

ORGAN-SPECIFIC EFFECTS ON METASTATIC TUMOUR GROWTH STUDIED IN VITRO

E. HORAK, D.L. DARLING and D. TARIN

Nuffield Department of Pathology, (University of Oxford), John Radcliffe Hospital, Oxford OX3 9DU

Keywords: Metastasis – Organ distribution – Cell survival –
           Microenvironment

INTRODUCTION

   Clinical and experimental observations in humans and several vertebrates have established that metastases from malignant neoplasms have predictable patterns of organ distribution relatable to the site and type of the primary tumour (Tarin et al. 1984; Juacaba 1983; Fidler & Nicolson 1976). For instance, metastases from carcinomas of the breast are commonly found in the bones, lungs, liver and brain but infrequently in other sites, although there is good evidence that cells released intravascularly arrive in the tumour-free organs (Tarin et al. 1984; Potter et al. 1983). These observations prompt the hypothesis that, whilst certain organs allow the survival and proliferation of tumour cells, others prevent their growth. The experiments reported below were designed to test whether the cells of normal organs can influence the growth and behaviour of tumour cells and, if so, to examine the mechanisms by which such effects are mediated.

MATERIALS AND METHODS

Animals, tumours and normal tissues

   Tumour cells obtained from 25 separate naturally-occurring mammary carcinomas in C3H/A^{vy} mice were studied. Tumour disaggregation, counting of cell numbers and assessment of cell viability were carried out as previously described (Tarin & Price 1979; 1981). Normal organs (lungs and livers) for preparation of organ-conditioned medium were obtained from tumour-free animals of the same strain.

Organs and organ-conditioned medium

Each batch of organ-conditioned medium was prepared from the lungs or livers of at least 6 mice.   The organs were finely minced with scalpel blades and homologous organ fragments pooled and weighed.   The fragments were then suspended, at a standard ratio of 0.0167 gm of tissue per ml of culture medium, in Minimum Essential Medium containing 10% foetal calf serum and incubated at 37°C for 24 hours.   The conditioned medium was then collected, spun at 900g and stored in 2 ml aliquots at -20°C.   The conditions for testing organ-conditioned medium were standardised at: 0.5 ml conditioned medium mixed with 1.5 ml fresh SMEM per culture dish seeded with 2.0×10^6 living tumour cells.   Controls consisted of cultures in SMEM alone, without organ-conditioned medium.   All cultures were set up in duplicate and incubated for 24 hours at 37°C, at the end of which time the numbers of surviving floating and attached cells (freed by trypsinisation) were counted.

Fibroblasts obtained from subcutaneous tissue of newborn mice of the same strain were used as non-neoplastic control cells.

Comparison of results - standardisation

The total numbers of surviving cells and the numbers attached to the substratum at 24 hours, in untreated cultures, differed from tumour to tumour.   Comparisons between treated and control cultures are therefore expressed as percentage deviations from the control value, which is expressed as a baseline of 100%, for each tumour.

Dialysis experiments

The organ-conditioned media were dialysed for 24 hours against fresh MEM and both the dialysate and the residue within the dialysing membrane were tested for activity on tumour cell cultures.   Compensation was made for dilution effects due to dialysis.   Cultures of the same tumours, both non-conditioned and conditioned with non-dialysed fluids, were used as controls.

RESULTS

For 9 of the 25 tumours, the number of surviving cells in lung-conditioned cultures exceeded 150% of the control value, whilst it fell below 50% of the control value in only 1 culture.   Thus in the remaining 15 cultures the total number of surviving cells did not differ significantly from the controls (a deviation of 50% being regarded as a conservative minimal level of significance). In 16 (64%) of the cultures treated with lung-conditioned medium (LUN-CM) the number of <u>attached</u> cells was augmented by more than 50% above the controls, whilst it decreased significantly with only 2 tumours. In the <u>liver-conditioned</u> cultures the number both of surviving and of attached cells consistently decreased substantially (Graph 1) frequently resulting in total cell death. It can also be seen in Graph 1 that for some tumours incrementation of <u>attachment</u> by LUN-CM is greater than incrementation of <u>cell survival</u> and that the effects on these two processes can, in other tumours, be divergent. As the results are expressed in <u>relative</u> values compared with the control, <u>changes</u> in cell attachment resulting from treatment with conditioned medium are sometimes greater than <u>changes</u> in total cell survival.

LUN-CM and LIV-CM both markedly decreased the number of surviving and attached normal fibroblasts, compared to control cultures (Graph 2).

The effects of the dialysis experiments are represented in Graph 3. The component in LUN-CM, mediating the protective effect on cell survival and attachment, was not dialysable but the mediator from liver causing cell degeneration and death was.

COMMENTS

These results show directly that the survival and attachment to the substratum, of normal and tumour cells <u>in vitro</u>, can be influenced by soluble components released by cells of normal organs. LIV-CM consistently kills cells from these murine mammary tumours, although the survival and attachment of cells from some mammary tumours is actually <u>promoted</u> by LUN-CM, which sometimes exerts a relatively stronger effect on attachment than on survival. In contrast, normal fibroblasts are inhibited by both LIV-CM and by LUN-CM.

The results agree with our earlier (<u>in vivo</u>) observations in which <u>murine</u> mammary tumour metastases occurred predominantly in the lungs and rarely in the liver (Juacaba et al. 1983), in spite of numerous tumour cells being detectable in that organ after intra-aortic inoculation (Potter et al. 1983).

Our results are preliminary and the study investigates only one possible factor influencing the metastatic cascade, i.e. the host organ microenvironment. However, the findings suggest mechanisms for the non-random distribution of metastases characteristic of each tumour type and indicate that circulating metastasis-competent cells are not necessarily invincible.

REFERENCES

Fidler, I.J. & Nicolson, G.L., 1976, Journal of the National Cancer
     Institute, 57, 1199.
Juacaba, S.F., Jones, L.D. & Tarin, D., 1983, Invasion Metastasis, 3, 208.
Juacaba, S.F., Horak, E., Price, J.E. & Tarin, D., 1984 (in preparation).
Potter, K.M., Juacaba, S.F., Price, J.E. & Tarin, D., 1983, Invasion
     Metastasis, 3, 221.
Tarin, D. & Price, J.E., 1979, British Journal of Cancer, 39, 740.
Tarin D. & Price, J.E., 1981, Cancer Research, 41, 3604.
Tarin, D., Price, J.E., Kettlewell, M.G.W., Souter, R.G., Vass, A.C.R. &
     Crossley, B., 1984, Cancer Research, 44, 3584.

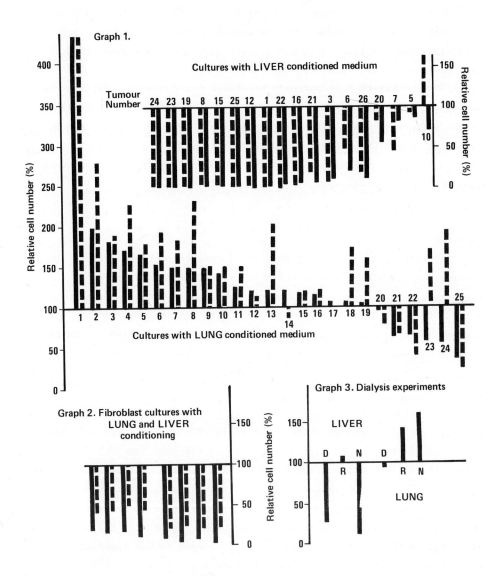

Legends: ▬▬▬: Surviving cells; ▬ ▬ ▬: Attached cells; N: conditioned medium, no dialysis;
          D: dialysate; R: residue within the dialysing membrane

ORGAN SPECIFICITY OF HUMAN MELANOMA

P.K. CHAUDHURI and B. CHAUDHURI

Section of Surgical Oncology, Dept. of Surgery, Loyola University
of Chicago at the Medical Center, Maywood, Illinois 60153,
Dept. of Pathology, Hinsdale Hospital, Hinsdale, Illinois, 60521

Keywords: human melanoma;   organ selectivity

INTRODUCTION

The most important feature of a malignant tumor is its ability to spread
to distant organs. A large body of literature exists on the mechanisms of
metastasis, and while the actual mechanism remains elusive, several theories
have been proposed (Fidler I.J. and Nicolson G.L. 1976; Hart I.R. and
Fidler I.J. 1980; Nicolson G.L. and Poste G.1982). Recently, several investigators have reported organ specific metastatic clones in animal tumor
models, (Nicolson G.L. 1978; Brunson K.W. et al 1978). The importance of
such organ specificity in understanding the mechanism of metastasis is
obvious, and detection of such organ specific clones in metastatic human
tumors may also be of therapeutic and prognostic importance.

As an initial step in evaluating the morphologic and biochemical
differences between different organ specific human melanoma clones, we
attempted to develop these clones from human melanoma tissue obtained from
different metastatic sites of a melanoma patient.

MATERIALS AND METHODS

Human melanoma tissues were obtained from a female patient with liver
metastasis, subcutaneous metastasis and small bowel metastasis. All tumors
were obtained during operation and cultured separately in tissue culture
flasks using MEM with 18% Fetal Calf Serum and antibiotics. Fibroblasts
were removed from the melanoma cells by culturing on 2% Agar medium. No
cloning of individual cell lines was attempted. After approximately 5-6
passages in tissue culture, cells were harvested for inoculation into athymic
mice.

Individual cell lines were characterized by cytosolic oestrogen
receptor assay and growth rate in vitro and in vivo.   A cell line obtained
from subcutaneous metastasis had oestrogen receptor (Rc 18.6 fmol/mg cyt
prot), and a cell line obtained from small bowel metastasis also had detectable oestrogen receptor (Rc 2.8 fmol/mg cyt protein).   However a cell line
obtained from liver metastasis had no detectable oestrogen receptor.   Also
the liver metastasis line exhibited the highest growth rate in vivo and in
vitro followed by the subcutaneous metastasis and small bowel metastasis.
The human origin of each cell line was verified by indirect immunofluorescence
using a monoclonal antibody to human cell surface receptor to transferrin
(Omary M.D. et al 1980).

To evaluate the organ specificity of human metastatic melanoma, an
athymic mouse model was used.   All mice were kept in groups of 5 per cage
in a filtered air environment of 12 hrs. light and 12 hrs. dark period.
All mice received sterile chow and sterile water ad lib.   3 to 4 week old
male mice were inoculated with 500,000 cells from cell line I and III (subcutaneous and liver metastasis respectively) in the proximal portion of
right hind limb.   All mice were examined daily and sacrificed 6 weeks
following injection.   Autopsies were performed to evaluate metastasis.   Any
liver metastases from cell line III were harvested, recultured and reinjected in a subsequent group of athymic mice and termed second generation.
This was repeated for seven generations.   Subcutaneous tumors from cell
line I were harvested, recultured and reinjected into athymic mice for 7
generations also.   Evidence of metastasis in any organ was sought in every
generation.   For cell line II (small bowel metastasis), a different approach
was used.   Initially 500,000 cells were injected intraperitoneally into a
group of mice.   Tumors from the surface of the small bowel were obtained
and injected subcutaneously in one group of 10 athymic mice and intraperitoneally in another group of 10 athymic mice.   After 6 weeks mice from
the subcutaneous injection group were evaluated for organ metastasis.
Tumor tissue from the small bowel of mice which had received intraperitoneal
injections were harvested and reinjected into two more groups of mice;
one group subcutaneously and the other group intraperitoneally and termed
generation 2.   The experiment was carried up to 5 generations.   The
incidence of metastasis was verified by histological examination.

RESULTS

A selection process followed a method previously described by other authors (Fidler I.J. and Nicolson G.L. 1976; Nicolson G.L. 1978) failed to demonstrate any organ specificity. A few generations of cell line I obtained from subcutaneous metastasis showed cells which were still capable of liver metastasis (Table 1). Cell line II obtained from small bowel metastasis failed to demonstrate any evidence of small bowel metastasis following subcutaneous injection, however one passage did demonstrate the ability to form liver metastases (Table 2). In contrast to cell line I and cell line II, every generation of tumor originally obtained from cell line III (liver metastasis), showed ability to form liver metastases in athymic mice. However, the incidence of metastasis and number of metastatic nodules (2 to 4) remained unchanged (Table 3).

Table 1. Incidence of metastasis of human melanoma obtained from subcutaneous tissue following subsequent passage in athymic mice.

Passage	Liver mets (# mets/#inj)	Lung mets (# mets/#inj)	Small bowel mets (# mets/#inj)	Kidney mets (# mets/#inj)
1	0/10	0/10	0/10	0/10
2	0/9	0/9	0/9	0/9
3	1/10	0/10	0/10	0/10
4	0/8	0/8	0/8	0/8
5	1/10	0/10	0/10	0/10
6	0/10	0/10	0/10	0/10
7	0/7	0/7	0/7	0/7

Table 2. Incidence of metastasis of human melanoma obtained from small bowel metastasis following subsequent passage in athymic mice.

Passage	Liver mets (# mets/# inj)	Lung mets (# mets/# inj)	Small bowel mets (# mets/# inj)	Kidney mets (# mets/# inj)
1	0/7	0/7	0/7	0/7
2	0/10	0/10	0/10	0/10
3	0/10	0/10	0/10	0/10
4	0/10	0/10	0/10	0/10
5	0/9	0/9	0/9	0/9

Table 3. Incidence of metastasis of human melanoma obtained from
liver metastasis following subsequent passage in athymic mice.

Passage	Liver mets (# mets/# inj)	Lung mets (# mets/# inj)	Small bowel mets (# mets/# inj)	Kidney mets (# mets/# inj)
1	2/10	0/10	0/10	0/10
2	1/9	0/9	0/9	0/9
3	3/10	0/10	0/10	0/10
4	2/10	0/10	0/10	0/10
5	2/10	0/10	0/10	0/10
6	1/8	0/8	0/8	0/8
7	1/9	0/9	0/9	0/9

DISCUSSION

In the present study, we attempted to demonstrate organ specific metastasis from human melanoma. Using an athymic mouse model, we failed to
obtain evidence of such clones in human melanoma. The study of human tumor
metastasis in vivo is difficult due to the lack of suitable models. Athymic
mice offer the best model despite several draw backs, e.g. the presence of
NK cells in older animals. Our work demonstrating a fairly high incidence of
metastasis of human melanoma in athymic mice (Chaudhuri P.K. et al 1981)
suggests that this model, although not ideal, is suitable for the study of
human tumor metastasis. The data obtained failed to demonstrate selectivity
and organ specificity of metastasis of human melanoma.

REFERENCES

Brunson, K.W., Beattie, G., Nicolson G.L., 1978, Nature 272, 543.
Chaudhuri, P.K., Walker, M.J., Beattie, C.W., Briele H.A., Das-Gupta, T.K.
    1981, In Phenotypic expression in pigment cells, Seiji M. (Ed).
    University of Tokyo Press, p 593.
Fidler, I.J., Nicolson, G.L. 1976, Journal of National Cancer Institute,
    57, 1199.
Hart, I.R., Fidler, I.J. 1980, Quarterly Review Biology, 55, 121.
Nicolson, G.L. 1978, Bioscience, 28, 241.
Nicolson, G.L., Poste, G. 1982 Current Problems in Cancer Volume VII, No.6.
Omary, M.D., Trowbridge I.S., Minowada J. 1980, Nature, 286, 888.

LYSOSOMAL ENZYME ACTIVITY IN PLASMA MEMBRANES OF MURINE TUMORS

B.F. SLOANE[1,2], J. ROZHIN[3], J.D. CRISSMAN[3] and K.V. HONN[2,4]

Departments of Pharmacology[1], Radiation Oncology[2], Pathology[3] and
Biological Sciences[4]

Wayne State University and Harper-Grace Hospitals, Detroit, MI 48201 USA

Keywords: cathepsin B, cysteine proteinase, glycosidase

INTRODUCTION

The ability of tumor cells to invade into host stroma has been
linked to enzymes released from tumor cells or associated with tumor cell
plasma membranes. There is suggestive evidence that activities of lysosomal proteinases (Sloane & Honn, 1984) and glycosidases (Dobrossy et
al., 1980) may correlate with tumor malignancy. Activity of a lysosomal
cathepsin B-like cysteine proteinase (CB) and a lysosomal glycosidase
β-N-acetyl-glucosaminidase (β-NAG) can be measured in culture medium of
B16-F1 and B16-F10 melanoma cells (Sloane et al., 1982). The presence
extracellularly of these enzymes suggests that they might also be
associated with the tumor cell plasma membrane. In this study we isolated lysosomal and plasma membrane fractions from murine melanomas and
murine liver and assayed fractions for activity of CB, β-NAG and cathepsin H (another lysosomal cysteine proteinase).

METHODS

Tumor lines

An amelanotic variant (B16a) of the B16 melanoma, the B16-F1 metastatic variant and the Cloudman melanoma were obtained from the Division
of Cancer Treatment (NCI) tumor bank and propagated in syngeneic mice as
previously described (Honn et al., 1984).

Subcellular fractionation

Normal livers and subcutaneous tumors were homogenized and fractionated by differential centrifugation as previously described (Sloane

et al., 1981). The light mitochondrial pellet was further fractionated
by density gradient centrifugation on 30% isoosmotic Percoll into a L-1
(density = 1.045 g/ml) and a L-2 (density = 1.07 g/ml) fraction.

Enzyme assays

CB and cathepsin H were assayed by a modification of our described
methods (Rozhin et al., 1985). β-NAG was assayed as previously described (Sloane et al., 1982). Protein was determined by the Bradford
procedure (Reed and Northcote, 1981) and Na^+, K^+-ATPase by the method
of Jorgensen (1974).

RESULTS

Murine liver and Cloudman, B16-F1 and B16a melanomas were fractionated into nuclear, heavy mitochondrial, light mitochondrial and supernatant fractions. Recovery of CB, β-NAG, cathepsin H and Na^+, K^+-
ATPase activities ranged from 81-118% for the four tissues. Recovery
of protein ranged from 87-98%. Distributions of the three lysosomal
hydrolases followed similar patterns. The purification achieved for
the lysosomal hydrolases and Na^+, K^+-ATPase was calculated by determining the relative specific activity (RSA) = specific activity/%
protein. The original homogenate would have a RSA of 1.0; therefore,
a RSA >1.0 indicates a purification of the enzyme in that fraction.
RSA values for the four enzymes in the light mitochondrial fractions
are given in Table 1.

Table 1. Relative specific activity of enzymes in light mitochondrial
fractions.

Enzyme	Tissue			
	Liver	Cloudman	B16-F1	B16a
Na^+, K^+-ATPase	2.3	4.1	2.6	3.6
CB	2.3	5.0	3.9	4.3
β-NAG	1.5	1.9	2.4	1.6
Cathepsin H	2.1	4.4	N.D.[a]	2.3

[a]N.D. = not determined.

The light mitochondrial fractions were further fractionated into
two fractions on Percoll gradients. The plasma membrane marker Na^+,K^+-
ATPase was localized primarily in the L-1 fraction (Figures 1 & 2); RSA
values ranged from 3.4 to 4.9. In contrast the lysosomal enzymes were
localized primarily in the L-2 fraction (Figures 1 & 2). RSA values in

L-2 ranged from 6.2 to 9.0 for CB, from 2.7 to 4.4 for β-NAG and from 5.0 to 16.4 for cathepsin H (Figure 2). Cathepsin H activity was not purified in the L-1 fraction, nor were CB and β-NAG activities in the L-1 fractions of liver and the Cloudman melanoma. However, in the B16-F1 and B16a melanomas both CB and β-NAG were associated with the plasma membrane fraction (L-1). The RSA values for CB were ~4.0 and for β-NAG were ~1.5. This association was not disrupted by treating the fractions with isotonic potassium acetate, suggesting that the enzymes were not merely trapped in or adsorbed to the L-1 fractions.

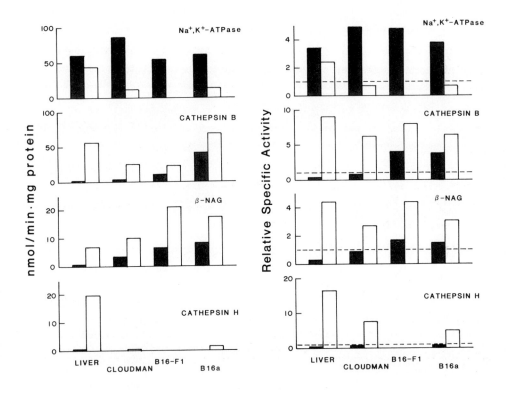

FIGURE 1. Specific activities of enzymes in plasma membrane (solid bars) and lysosomal (open bars) fractions of murine liver and melanomas.

FIGURE 2. Relative specific activities (RSA) of enzymes in plasma membrane (solid bars) and lysosomal (open bars) fractions of murine liver and melanomas. RSA = specific activity/% protein; RSA = 1.0 or equivalent to the original homogenate is indicated by the dashed line.

DISCUSSION

Pietras and Roberts (1981) have established that CB activity is associated with the plasma membrane of neoplastic cervical epithelial cells yet not that of normal cervical epithelial cells. However, Koppel et al. (1984) reported that the % of plasma membrane CB activity is less in a metastatic sarcoma variant than a non-metastatic variant. In the present study, we established that activities of CB and β-NAG were associated with plasma membranes in the two tumors which metastasize to the lung, either upon tail-vein injection (B16-F1, B16a) or spontaneously (B16a). In contrast, activities of CB and β-NAG were not associated with plasma membranes in a normal tissue (liver) and an essentially non-metastatic tumor (Cloudman). This could be of importance in metastatic ability since membrane-associated enzymes may possess hydrolytic activity when free enzymes would not. For example, proteinase inhibitors have been shown to be less effective against membrane-associated proteinases than free proteinases (Steven et al., 1982). Membrane associated tumor cell hydrolases such as CB and β-NAG thus may enable tumor cells to invade into host stroma despite the presence of extracellular inhibitors.

REFERENCES

Dobrossy, L., Pavelic, Z.P., Vaughn, M., Porter, N., & Bernacki, R.J., 1980, Cancer Research, 40, 3281.

Honn, K.V., Onoda, J.M., Diglio, C.A., Carufel, M.M., Taylor, J.D. & Sloane, B.F., 1984, Clinical and Experimental Metastasis, 2, 61.

Jorgensen, P.L., 1974, Methods in Enzymology, 32B, 277.

Koppel, P., Baici, A., Keist, R., Matzku, S., & Keller, R., 1984, Experimental Cell Biology, 52, 293.

Pietras, R.J. & Roberts, J.A., 1981, Journal of Biological Chemistry, 256, 8536.

Reed, S.M. & Northcote, D.H., 1981, Analytical Biochemistry, 116, 53.

Rozhin, J., Crissman, J.D., Honn, K.V. & Sloane, B.F., 1985, Submitted.

Sloane, B.F. & Honn, K.V., 1984, Cancer Metastasis Reviews, in press.

Sloane, B.F., Dunn, J.R. & Honn, K.V., 1981, Science, 212, 1151.

Sloane, Honn, K.V., Sadler, J.G., Turner, W.A., Kimpson, J.J. & Taylor, J.D., 1982, Cancer Research, 42, 980.

Steven, F.S., Griffin, M.M. & Itzhaki, S., 1982, European Journal of Biochemistry, 126, 311.

BIOCHEMICAL IDENTIFICATION OF MEMBRANE PROTEINS AND MOLECULAR CLONING OF ENCODING GENES THAT DETERMINE THE METASTATIC PHENOTYPE OF ESb LYMPHOMA CELLS

P. ALTEVOGT, B. HECKL-ÖSTREICHER, H.P. SCHMITT[+] and V. SCHIRRMACHER
Institute for Immunology and Genetics and [+]Experimental Pathology,
Deutsches Krebsforschungszentrum, D-6900 Heidelberg, Federal Republic
of Germany

Keyword: 2D gel electrophoresis, microinjection, cDNA cloning, metastasis
        genes

INTRODUCTION

The term "metastatic phenotype" is frequently used to refer to special
functional and structural properties of metastatic tumor cells. What these
properties really reflect in molecular terms is far from being understood.
Since metastasis of tumor cells is a multistep process it can be assumed
that various genetic and epigenetic changes occur in tumor cells on their
way to becoming metastatic.

Many of the properties defining the metastatic phenotype can be linked
to the cell surface or to secreted cellular products. Thus, there seems to
be a requirement for a specific state of gene activation. In order to
investigate this we have studied cell surface changes associated with
increased metastatic capacity using two distinct sublines of a murine T
lymphoma (Eb/ESb) (Schirrmacher et al. 1982). Here we show that these cell
types differ in the protein composition of the plasma membrane. We also
describe our attempts to clone genes from metastatic ESb cells that are
necessary for their metastatic behaviour.

MATERIAL AND METHODS

1. 2D gel mapping

Membrane proteins of ^{35}S-Methionine labelled cells were prepared using
a stepwise sucrose gradient. 5´Nucleotidase was used as PM marker and the
purification resulted in a 37fold enrichment over total cell homogenate.
PM preparations from ESb clone 18.1, Eb clone 34.2 and normal DBA/2 ConA

blasts were compared by 2D gel electrophoresis using IEF in the first
dimension and SDS-PAGE in the second (Altevogt and Schirrmacher 1984).

2. mRNA-isolation and microinjection of oocytes

Total mRNA was isolated by the Guanidinium/CsCl method (Maniatis et al.
1982). Poly A + mRNA was selected on oligo dT cellulose. 50 nl/oocyte of
poly A + mRNA (1ug/ul) in Barth's medium containing 40 uCi ^{35}S-Methio-
nine/ul were injected in groups of 10 Xenopus laevis oocytes. Control
groups received Medium alone plus radioactive label. The oocytes were
incubated for 24 hrs at 25°C then the medium was removed and oocyte
homogenates were prepared in 10 mM Tris/HCl pH 7.0 containing 1M NaCl,1%
Triton X 100 plus protease inhibitors. Homogenates were centrifuged for 2
min in an Eppendorf centrifuge and the transparent interphase was collected. Aliquots from homogenates and incubation medium were prepared for
SDS-PAGE analysis.

3. cDNA cloning

Single and double stranded cDNA's were prepared from poly A + mRNA of
ESb using standard procedures (Maniatis et al. 1982). Double stranded cDNA
was sized by Agarose gel electrophoresis and 0.5-2 kb species were cloned
into pUC8. Transformed bacterial colonies were screened on replica filters
by the high density colony hybridization method (Hanahan and Meselson
1980) using end labelled poly A + mRNA from ESb and nonmetastatic Eb
cells.

RESULTS AND DISCUSSION

1. 2D gel mapping of PM proteins

Plasma membranes were isolated from biosynthetically labelled tumor
cells and syngeneic ConA blasts and analyzed by 2D gel mapping. The 2D gel
pattern from low metastatic Eb cells revealed 169 spots; those from high
metastatic ESb cells 203 spots; and those from ConA T lymphoblasts 248
spots. Due to the IEF conditions used this analysis did not include the
very basic proteins. Of the 169 Eb spots about 60% were also detected on
gels from ESb cells. There were some protein spots noted that were
specific for either Eb or ESb cells. On the whole the ESb spot pattern
contained approximately 50 additional spots compared to Eb. About 41 (82%)
of the 50 new spots from ESb type cells were also detected on normal

syngeneic ConA T lymphoblasts. We conclude that many of the new plasma membrane proteins expressed by the high metastatic variant seem to represent differentiation or activation related proteins of normal cells rather than being tumor cell specific. A more detailed discussion about these findings has been published recently (Altevogt and Schirrmacher 1984).

2. Characterisation of ESb mRNA and cDNA cloning

The influence of particular new proteins on the biological properties of tumor cells is difficult to study at the protein level. We therefore decided to study the expressed genes of metastatic ESb tumor cells. Poly A + mRNA was isolated from both tumor lines and their in vitro translation studied in Xenopus oocytes. As seen in Fig. 1 mRNA's from both cell types are efficiently translated by the oocytes. The SDS-gel pattern of transla-ted proteins are very similar and do not reflect the differences as discussed above for membrane proteins. This is most likely due to the fact

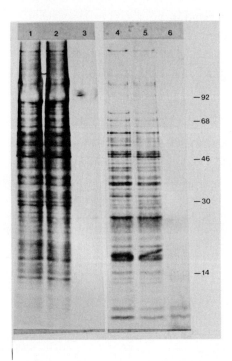

Figure 1.   35S-Methionine labelled translation products of Xenopus oocytes injected with poly A + mRNA from Eb (lanes 1,4), ESb (lanes 2,5) or controls without mRNA. Lanes 1-3: oocyte homogenates, lanes 4-6: oocyte culture medium.

that high abundant mRNA species are shared by both types of cells whereas mRNA´s for membrane proteins comprise only a minor pool of total poly A + mRNA. Different pattern of proteins can be noted between translated proteins isolated from the oocyte culture medium and those of the oocyte homogenate. It is likely that normally secreted cellular proteins are also secreted by the oocytes.

Double stranded cDNA was prepared from ESb mRNA, sized and cloned into pUC8. 3400 bacterial colonies of our initial library were identified as carrying ESb cDNA inserts. By differential screening on replica filters using labelled mRNA from ESb and Eb we have so far identified 44 colonies that gave signals with ESb mRNA only. We are presently extending our library in order to identify more bacterial clones carrying ESb specific inserts.

What can be done with plasmids containing cDNA inserts of a metastatic tumor? It is clear that these plasmids can be screened for genes that are important for the metastatic phenotype of ESb tumor cells. This should be possible by means of transfection into suitable low metastatic recipient cells and in vivo screening of positive transfections for altered metastatic potential. Despite the manifold technical difficulties and the complexity of the metastatic process itself we hope that such an approach will be useful to dissect the genetic requirements of the metastatic phenotype.

Altevogt, P. & Schirrmacher, V., 1984, European Journal of Cancer & Clinical Oncology, 20, 1155-1162.
Schirrmacher, V., Fogel, M., Rußmann, E., Bosslet, K., Altevogt, P. & Beck, L., 1982, Cancer Metastasis Reviews 1, 241-274.
Mariatis, T., Fritsch, E.F. & Sambrook, J., 1982, Cold Spring Harbor Laboratory.
Hanahan, O. & Meselson, M., 1980, Gene 10, 63.

ENHANCED SPONTANEOUS METASTATIC CAPACITY OF MOUSE MAMMARY CARCINOMA CELLS
TRANSFECTED WITH H-RAS

S.A. ECCLES[1], C.J. MARSHALL[2], K. VOUSDEN[2], & H.P. PURVIES[1]
[1]Section of Tumour Immunology, Institute of Cancer Research, Sutton, U.K.
[2]Section of Cell and Molecular Biology, Institute of Cancer Research,
London, U.K.

Keywords: Ras oncogene; mammary adenocarcinoma; transfection

INTRODUCTION

   MT1 clone 5/7 retains many of the properties of its parent mouse mammary
tumour (Barnett & Eccles, 1984) it is of epithelial morphology in vitro,
non-immunogenic, and in vivo produces well-differentiated adenocarcinomas
from which spontaneous metastasis is rare, and confined to the lungs.

   It had previously been shown (Vousden & Marshall, 1984) that the appearance of an activated C-Ki-ras gene in late passages of a murine T-Lymphoma
paralleled the acquisition of spontaneous metastatic potential. MT1 clone
5/7 was found, like the early passage, non-metastatic lymphoma, to lack
activated ras genes, based on the inability of DNA from these cells to
transform N1H-3T3 cells. We therefore were able to examine directly
whether the introduction of cloned mutant ras genes would influence the
growth and spontaneous metastasis of this carcinoma in syngeneic hosts.

METHODS
In vitro

   The c-Ha-ras-1 gene cloned from EJ/T24 cells (Goldfarb et al. 1982; Shih
& Weinberg, 1982) was inserted into BamH1 site of pSV2Neo vector of
Southern and Berg (Southern & Berg, 1982) to generate a plasmid designated
pSV2Neo-EJ. Clone 5/7 cells were then transfected with pSV2Neo or pSV2Neo-
EJ using the calcium phosphate co-precipitation technique. Selection for
transfectants was carried out in 1mg/ml G418 (neomycin). Three independent
G418^r cell clones arising from transfection with pSV2Neo-EJ (Clones EJ 11,
12 and 15) and three from pSV2Neo transfections (Neo 13, 14, and 16) were
isolated for further analysis. Cell lines were expanded in DMEM + 10% FCS
and released from tissue culture flasks using 0.1% trypsin in PBS-EDTA.

In vivo

Local growth and spontaneous metastasis. 10^5 cells of each of the 3 Neo
clones, 3 EJ clones and the parental clone 5/7 were injected s.c. into the
midflank of groups of 12 syngeneic female mice 10-12 weeks old. The tumours
were surgically excised at a mean diameter of 9-10 mm (33-37 days later)and
weighed. Mice were observed for a further 120 days. Those showing symptoms
of metastatic disease were killed and autopsied, and at the end of the
experiment survivors were killed and similarly examined. Suspected
metastatic deposits were confirmed histologically.

Lung colonisation potential. The ability of the cell lines to colonise
the lungs of syngeneic mice was determined following their i.v. inoculation.
10^5 cells of each line were injected into groups of 5 mice. The results
were recorded as survival time, lung weight, and number of tumour colonies
on the surface of Bouins-fixed lungs.

RESULTS

All mice inoculated s.c. with 10^5 cells of each type developed tumours,
and although there was a tendency towards increased growth rate in the EJ
clones neither the individual nor pooled values (EJ $\bar{x}$) were significantly
different from each other, the Neo clones or clone 5/7 (Table 1.)

Table 1. Growth rate of tumour cell lines s.c.

Cell line	Growth rate (mgm/day ± s.e.)	
Neo 13	12.30 ± 2.78)	
Neo 14	12.30 ± 3.38)	11.80 ± 2.94
Neo 16	10.80 ± 3.03)	(Neo $\bar{x}$)
EJ 11	14.90 ± 3.98)	
EJ 12	12.90 ± 2.30)	14.70 ± 3.21
EJ 15	16.30 ± 4.04)	(EJ $\bar{x}$)
Clone 5/7	12.90 ± 6.70	

Following surgical excision of the tumours, 90% of mice remained tumour-
free in the clone 5/7 group, whereas only $^1/_{36}$ mice survived excision of EJ
clones, with median survival times (MST) of 47-67 days. Although the Neo
groups also developed more metastatic disease than the control group, this
was significantly less frequent than in the EJ groups. (17 long-term
survivors, MST of non-survivors 73-83 days). (Figure 1.)

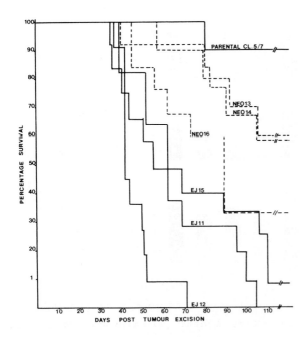

Figure 1. Survival of mice following surgical excision of clone 5/7 and Neo and EJ transfected cells.

All deaths scored were due to metastasis.

Table 2. Organ distribution of spontaneous metastasis of Neo and EJ clones.

SITE	% ANIMALS WITH METASTASIS							
	EJ 11	EJ 12	EJ 15	EJ $\overline{X}$	NEO 13	NEO 14	NEO 16	NEO $\overline{X}$
LUNG	100	92	67	88	18	25	33	26
LIVER	9	8	8	8				
KIDNEY							17	6
ADRENAL	36	17		18	9			3
OVARY	55	25	25	35	9		17	12
CNS	9	17	33	18		8	17	9
P.LN	55	58	42	53				
V.LN	45	50	25	41				
BONE					18		8	9
MUSCLE			8	3		8		3
OTHER	9	25	17	18		17	17	12

Key: P.LN and V.LN - peripheral and visceral lymph nodes.

Both Neo and EJ cells, unlike the parental clone 5/7, produced extra-pulmonary metastases, but the frequency was much greater in the EJ groups. (Table 2). Nearly 90% of mice in the EJ groups developed metastases at more than one site; the involvement of 3-5 organs was a common occurrence. In contrast, of the 'Neo' mice that died of metastases, in only 16% was more than one organ involved. Also notable was the lack of lymphatic metastasis in the Neo groups compared with incidences of 40-50% in the EJ groups.

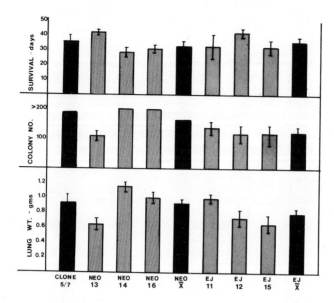

Figure 2. Lung colonisation potential of clone 5/7 and Neo and EJ transfected cells.

Individual clones varied in their ability to grow in mouse lung, but none had a significantly enhanced colonisation potential compared with clone 5/7 (fig. 2). Thus the observed differences in spontaneous metastasis do not merely reflect differences in growth rate (Table 1) or clonogenic capacity of the cells.

DISCUSSION

We have shown that introduction of a transforming C-Ha-ras-1 oncogene into mouse mammary carcinoma cells leads to a significant increase in the incidence, distribution and rate of appearance of spontaneous metastases compared with pSV2Neo or non-transfected controls. The 3 EJ clones, and representative metastases, were shown to contain the oncogene by Southern blotting using the 2.9Kb Sst1 fragment of c-Ha-ras-1 as a probe, and to express the c-Ha-ras-1 encoded p21 protein - (unpublished observations). These results therefore are in accord with our previous observations (Vousden & Marshall, 1984) and suggest that sequential activation of cell-ular oncogenes can contribute to tumour progression and the acquisition of metastatic capacity.

REFERENCES
Barnett, S.C. & Eccles, S.A. 1984. Clinical & Experimental Metastasis, 2,15.
Goldfarb, M., Shimizu, K., Perucho, M., & Wigler, M., 1982. Nature 296, 404.
Shih, C., & Weinberg, R.A., 1982. Cell 29, 161.
Southern, P.J. & Berg, P., 1982. Journal of Molecular and Applied Genetics
   1. 327.
Vousden, K.H., & Marshall, C.J., 1984. The European Molecular Biology
   Organisation Journal 3, 913.

METASTATIC VARIANTS GENERATED BY SOMATIC CELL FUSION FOLLOWED BY CHROMOSOME SEGREGATION AND GENETIC REARRANGEMENT

V. SCHIRRMACHER[1], L. LARIZZA[2], L. GRAF[1], C. A. WALLER[1], M. KRAMER[1], and E. PFLÜGER[1]

[1] Institut für Immunologie und Genetik, Deutsches Krebsforschungszentrum, D-6900 Heidelberg, FRG

[2] Institute of General Biology, University of Milano, Faculty
of Medicine, I-20133 Milano, Italy

Keyword: cell fusion; metastatic capacity; invasiveness

INTRODUCTION

Tumor cell populations displaying metastatic properties
often show increased ploidy levels, chromosome duplications
and gene amplifications. The acquisition of higher gene
dosages by tumor cells can be achieved by various mechanisms.
Endoreduplication or somatic hybridisation either between
tumor cells or between tumor and host cells could all lead to
an increase of genetic variability and instability since they
may trigger a polyploidisation-segregation cycle. Evidence for
in vivo fusion of tumor and normal host cells has been
reported in different tumor systems. Tumor host hybrids with a
higher degree of malignancy have been observed, however, only
following substantial chromosome segregation (De Baetselier et
al. 1981; Kerbel et al 1984). Such segregational mechanisms
may bring about homozygosity or heterozygosity of recessive
alleles in tumor host hybrids thus leading to their expression. The chromosome dynamics observed in tumor host
hybrids may also lead to extensive chromosome rearrangements
which may cause, for instance, altered oncogene activity (for
review see Larizza & Schirrmacher 1984).

We here report about the acquisition of high metastatic
capacity after in vitro hybridisation of a low metastatic
tumor line with a bone-marrow derived macrophage. The characteristics of two highly metastatic hybrid lines will be
described.

METHODS
Cells and hybridisation
The low metastatic T-cell lymphoma Eb (Schirrmacher et. al.
1979) was made thioguanine resistant without mutagenesis by
stepwise procedure of culture in the presence of increasing
concentrations of thioguanine. As fusion partner we chose in
vitro differentiated macrophages derived from the bone-marrow
of syngeneic adult DBA/2 mice precultured for 15 days in
L-cell conditioned medium. Tumor macrophage fusions were
performed with polyethyleneglycol (PEG), MW 1000, (Merck,
Darmstadt, FRG) by a modified procedure of the method used for
fusing lymphocytes with attached cells in monolayer (Brahe &
Serra 1981). Details are described elsewhere (Larizza et al.
1984a).

Analysis of cell surface marker expression
The expression of differentiation antigens from T-cells or
macrophages and of class I and class II major histocompatibility antigens on the hybrid cells was investigated using
three different techniques: 1. indirect immune fluorescence
staining and cytofluorographic analysis, 2. complement
dependent cytotoxicity as measured by 51 chromium release and
3. immunoprecipitation and SDS-PAGE analysis. All methods have
been described in detail elsewhere (Larizza et al. 1984b).

RESULTS AND DISCUSSION
Hybridisation of drug marked Eb cells (Eb TGR) with
syngeneic bone-marrow derived macrophages resulted in the
establishment of two HAT medium resistant lines, Eb-F1 and
Eb-F2 which could be stabilized in tissue cultures 60 days
after fusion. These lines showed a plastic adhesiveness which
was intermediate between that of the parental tumor line
(non-adherent) and that of the macrophages (strongly adherent). The two lines also showed a highly increased activity
of a neutral protease as tested with a chromogenic substrate
while the parental line was very low.

The in vitro invasive capacity of the new tumor lines was
investigated using two new invasion assays. One is an endothe-

lial monolayer penetration assay in a Boyden Chamber. The
other assay uses rotation mediated brain cell microspheres as
a substrate for invasion by radioactively labelled tumor cells
(Schirrmacher et al. 1982). In both assays the two hybrid
lines showed a significant increase in invasive activity as
compared to the parental tumor line. Mice inocculated with the
parental line developed large primary tumors and died after
about 6 weeks without overt metastases. In contrast, mice
inoculated with Eb-Fl or Eb-F2 cells died after only 10 to
14 days with small primary tumors and metastases in liver,
lung and spleen. From several sub-clones of the lines tested
most showed high metastatic activity while one showed only
intermediate metastatic capacity.

Evidence for the hybrid nature of the two cell lines was
obtained by a cytogenetic analysis of G-banded metaphase
chromosomes. It rests primarily on the presence of normal
chromosomes of No. 12 which were never found in the parental
lymphoma line and which co-existed in the hybrids with the two
abnormal forms of No. 12 chromosomes of the parental lymphoma
line (Larizza et al. 1984b). Apart from the additional normal
12 chromosomes the hybrid lines carried several new marker
chromosomes not found in the parental Eb TGR cells.

The two hybrid lines were found to express several new cell
surface markers which were not found on the parental Eb TGR
cells. 1. Mac-1. The macrophage antigen Mac-1 could be
visualised by indirect immunofluorescence and could be
correctly identified by immunoprecipitation and SDS-PAGE
analysis. 2. Class II major histocompatibility antigens. I-A^d
and I-E^d antigens as well as the invariant chain of class II
MHC antigens was detected with the help of monoclonal antibodies, immunoprecipitation and 2D gel electrophoresis. 3. Fc
receptors. The hybrid lines were found to form rosettes with
antibody-coated erythrocytes while Eb TGR cells were negative.

All the new surface markers (Mac-1, class II MHC, Fc-
receptors) can be considered as phenotypic traits derived from
the normal cell fusion partner, most likely a macrophage. They
could all be identified on a macrophage tumor line but were
not expressed by various T cell lymphomas.

We have thus shown that fusion of a low metastatic tumor
line with a bone-marrow derived normal host cell (macrophage)
followed by intensive chromosome segregation and rearrangements can lead to the generation of high metastatic tumor
variants. Such metastatic variants may not always be recogni-
zable as hybrids because of the intensive chromosome segregation. In such situations monoclonal antibodies against
defined differentiation antigens may be very useful additional
tools to detect such fusion derived tumor variants. The highly
increased metastatic capacity in the hybrids may be due to the
observed changes in functional characteristics, such as
adhesiveness, motility and invasive capacity.

Brahe, C., & Serra, A., 1981, Somatic Cell Genetics, 7, 109.
De Baetselier, P., Gorelik E., Eshhar, Z., Ron, Y., Katzav,
    S., Feldman, M. & Segel, S., 1981, Journal of the National
    Cancer Insitute, 67, 1079.
Kerbel, R. S., Largarde, A. E., Dennis, J. W., Nestel. F. P.,
    Donaghue, T. P., Siminovitch, L. & Fulchiguoni-Latand, M.
    C., 1984, in: Cancer Invasion and Metastasis: Biological
    and therapeutic aspects, edited by Nicolson & G. L. Milas,
    L. (Raven Press, New York), p. 47.
Larizza, L. & Schirrmacher V., 1984, in: Cancer Metastasis
    Reviews (in the press).
Larizza, L., Schirrmacher, V., Graf, L., Pflüger, E., Peres-
    Martinez, M. & Stöhr, M., 1984a, International Journal of
    Cancer (in the press).
Larizza, L., Schirrmacher, V. & Pflüger, E., 1984b, Journal of
    Experimental Medicine (in the press).
Schirrmacher, V., Waller, C. & Vlodavsky, I., 1982, in: B and T
    cell tumors, edited by Vitetta, E. (Academic Press), p.
    307.

HETEROGENEITY, STABILITY AND SELECTION IN METASTATIC CELLS

S.R. CLARK and E. SIDEBOTTOM
Sir William Dunn School of Pathology, Oxford, England

Keyword: Metastasis. Selection. Heterogeneity. Clonal morphology

INTRODUCTION

Accumulating evidence supports the notion that malignant tumours may consist of distinct subpopulations of cells (Owens et al. 1982).

The tumour cell systems used to investigate metastasis are often hetero-geneous (Fidler & Hart, 1982; Weiss, 1983) and it would be valuable to find markers which are stable and can discriminate between variants which differ in their behaviour in vivo. Relationships between cell shape and control of cell growth (Folkman & Moscona, 1978; Raz & Ben-Zeev, 1983) and between clonal morphology in suspension and colonization potential (Cifone, 1981) have been described. However, these in vitro phenotypes were unstable and could not be selected on repeated passage.

We have previously shown how genetic instability induced in a metastatic mouse melanoma by cell fusion can lead to a reduction in metastasis (Side-bottom & Clark, 1983). We describe here heterogeneity for clonal morphology that is maintained in a highly metastatic mouse melanoma cell line. The characters are surprisingly stable during growth in vivo and in vitro and there are correlations between morphology and tumorigenicity and metastasis.

METHODS

The cells used were the highly metastatic mouse melanoma hybrid line F87C16T2 (6T2) whose isolation and properties have already been described (Sidebottom & Clark, 1983). Cloning was carried out by plating appropriate cell suspensions into 96 well tissue culture plates. Clonal morphology was scored after 6 days growth when 3 distinct clonal types were identified: tight, intermediate and loose. Tight clones had a smooth, clearly deline-ated periphery which enclosed compact epithelial-like cells (Fig. 1a).

Loose clones had no clear periphery and an interior containing substantial intercellular spaces (Fig. 1c). The intermediate clones showed mixed characteristics of the other two types (Fig. 1b).

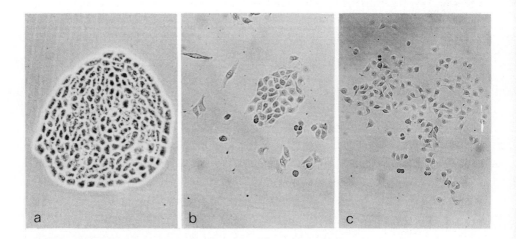

Figure 1.   Clonal morphology of F87C16T2 cells. (a) Tight, (b) Intermediate, (c) Loose.

Tight or loose clones were located in wells containing a single clone and allowed to grow for a further 4 days. The cells were then removed with trypsin/EDTA and either recloned directly, injected into a mouse or used to establish a bulk culture.

To assay for tumorigenicity and metastasis individual dissociated clones or 5×10^4 cells from bulk cultures were injected subcutaneously into new born (<5 days) sublethally irradiated (4 Gy) histocompatible mice. Animals were sacrificed when death was impending due to tumour load so as to maximise the probability of observing metastases.

RESULTS

The results of cloning 6T2 cells in one experiment are shown in table 1. 67% of the clones were loose, 14% tight and the remainder intermediate. Recloning from a loose clone (second cloning, table 1) increased the proportion of loose clones to 98%. Recloning from a tight

clone increased their proportion to 85% (table 1). A third round of
cloning from either two loose or two tight clones showed that the phenotypes were stable under selective clonal conditions.

The effect of transferring clones into tissue culture flasks for
routine culture was monitored. After 25 passages the tight cells (IG8)
produced 79% tight and 6% loose colonies, and the loose cells (IG3)
produced 77% loose and 8% tight colonies.

Table 1. Selection by sequential cloning

Colony type[1] formed	First cloning from 6T2	Second cloning from		Third cloning from			
		L	T	L	L	T	T
L	67	98	1	97	90	0	0
I	19	1	14	3	10	21	26
T	14	1	85	0	0	79	74

[1] L, Loose; I, Intermediate; T, Tight

When injected into mice all the clones and cell lines gave primary
tumours (table 2). From the time of sacrifice it is evident that the
tight clones and their cell lines produced slower growing tumours than
the loose clones and cell lines. They also differed in the extent to
which they produced metastases. Fewer secondary lung deposits are seen
in mice injected with tight clones and cell lines than in those injected
with loose clones and cell lines.

Table 2. Tumorigenicity and metastasis of tight and loose clones and cell
lines.

Cells inoculated	Tumour take	Day mice killed	Mice with 2° tumours	Extent of[1] metastases
Tight clones	11/11	35–85	7/11	+
Loose clones	9/9	19–33	6/9	+/++++
Tight cell line (IG8)	26/26	29–47	9/26	+/++
Loose cell line (IG3)	20/20	14–18	18/20	++/++++

[1] Semiquantitative scale from + (<6 lung deposits) to ++++ (approx. 100).

To determine whether these morphological phenotypes were stable and
if there was selection for the faster growing loose cells in vivo cell
suspensions were prepared directly from the primary and secondary tumours
of mice injected with either IG8 or IG3 cells. Cloning the dissociated
tight cell tumours resulted in a majority of tight clones and a small

percentage of loose ones. Similarly loose cell tumours produced a large
majority of loose clones and no tight ones at all (table 3). This demon-
strates that the ability of these cell lines to produce either tight
or loose clones is conserved during the growth of the primary tumour
and also during subsequent steps leading to metastasis.

Table 3. Direct cloning of primary and secondary tumours.

Injected cell line	Tumours	% Colonies formed on cloning		
		T	I	L
Tight	1°	79	17	5
	2°	67	29	4
Loose	1°	0	9	91
	2°	0	7	93

1° = Primary tumour; 2° = Secondary lung tumours.

These results demonstrate that repeated clonal selection does not
necessarily lead to a reduction in metastatic ability, and that the
phenotypes we have selected for can be maintained both in vivo and in
vitro. We have evidently been able to differentiate between metastatic
variants on the basis of clonal morphology in this system. It appears
that the tight cells only metastasize at a low rate compared to the loose
cells. Despite the considerable difference in growth rates in vivo there
is no evidence of selective overgrowth in the primary or secondary tumours
by any loose cells existing in the tight cell population.

To find out if the differences in tumorigenicity and metastasis are
a result of greater selection against IG8 than IG3 cells we are investigating the growth kinetics of these cell lines in vivo.

REFERENCES
Cifone, M.A., 1981, Experimental Cell Research, 131, 435.
Fidler, I.J. & Hart, I.R., 1982, Science, 217, 998.
Folkman, J. & Moscona, A., 1978, Nature (London), 273, 345.
Owens, A.H., Coffey, D.S. & Baylin, S.B. (Editors) 1982, Tumor cell
    heterogeneity. Origins and implications. Bristol-Myers Cancer
    Symposia Vol.4, Academic Press.
Raz, A. & Ben-Zeev, A., 1983, Science, 221, 1307.
Sidebottom, E. & Clark, S.R., 1983, British Journal of Cancer, 47, 399.
Weiss, L., 1983, Invasion Metastasis, 3, 193.

AUTHOR INDEX

SUBJECT INDEX

Adjuvant chemotherapy
- breast cancer   93
- nasopharyngeal cancer
  89
- small cell lung cancer
  97
see also chemotherapy
Adrenal
- metastases   187
- tumour colonies   113,
  191
Adriamycin   13, 93, 97,
  179, 203
Aminobenzamide   125
Amnion   243
Angiogenesis   207
Anticoagulants   73, 77,
  207, 339
Antigens
- of colorectal ca.   21
- H-2   355
Antimetastatic drugs   25,
  129
Athymic animals   207, 323
  355, 373
Autochthonous tumours
  see: cancer (experimental)
AVCF combined therapy   93

B16 Melanoma
  see: cancer (experimental)
Bacteriocins   133
BCNU   137
Biological response
  modifiers   149, 153, 157
Bleomycin   89, 125
Bone metastases   33, 85, 385

Brain
- metastases   127, 385
- microsphere assay   331
Brown fat   191

Calcium
- calcification   107
- calmodulin antagonists
  295
- channel blockers   259
Cancer (clinical)
- breast   29, 33, 61, 93
  101
- colorectal   13, 17, 21
  41, 323
- lung   1, 5, 25, 97
- melanoma   45, 49, 73
- nasopharyngeal   89
Cancer (experimental)
- autochthonous   153,
  307, 369
- ASCA-SG   227
- bladder   247
- carcinoma
  - LMC1   187
  - MCA-4   227
  - MCA-35   227
  - MCA-K   227
  - Walker 255   81, 259,
    263
- colorectal DHD-K12-TR
  57
- fibrohistiocytoma P77
  145
- glioma C6   279

401